16

CURRENT CLINICAL TOPICS IN INFECTIOUS DISEASES

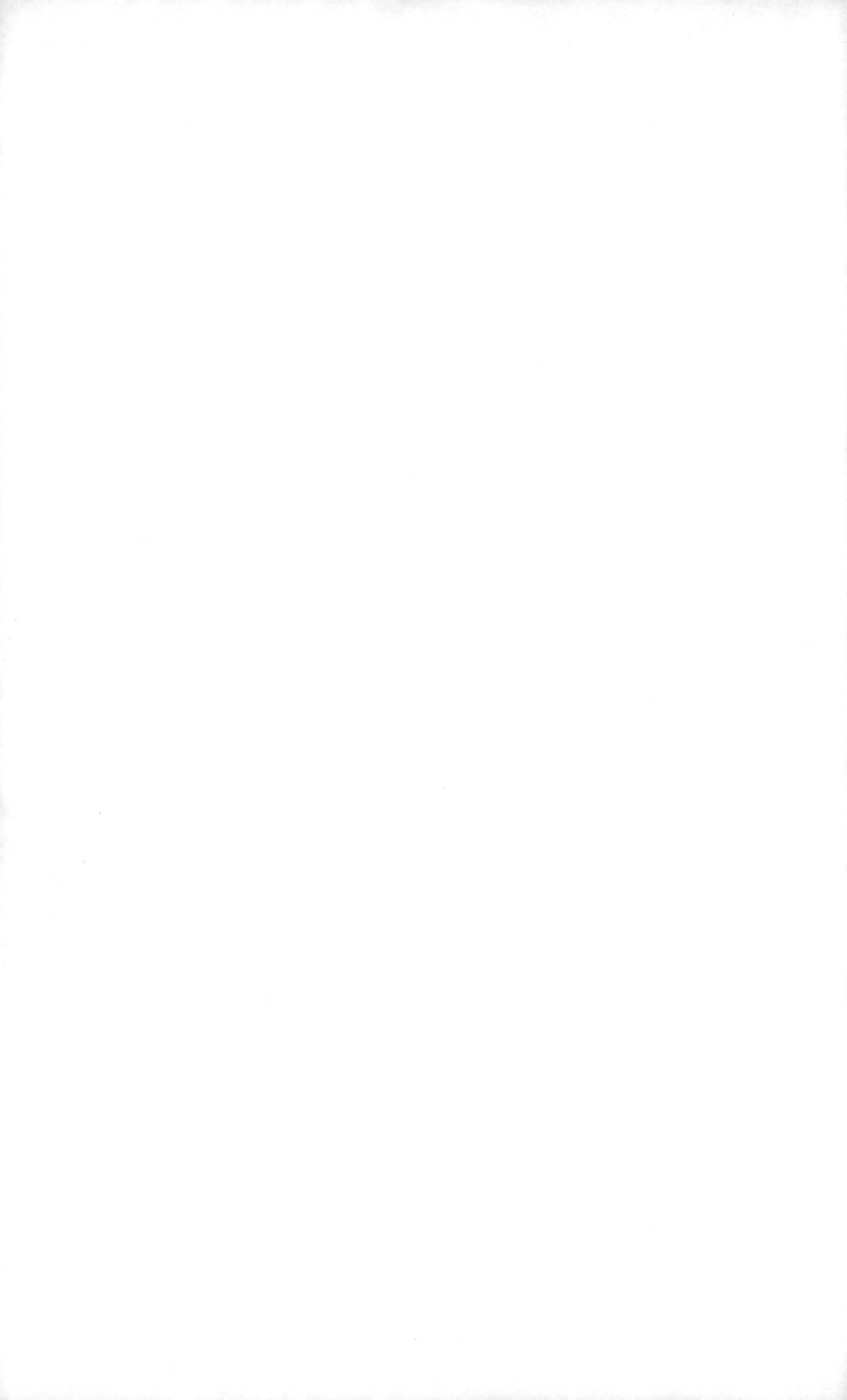

16

CURRENT CLINICAL TOPICS IN INFECTIOUS DISEASES

Edited by

JACK S. REMINGTON, MD

Professor of Medicine
Division of Infectious Diseases and Geographic Medicine
Stanford University School of Medicine
Marcus A. Krupp Research Chair
Chairman, Department of Immunology and Infectious Diseases
Research Institute
Palo Alto Medical Foundation
Palo Alto, California

MORTON N. SWARTZ, MD

Chief, James Jackson Firm, Medical Services
Infectious Disease Unit
Massachusetts General Hospital
Boston, Massachusetts

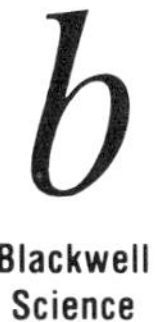

Blackwell
Science

BLACKWELL SCIENCE

Editorial offices:

238 Main Street, Cambridge, Massachusetts 02142, USA
Osney Mead, Oxford OX2 0EL, England
25 John Street, London WC1N 2BL, England
23 Ainslie Place, Edinburgh EH3 6AJ, Scotland
54 University Street, Carlton, Victoria 3053, Australia
Arnette Blackwell SA, 1 rue de Lille, 75007 Paris, France
Blackwell Wissenschafts-Verlag GmbH
Kurfurstendamm 57, 10707 Berlin, Germany
Feldgasse 13, A-1238 Vienna, Austria

Distributors:

USA
Blackwell Science, Inc.
238 Main Street
Cambridge, Massachusetts 02142
(Telephone orders: 800-215-1000 or 617-876-7000)

Canada
Copp Clark, Ltd.
2775 Matheson Blvd. East
Mississauga, Ontario, Canada L4W 4P7
(Telephone orders: 800-263-4374 or 905-238-6074)

Australia
Blackwell Science Pty Ltd
54 University Street
Carlton, Victoria 3053
(Telephone orders: 03-347-0300
fax: 03-349-3016)

Outside North America and Australia
Blackwell Science, Ltd.
c/o Marston Book Services, Ltd.
P.O. Box 87
Oxford OX2 0DT
England
(Telephone orders: 44-1865-791155)

Acquisitions: Victoria Reeders
Development: Kathleen Broderick
Production: Michelle Choate
Manufacturing: Karen Feeney
Printed and bound by Braun-Brumfield Inc.

Printed in the United States of America
96 97 98 99 5 4 3 2 1

Notice: The indications and dosages of all drugs in this book have been recommended in the medical literature and conform to the practices of the general medical community. The medications described do not necessarily have specific approval by the Food and Drug Administration for use in the diseases and dosages for which they are recommended. The package insert for each drug should be consulted for use and dosage as approved by the FDA. Because standards of usage change, it is advisable to keep abreast of revised recommendations, particularly those concerning new drugs.

Library of Congress Cataloging in Publication Data

The Library of Congress has cataloged this serial publication as follows:

Current clinical topics in infectious diseases.
1-
New York, McGraw-Hill Book Co.,
c1980–1988
Boston, Blackwell Science, Inc.
c1989–
v. ill. 25 cm
Annual.
Key title: Current clinical topics in
infectious diseases, ISSN 0195-3842.
I. Communicative diseases—Periodicals.
DNLM: 1. Communicable Diseases—Periodicals. W 1 CU786T
RC111.C87 616.9'05 80-643590
ISBN 0-86542-477-2

Contents

Preface

As literature in the field of infectious diseases has increased in complexity and volume, a need has become evident for timely, concise summaries and critical commentaries on subjects pertinent to the student and practitioner of medicine, the specialist in infectious diseases, and those in allied fields. It is our intention that this series provide the reader with a true update of information in very specific areas of infectious diseases that require reevaluation.

Each author was requested to confine his or her chapter to a relatively narrow subject, to deal only with contemporary questions and problems, to gather and synthesize the information on recent advances that is often spread diffusely among numerous journals, to offer critical evaluation of this information, to place the information into perspective by defining its present status, and to point out deficiencies in the information and thereby indicate directions for further study. All of this was to be done within the most rigid deadlines to ensure that the chapters be written and published in less than a year. We are extremely grateful to the contributing authors, each of whom is a recognized authority in their particular field, for consenting to undertake such an admittedly difficult task.

Current Clinical Topics in Infectious Diseases: 16 is the sixteenth volume of a series that is published annually. Each text in the series consists of updates of a variety of subjects covering the wide scope of clinical infectious disease problems, including bacteriology, mycology, virology, parasitology, and epidemiology.

JACK S. REMINGTON
MORTON N. SWARTZ

Contributors

Anthony Adamis, MD
Assistant Professor of Ophthalmology
Harvard Medical School
Attending Surgeon
Massachusetts Eye and Ear Infirmary
Boston, Massachusetts

M. John Albert, PhD
Head, Department of Laboratory Research
International Center for Diarrheal Disease Research
Dhaka, Bangladesh

Ann Sullivan Baker, MD
Associate Professor of Medicine (Ophthalmology)
Harvard Medical School
Director, Infectious Diseases
Massachusetts Eye and Ear Infirmary
Boston, Massachusetts

Richard T. D'Aquila, MD
Assistant Professor of Medicine
Harvard Medical School and Massachusetts General Hospital
Boston, Massachusetts

Paul T. Davidson, MD
Director of Tuberculosis Control
Los Angeles County Department of Health Services
Director of TB Control
Clinical Professor of Medicine
University of Southern
California School of Medicine
Los Angeles, California

Jacqueline E. Dawson, MS
Research Microbiologist
Viral and Rickettsial Zoonoses Branch
National Center for Infectious Diseases
Centers for Disease Control
United States Public Health Services
Atlanta, Georgia

Oscar H. Del Brutto, MD
Head, Neurology Department
Hospital Luis Vernaza
Guayaquil, Equador

David W. Denning, MRCP, MRCPath, DCH
Senior Lecturer, Infectious Diseases
University of Manchester School of Medicine
Honorary Consultant in Medicine
North Manchester General and Hope Hospitals
Manchester, United Kingdom

Marlene Durand, MD
Instructor
Harvard Medical School
Clinical Assistant in Medicine
Massachusetts General Hospital
Boston, Massachusetts

George M. Eliopoulos, MD
Associate Professor of Medicine
Harvard Medical School
Assistant Chairman
Department of Medicine
Deaconess Hospital
Boston, Massachusetts

Ferric C. Fang, MD
Assistant Professor of Medicine, Microbiology and Pathology
Director, University Hospital Clinical Microbiology Laboratory
University of Colorado Health Sciences Center
Denver, Colorado

Hanh Quoc Le, MD
Associate Director of Tuberculosis Control
Los Angeles County Department of Health Services
Los Angeles, California

Nancy E. Madinger, MD
Assistant Professor of Medicine and Pathology
Associate Director, University Hospital Clinical Microbiology Laboratory
University of Colorado Health Sciences Center
Denver, Colorado

Daniel M. Musher, MD
Professor of Medicine
Professor of Microbiology and Immunology
Chief of Infectious Diseases
Baylor College of Medicine
Chief, Infectious Disease Section
Veterans Affairs Medical Center
Houston, Texas

Jeffrey Parsonnet, MD
Associate Professor of Medicine and Microbiology
Dartmouth Medical School
Attending Physician
Infectious Diseases Unit
Dartmouth-Hitchcock Medical Center
Lebanon, New Hampshire

Andrea M. Prevan, DO
Postdoctoral Fellow
Department of Medical Microbiology
Creighton University School of Medicine
Omaha, Nebraska

Jack S. Remington, MD
Professor of Medicine
Division of Infectious Diseases and Geographic Medicine
Stanford University School of Medicine
Marcus A. Krupp Research Chair
Chairman, Department of Immunology and Infectious Diseases
Research Institute
Palo Alto Medical Foundation
Palo Alto, California

Gustavo C. Roman, MD
Neurologist
International Spinal Neurosurgical Clinic, University of Texas at San Antonio
San Antonio, Texas

R. Bradley Sack, MD, ScD
Professor of International Health
Johns Hopkins University School of Hygiene and Public Health
Baltimore, Maryland

Christine C. Sanders, PhD
Professor of Medical Microbiology
Director, Center for Research in Anti-Infectives and Biotechnology
Creighton University School of Medicine
Omaha, Nebraska

W. Michael Scheld, MD
Professor of Internal Medicine and Neurosurgery
Associate Chair for Residency Programs
Director, Residency Program in Internal Medicine
University of Virginia Health Sciences Center
Charlottesville, Virginia

A. Kasem Siddique, MBBS, MPH
Senior Scientist
Community Health Division
International Centre for Diarrheal Disease Research
Dhaka, Bangladesh

Julio Sotelo, MD
Head, Research Division
National Institute of Neurology and Neurosurgery
Mexico City, Mexico

Steven J. Spindel
Senior Fellow
Infectious Disease Section
Baylor College of Medicine
Houston, Texas

Morton N. Swartz, MD
Chief, James Jackson Firm, Medical Services
Infectious Disease Unit
Massachusetts General Hospital
Boston, Massachusetts

Kenneth S. Thomson, PhD
Assistant Professor of Medical Microbiology
Associate Director, Center for Research in Anti-Infectives and Biotechnology
Creighton University School of Medicine
Omaha, Nebraska

Allan R. Tunkel, MD, PhD
Associate Professor of Medicine
Medical College of Pennsylvania and Hahnemann University School of Medicine
Philadelphia, Pennsylvania

Richard P. Wenzel, MD, MSc
Professor and Director
Department of Internal Medicine
Division of General Medicine, Clinical Epidemiology and Health Services Research
The University of Iowa College of Medicine
Iowa City, Iowa

R. Todd Wiblin, MD
Fellow Associate
Department of Internal Medicine
Division of General Medicine, Clinical Epidemiology and Health Services Research
The University of Iowa College of Medicine
Iowa City, Iowa

Other Volumes in the Series

CURRENT CLINICAL TOPICS IN INFECTIOUS DISEASES 1

The Role of CT Scanning in Diagnosis of Infections of the Central Nervous System
Staphylococcus aureus Bacteremia
Cytomegalovirus Infection in Transplant and Cancer Patients
Diagnosis and Management of Meningitis Due to Gram-Negative Bacilli in Adults
Infection Prevention during Granulocytopenia
Infant Botulism
The Role of Surgery in Infective Endocarditis
Treatment of Bacterial Infections of the Eye
Giardiasis: The Rediscovery of an Ancient Pathogen
Legionnaires Disease
Antibiotic-Associated Diarrhea
Antibiotic-Resistant Pneumococci
The Cancer Patient with Fever and Pulmonary Infiltrates: Etiology and Diagnostic Approach
Q Fever: An Update

CURRENT CLINICAL TOPICS IN INFECTIOUS DISEASES 2

Acute Epiglottitis, Laryngitis, and Croup
Urinary Tract Infections in the Female: A Perspective
Treatment of Cryptococcal, Candidal, and Coccidiodal Meningitis
Bacteriology, Clinical Spectrum of Disease, and Therapeutic Aspects in Coryneform Bacterial Infection
Rocky Mountain Spotted Fever: A Clinical Dilemma
The Doctor's Dilemma: Have I Chosen the Right Drug? An Adequate Dose Regimen? Can Laboratory Tests Help in My Decision?
Shock in Gram-Negative Bacteremia: Predisposing Factors, Pathophysiology, and Treatment
The Management of Patients with Mycotic Aneurysm
A Review of the "New" Bacterial Strains Causing Diarrhea
Endocarditis Complicating Parenteral Drug Abuse
The Cephalosporins and Cephamycins: A Perspective
The Diagnosis and Treatment of Gangrenous, and Crepitant Cellulitis
Management of Acute and Chronic Otitis Media

CURRENT CLINICAL TOPICS IN INFECTIOUS DISEASES 3

Sexually Transmitted Enteric Disease
Nucleotide Derivatives and Interferons as Antiviral Agents

Prophylaxis and Treatment of Malaria
Guillain-Barré Syndrome
Newer Antifungal Agents and Their Use, Including an Update on Amphotericin B and Flucytosine
Role of Ultrasound and Computed Tomography in the Diagnosis and Treatment of Intraabdominal Abscess
Treatment of Infections Due to Atypical Mycobacteria
Combination of Single Drug Therapy for Gram-negative Sepsis
Deep infections Following Total Hip Replacement
Treatment of the Child with Bacterial Meningitis
Diagnosis and Management of Meningitis Associated with Cerebrospinal Fluid Leaks
Prophylactic Antibiotics for Bowel Surgery
Infections Associated with Intravascular Lines
Diagnosis and Treatment of Cutaneous Leishmaniasis
Candida Endophthalmitis

CURRENT CLINICAL TOPICS IN INFECTIOUS DISEASES 4

Diagnosis and Management of Septic Arthritis
Kawasaki's Disease
A Critical Review of the Role of Oral Antibiotics in the Management of Hematogenous Osteomyelitis
When Can the Infected Hospital Employee Return to Work?
Endocardiography and Infectious Endocarditis
Orbital Infections
The Use of White Blood Cells Scanning Techniques in Infectious Disease
Antimicrobial Prophylaxis in the Immunosuppressed Cancer Patient
The Diagnosis of Fever Occurring in a Postpartum Patient
Management at Delivery of Mother and Infant When Herpes Simplex, Varicella-Zoster, Hepatitis, or Tuberculosis Have Occurred during Pregnancy
"Nonspecific Vaginitis," Vulvovaginal Candidiasis, and Trichomoniasis: Clinical Features, Diagnosis and Management
Radionuclide Imaging in the Management of Skeletal Infections
Comparison of Methods for Clinical Quantitation of Antibiotics?
What Is the Clinical Significance of Tolerance to *B*-lactam Antibiotics?
A Critical Comparison of the Newer Aminoglycosidic Aminocyclitol
The Third Generation Cephalosporins

CURRENT CLINICAL TOPICS IN INFECTIOUS DISEASES 5

Prostatitis Syndromes
Staphylococcus epidermidis: The Organism, Its Diseases, and Treatment
Management of Nocardia Infections
Current Issues in Toxic Shock Syndrome
Isolation and Management of Contagious, Highly Lethal Diseases
Nutrition and Infection
Infections Associated with Hemodialysis and Chronic Peritoneal Dialysis
New Perspectives on the Epstein-Barr Virus in the Pathogenesis of Lymphoproliferative Disorders
Staphylococcal Teichoic Acid Antibodies
Current Status of Granulocyte Transfusion Therapy
Infections Associated with Intrauterine Devices
Hospital Epidemiology: An Emerging Discipline
The Viridians Streptococci in Perspective
Current Status of Prophylaxis for *Haemophilus influenzae* Infections
Acute Rheumatic Fever: Current Concepts and Controversies

CURRENT CLINICAL TOPICS IN INFECTIOUS DISEASES 6

The Acquired Immunodeficiency Syndrome
Health Advice and Immunizations for Travelers
Travelers' Diarrhea: Recent Developments
Bacterial Adherence and Anticolonization Vaccines

Serum Bactericidal Test: Past, Present and Future Use in the Management of Patients with Infections
Lyme Borreliosis
The Role of MR Imaging in the Diagnosis of Infections of the Central Nervous System
Imipenem and Aztreonam: Current Role in Antimicrobial Therapy
Progressive Multifocal Leukoencephalopathy
Campylobacter pylori: Its Role in Gastritis and Peptic Ulcer Disease
Nucleic Acid Probes in Infectious Diseases
Norfloxacin, Ciprofloxacin, and Ofloxacin: Current Clinical Roles
Liposomes in Infectious Disease: Present and Future
Antibiotic Prophylaxis: Non-abdominal Surgery
Prevention of *Haemophilus influenzae* Type b Disease: Vaccines and Passive Prophylaxis

CURRENT CLINICAL TOPICS IN INFECTIOUS DISEASES 11

The Chlamydial Pneumonias
Human Immunodeficiency Virus (HIV)-Associated Pneumocystosis
Fever of Unknown Origin—Reexamined and Redefined
Echinococcal Disease
The Epidemiology of AIDS: A Decade of Experience
Antibiotic Resistance Among Enterococci: Current Problems and Management Strategies
Intraocular Infections: Current Therapeutic Approach
Bronchiectasis: A Current View
Infection of Burn Wounds: Evaluation and Management
Colonic Diverticulitis: Microbiologic, Diagnostic, and Therapeutic Considerations
Echocardiography in the Management of Patients with Suspected or Proven Endocarditis
The Clinical Spectrum of Human Parvovirus B19 Infections

CURRENT CLINICAL TOPICS IN INFECTIOUS DISEASES 12

Viral Aseptic Meningitis in the United States: Clinical Features, Viral Etiologies, and Differential Diagnosis
Aeromonas Species: Role as Human Pathogens
Neurologic Complications of Bacterial Meningitis in Children
Purulent Pericarditis
Diagnosis and Management of Infections of Implantable Devices Used for Prolonged Venous Access
Pancreatic Abcess and Infected Pseudocyst: Diagnosis and Treatment
Approach to the Febrile Traveler Returning from Southeast Asia and Oceania
Management of Septic Shock: New Approaches
The Increasing Prevalence of Resistance to Antituberculosis Chemotherapeutic Agents: Implications for Global Tuberculosis Control
Use of Immune Globulins in the Prevention and Treatment of Infections
Mycobacterium avium Complex in AIDS
Hepatitis B Immunization: Vaccine Types, Efficacy, and Indications for Immunization
Therapy of Cytomegalovirus Infections with Ganciclovir: A Critical Appraisal
Evaluation of Cryptic Fever in a Traveler to Africa

CURRENT CLINICAL TOPICS IN INFECTIOUS DISEASES 13

The Pathogenesis, Prevention, and Management of Urinary Tract Infection in Patients with Spinal Cord Injury
Epidemiologic Considerations in the Evaluation of Undifferentiated Fever in Traveler Returning from Latin America or the Caribbean
Fever in a Recent Visitor to the Middle East
Fluconazole and Intraconazole: Current Status and Prospects for Antifungal Therapy
Genital Warts: Diagnosis, Treatment, and Counseling for the Patient
Varicella in a Susceptible Pregnant Woman
Evaluation and Treatment of Patients with Prior Reactions to *B*-Lactam Antibiotics
Periodontal Disease: Gingivitis, Juvenile Periodontis, Adult Periodontis

Diagnosis and Management of Perianal and Perirectal Infection in the Granulocytopenic Patient
Hemolytic Uremic Syndrome: Clinical Picture and Bacterial Connection
Clinical Features and Treatment of Infection Due to Myobacterium Fortuitum/Chelonae Complex
Fish and Shellfish Poisoning
Management of Infectious Complications Following Liver Transplantation
The Management of Cryptococcal Disease in Patients with AIDS
Magnetic Resonance Imaging Update on Brain Abscess and Central Nervous System Aspergillosis
Prophylaxis and Treatment of Infection in the Bone Marrow Transplant Recipient
Toxoplasmosis in the Non-AIDS Immunocompromised Host

CURRENT CLINICAL TOPICS IN INFECTIOUS DISEASES 14

Foot Infections in Diabetes: Evaluation and Management
Splenic Abcess: Pathogenesis, Clinical Features, Diagnosis, and Treatment
Azithromycin and Clarithromycin
Biologic and Geographic Factors in Prevention and Treatment of Malaria
Automated Antimicrobial Susceptibility Testing: What the Infectious Diseases Subspecialist Needs to Know
Hepatitis C Virus and Chronic Liver Disease
Nodular Lymphangitis: Clinical Features, Differential Diagnosis, and Management
Human Herpesvirus 6
Methicillin-Resistant *Staphylococcus aureus:* The Persistent Resistant Nosocomial Pathogen
How Vaccines Are Developed
Bacillary Angiomatosis and *Rochalimaea* Species
Prevention of Human Immunodeficiency Virus Infection among Hospital Personnel
Cytokine Therapy of Infectious Diseases
Intelligent Dosing of Antimicrobials
Ethical Issues in Infectious Diseases

CURRENT CLINICAL TOPICS IN INFECTIOUS DISEASES 15

When and How to Treat Serious Candidal Infections: Concepts and Controversies
An Approach to Acute Fever and Rash (AFR) in the Adult
Prophylaxis in Bowel Surgery
Update on Diagnosis of *Clostridium difficile*-Associated Diarrhea
Brucellosis: Current Epidemiology, Diagnosis, and Management
Chancroid: New Developments in an Old Disease
Cholangitis: Pathogenesis, Diagnosis, and Treatment
Septic Thrombophlebitis of Major Dural Venous Sinuses
Acute and Chronic Mastoiditis: Clinical Presentation, Diagnosis, and Management
Enteropathogenic and Enteroaggregative Strains of *Escherichia coli:* Clinical Features of Infection, Epidemiology, and Pathogenesis
BCG Immunization: Review of Past Experience, Current Use, and Future Prospects
Immunization in Adults in the 1990s
Outpatient Management of HIV Infection in the Adult: An Update
Antimicrobial Prophylaxis in Patients Undergoing Solid Organ Transplantation

To our fellows

Nonmenstrual Toxic Shock Syndrome: New Insights into Diagnosis, Pathogenesis, and Treatment

JEFFREY PARSONNET

Toxic shock syndrome (TSS) is a clinical diagnosis defined by the presence of high fever, hypotension, rash, multiple organ-system dysfunction, and desquamation during convalescence (Table 1.1) (1,2). Although best known for its association with menstruation and tampon use, more cases of TSS occur in settings other than during menstruation. TSS is caused by toxigenic strains of *Staphylococcus aureus*, although *Streptococcus pyogenes* can cause an indistinguishable syndrome. When recognized early, before development of serious end-organ damage, TSS carries low rates of mortality and long-term sequelae. The challenge for physicians, therefore, is to consider and recognize TSS in diverse clinical settings, particularly when a primary site of infection is inapparent or the clinical presentation is not classic.

The true incidence of TSS is difficult to define, and this is especially true of nonmenstrual TSS. Although it remains a reportable disease, TSS is significantly underreported on the basis of passive surveillance alone, particularly when product liability is not perceived to be an issue, as in most cases of nonmenstrual disease. Active and passive surveillance by the Centers for Disease Control and Prevention has shown an incidence of roughly one case per 100,000 people in the United States, with only modest geographic differences in incidence. The author's personal experience, however, suggests that the true figure is higher. A full awareness of the epidemiology and varied manifestations of TSS results in increased recognition of this disease and enables the physician to institute appropriate therapy promptly.

Certain aspects of the diagnosis and treatment of nonmenstrual TSS are inherently complex and are emphasized in this review. A discussion of the differential diagnosis of TSS, including streptococcal toxic shock-like syndrome (TSLS) and Kawasaki syndrome, and of pitfalls in establishing a diagnosis of TSS are included. New treatment strategies are recommended on the basis of the author's and others' clinical experiences (in the absence of controlled studies), as well as data generated in the laboratory.

Table 1.1. Case Definition of Toxic Shock Syndrome

- Fever: temperature ≥38.9°C (102°F)
- Rash: typically a diffuse macular erythroderma
- Hypotension: systolic blood pressure ≤90 mm Hg for adults or below fifth percentile by age for children <16 yr of age; orthostatic drop in diastolic blood pressure ≥15 mm Hg, orthostatic syncope, or orthostatic dizziness
- Multisystem disease, consisting of three or more of the following:
  Gastrointestinal: vomiting or diarrhea at onset of illness
  Muscular: severe myalgias or CPK at least twice upper limit of normal
  Mucous membrane: vaginal, oropharyngeal, or conjunctival hyperemia
  Renal: blood urea nitrogen or creatinine at least twice the upper limit of normal, or pyuria (≥5 leukocytes per high-power field) in the absence of urinary tract infection
  Hepatic: total bilirubin or serum transaminase at least twice the upper limit of normal
  Hematologic: platelets ≤100,000/mm^3
  Central nervous system: disorientation or alterations in consciousness without focal neurologic signs when fever and hypotension are absent
- Desquamation: 1 to 2 wk after onset of illness
- Absence of other possible causes of illness, including negative results on the following tests, if obtained: blood, throat, or cerebrospinal fluid cultures (blood culture may be positive for *S. aureus*); rise in titer to agents of Rocky Mountain spotted fever, leptospirosis, or rubeola

Reproduced by permission from Reingold AL, Hargrett NT, Shands KN, et al. Toxic shock syndrome surveillance in the United States, 1980 to 1981. Ann Intern Med 1982;96:875–880.

EPIDEMIOLOGY

Predisposing Factors

TSS develops when a person becomes colonized or infected with a toxigenic strain of *S. aureus* in the absence of a protective level of antibody to that toxin. The most common TSS toxin is TSST-1, which causes almost all cases of menstrual TSS and the majority of cases of nonmenstrual TSS (3,4). TSST-1 is produced by roughly 20% of all strains of *S. aureus*, but only a small percentage of people who are colonized or infected develop TSS (because of immunity to the toxin). TSST-1 is made only by *S. aureus* but is closely related to other members of a family of staphylococcal and streptococcal toxins; this family includes the staphylococcal enterotoxins, which are best known for causing food poisoning, and the streptococcal pyrogenic exotoxins, which cause scarlet fever. The most common alternative TSS toxin is enterotoxin B (SEB), which has been reported to cause 20% to 40% of cases of nonmenstrual TSS (5,6); the other enterotoxins have also been implicated, to a lesser degree (7).

Most people are either intermittently or persistently colonized with *S. aureus* at one or more mucosal or cutaneous sites. At any given time, 10% to 20% of adults harbor *S. aureus* at a mucosal surface. Factors influencing the rate of carriage of *S. aureus* include the presence of chronic skin lesions, injecting drug use, habitation or employment in a health-care facility, hemodialysis, and other conditions. Vaginal colonization with *S. aureus* increases significantly during menstruation, from 7% in premenarchial and postmenarchial women who are not menstruating to 33% among menstruating women (Parsonnet J, unpublished data, 1994). At any given time, between 1% and 4% of healthy individuals, without risk factors for colonization, harbor a TSST-1–producing strain of *S. aureus* at a cutaneous or mucosal site.

Most adults have a protective level of antibody to TSST-1 (as well as to the staphylococcal enterotoxins) (8,9). The percentage of children with antibody rises rapidly between the ages of 6 months, by which time maternal antibody has waned, and 10 years, by which time 60% to 80% of children have protective antibody. The basis for this high rate of seroconversion is not well understood. Mucosal colonization with a toxigenic strain of *S. aureus* is probably immunizing, but subclinical infection or mild cases of illness are probably responsible for some, or possibly many, episodes of seroconversion. For reasons that are also not understood, some otherwise healthy adults never develop antibody, despite documented infection with a toxigenic strain. It is in this setting that recurrent TSS occurs, as discussed below.

Clinical Settings

The clinical settings for nonmenstrual TSS are innumerable and have been reviewed previously (10). A general system for classifying such cases is shown in Table 1.2. In addition to colonization with *S. aureus* and an absence of antibody to toxin, a superimposed factor of some kind usually contributes to development of TSS. This would include the presence of a foreign body at a mucosal surface, such as nasal packing, a barrier contraceptive, or a tampon; a surgical or traumatic wound, providing a nidus for bacterial multiplication and absorption of toxin; devitalized tissue, such as endometrial detritus after childbirth; or an impairment of host defenses, as seen after influenza or varicella. TSS may also accompany simple colonization of the upper respiratory tract (e.g., pharyngitis) (11) or of the lower genital tract (e.g., vaginitis), but such cases tend to be mild.

TSS can occur in association with colonization or infection of the female genital tract in the absence of tampon use. Numerous cases have been reported as having occurred during menstruation without tampon use (12–16). Both the contraceptive diaphragm and sponge have been shown to increase the risk of TSS, with the risk being comparable with that of tampons (17,18). Postpartum TSS occurs after both vaginal and cesarean delivery; in the latter setting, the site of the staphylococcal infection can be either the endometrium (i.e., an ascending infection) or infection of the surgical wound (10). Nonmenstrual TSS can also occur in the setting of a variety of other gynecologic conditions, such as vaginal lacerations, which serve as a nidus for bacterial multiplication and absorption of toxin.

Table 1.2. Clinical Epidemiology of Toxic Shock Syndrome

I. TSS associated with staphylococcal colonization or infection of the genitourinary tract.
   A. TSS associated with menstruation
      1. Tampons in use
      2. Tampons not in use
   B. TSS associated with use of barrier contraceptives
      1. Contraceptive diaphragm
      2. Contraceptive sponge
   C. TSS in the puerperium
      1. Vaginal delivery
      2. Cesarean delivery
   D. Miscellaneous: septic abortion, pelvic surgery, vaginal trauma
II. TSS associated with staphylococcal colonization or infection at other sites.
   A. Skin and soft tissue infections
      1. Superinfection of existing skin lesions: varicella, herpes zoster, burns, insect bites, paronychia, etc
      2. Primary staphylococcal infections: folliculitis, carbuncle, cellulitis, mastitis
   B. Respiratory tract infections
      1. Upper tract infections: sinusitis, pharyngitis, tracheitis, rhinoplasty with nasal packing
      2. Pneumonia (e.g., postinfluenza superinfection)
   C. Musculoskeletal infections: osteomyelitis, prosthetic joint infections, septic arthritis, bursitis, etc
   D. Miscellaneous surgical wound infections

TSS may occur as a consequence of infection of the upper or lower respiratory tract. Numerous cases have been reported in children and adults as a complication of sinusitis (19–21). Surgical procedures requiring postoperative nasal packing, such as rhinoplasty, appear to put patients at particular risk (22–26). Although *S. aureus* is not perceived to be a common cause of pharyngitis, the author has seen numerous children with TSS from whom pure cultures of *S. aureus* were obtained from pharyngeal exudate. Lower respiratory infection, frequently diagnosed as tracheitis in children and bronchitis or pneumonia in adults, results in the most serious cases associated with respiratory colonization (27–30). Particularly noteworthy are clusters of cases associated with outbreaks of influenza (31–33); elderly institutionalized patients appear to be at special risk, presumably as a consequence of higher rates of staphylococcal colonization and pneumonia after influenza and possibly of waning immunity to the TSS toxins.

A wide variety of skin and soft tissue infections may result in TSS. The most common of these are superinfected skin lesions, such as burns and vesicular lesions (including varicella and shingles). Because children often lack antibody, they are at particular risk of developing nonmenstrual TSS under such circumstances. A typical scenario would be that of a child with low-grade fever and a vesicular rash who, after several days of illness, suddenly develops high fever, an erythematous rash, and gastrointestinal or flu-like symptoms. It must be emphasized that the site of staphylococcal infection may be relatively benign in appearance, which requires physicians to have a high index of suspicion when faced with such a patient.

TSS may complicate a wide variety of other soft tissue infections, both primary and secondary. Tabulation of such conditions would serve little purpose other than to provide the basis for additional case reports of "first-ever" occurrences. Of paramount importance is that physicians consider the diagnosis for patients with some combination of suggestive signs and symptoms, particularly when a foreign body is in place or a patient has a higher than usual risk of staphylococcal infection.

CLINICAL MANIFESTATIONS

The clinical manifestations of nonmenstrual TSS are essentially the same as those of menstrual TSS (2,34). The case definition calls for a temperature of 38.9°C (102°F). The rash is most often described as a "sunburn-like" erythroderm and may be diffuse or limited to the face, trunk, or extremities. It may be prominent or subtle; it may also be evanescent, appearing and disappearing before presentation or appearing only after other manifestations of illness are fully established. A systolic blood pressure of less than 90 mm Hg is classic, but this criterion can be fulfilled by demonstration of orthostatic hypotension or a compelling history of orthostatic dizziness. Involvement of three or more organ systems is required, but individual profiles of organ involvement are varied and unpredictable. Gastrointestinal symptoms often predominate, but a flu-like presentation is also common, with prominent arthralgias and myalgias. The creatine phosphokinase is elevated in two thirds of cases, and overt rhabdomyolysis is not uncommon. Common manifestations of multi-system illness include the following: hyperemic mucous membranes; pulmonary edema, which often becomes apparent after fluid resuscitation; renal dysfunction, as manifested by azotemia, oliguria, and pyuria; nonspecific abnormalities of liver function and jaundice; hypocalcemia, which may be life threatening in severity; and thrombocytopenia. In advanced cases there may be intense vasoconstriction resulting in acral cyanosis or gangrene.

Desquamation, one of the hallmarks of TSS, does not begin until at least the fifth day of illness, a point that warrants emphasis. This process may involve just the fingers and toes or large areas of the extremities, trunk, and face. A late rash, occurring one to three weeks after the onset of illness, is occasionally seen, the pathogenesis of which remains uncertain. Reversible alopecia and loss of finger and toenails occur in a modest percentage of patients several months after the acute illness.

The question frequently arises as to whether patients may experience a *forme fruste* of TSS, in which there is compelling epidemiologic, clinical, and laboratory evidence to support the diagnosis but not all of the criteria are met. By definition, it is inappropriate to use the expression *TSS* to describe such an illness, but the author believes that mild cases of staphylococcal toxin-mediated disease do occur, possibly with considerate frequency. In the author's experience, an attenuated illness may be seen when TSS is associated with staphylococcal colonization, in the absence of true infection. Rapidly developing antibody may also result in an abbreviated or attenuated illness, although this is certainly the exception.

The diagnosis of nonmenstrual TSS in children may be especially problematic; the case definition is not as easily applied to this population as to adults. First, the systolic blood pressure of healthy young children is normally less than 90, and documenting a child's pressure less than the fifth percentile by age may be difficult. Second, young children may be unable to characterize symptoms that, in adults, may help define multiple organ-system dysfunction. Third, children may be physiologically more resilient, resulting in a lower incidence of complications such as renal insufficiency and adult respiratory distress syndrome (ARDS). Finally, there is among children a higher incidence of diseases that are difficult to distinguish from TSS, most notably Kawasaki syndrome and scarlet fever. In the author's opinion, mild cases of TSS (to sidestep the semantic inconsistency) frequently go unrecognized as such and are probably as common as full-blown disease, in which all criteria are met.

PATHOGENESIS

The most common TSS toxin is TSST-1, which causes almost all cases of menstrual TSS and 60% to 80% of cases of nonmenstrual TSS (3,4). TSST-1, which is caused only by *S. aureus*, has a molecular weight of 22,000 to 24,000. It is closely related to the staphylococcal enterotoxins and the streptococcal pyrogenic exotoxins (scarlet fever toxins), although there is not significant serologic cross-reactivity between TSST-1 and these toxins. About 20% of all clinical isolates of *S. aureus* produce TSST-1. Production of TSST-1 is regulated by a gene known as *agr* (35,36); strains possessing this gene produce TSST-1 constitutively, but the amount of TSST-1 produced varies over a wide range.

A variety of physicochemical factors is known to influence production of TSST-1. These include pH, with toxin production being greatest between pH 6 and 8; oxygen concentration, with little toxin produced at a Po_2 of less than 5 mmHg; concentration of CO_2, which increases TSST-1; and concentration of divalent cations, particularly magnesium (37–40). During menstruation, the vaginal pH changes from one of acidity to one of neutrality, and oxygen dissolved in menstrual fluid or introduced by a foreign body, such as a barrier contraceptive or a tampon, changes the environment from anaerobic to aerobic. These requirements for optimal production of TSST-1 may explain why nonmenstrual TSS is rarely seen in association with visceral abscesses, which are likely to be anaerobic and acidic in nature. Optimal conditions for production of TSST-1 may, however, be attained in a variety of nonmenstrual clinical settings (19).

TSST-1 and the alternative TSS toxins (of which SEB is the most common) are members of a family of bacterial exoproducts known as "superantigens" (41–43). These toxins interact with cells of the immune system by binding directly to MHC class II molecules, HLA-DR, -DP, and -DQ, which are present in large numbers on monocytes, macrophages, and B cells. The MHC-toxin complex then interacts with T lymphocytes bearing specific variable regions on the β subunit of the T-cell receptor. This interaction, which may involve a large percentage of T cells and is not dependent on specific recognition of the toxin, results in polyclonal T-cell proliferation (hence, the expression "superantigen") and initiation of a cascade of release of endogenous mediators of inflammation.

Use of the word "toxin" to describe TSST-1 is something of a misnomer, as this protein is not particularly toxic to human cells. Rather, TSST-1 appears to cause fever, hypotension, and multisystem disease by inducing production and release of endogenous mediators of inflammation (44). Although the relative importance of the individual cytokines remains the subject of ongoing research, it is clear that TSST-1 is a potent inducer of interleukin-2 production by lymphocytes and of interleukin-1 and tumor necrosis factor production by monocytes and macrophages (45–50). The diverse pathophysiologic effects of these cytokines in septic shock and TSS, and potential strategies directed against them, have recently been reviewed (51). TSST-1 itself has a relatively short serum half-life (52).

Neutralization of TSST-1 by administration of monoclonal or polyclonal antibody can bring about rapid reversal of early shock in animal models (52,53) and, by anecdotal report, in people with TSS (54). Once established, however, the cascade of endogenous mediators takes on a life of its own, resulting in hypoperfusion and end-organ damage—acute tubular necrosis, ischemic liver disease, ARDS, rhabdomyolysis, digital necrosis, and so on. The pace and severity of a patient's illness is difficult to predict at the time of presentation, but the duration of toxemia and severity of hypoperfusion are probably predictors of serious sequelae. Accordingly, rapid measures to eliminate circulating toxin and maintain organ perfusion are the cornerstones of therapy.

Several characteristic features of TSS merit special mention. The basis for the rash, which is variable in appearance but is most commonly a diffuse erythroderm, remains uncertain. Hypocalcemia, an almost invariable feature of TSS, reflects both a decrease in ionized calcium and a decrease in serum albumin concentration (55). Hypoalbuminemia is a nonspecific reaction to high levels of endogenous mediators, such as interleukin-1. Several explanations have been offered for the decrease in ionized calcium, such as high calcitonin levels, an inadequate parathyroid response, and massive influx of calcium into cells (55–57). The actual mechanism remains a matter of conjecture, however. Cardiac dysfunction (58–61), including arrhythmias, hypokinesis, and cardiac arrest, most likely reflects the effects of myocardial depressant substances (such as tumor necrosis factor) and electrolyte disturbances, but this too requires further study.

DIAGNOSIS

Differential Diagnosis

TSS is relatively easy to diagnose once a patient has developed desquamation; this does not occur, however, until 7 to 14 days after the onset of illness. The differential diagnosis at the time of presentation may be narrow or broad, depending on whether the pathognomonic features of full-blown disease are apparent. It would be a daunting proposition to review the broadest list of diagnoses associated with fever and rash. In evaluating a patient with serious manifestations of illness, however, the author has found it most helpful to consider the following entities.

Group A Streptococcal Infection *S. pyogenes* produces exotoxins that are closely related to TSST-1 and are capable of causing an illness that is indistinguishable, on clinical grounds, from staphylococcal TSS (62–64). A variety of terms have been used to describe this syndrome, including streptococcal TSS, TSLS, toxic strep syndrome, and others. A working case definition of streptococcal TSS has been derived (65). Cases are defined as the presence of hypotension plus two or more of the following: renal impairment; hepatic dysfunction; coagulopathy; ARDS; a generalized erythematous rash that may desquamate; and soft tissue necrosis, including necrotizing fasciitis or myositis. A case is called "confirmed" if group A streptococcus is isolated from a normally sterile site and "probable" if the organism is isolated from a nonsterile site, such as the throat, vagina, respiratory tract, or skin lesions. The primary site of infection is most often skin, soft tissues, or mucous membranes, although a definite portal of entry cannot be ascertained in some patients. Cases have been reported to occur in association with streptococcal pharyngitis alone (i.e., without bacteremia or evidence of disseminated infection) (66). The illness may begin as a flu-like syndrome, with fever, chills, myalgia, and gastrointestinal symptoms, or as localized pain at the site of infection. As with TSS, hypotension is a defining criterion of TSLS. Rash and desquamation are less common in streptococcal than in staphylococcal TSS, whereas cellulitis and fasciitis suggest a streptococcal etiology. The frequency of various manifestations of TSLS have recently been reviewed (67).

The emergence of streptococcal TSS (or TSLS) as a widely recognized phenomenon most likely reflects changes, over the past decade, in the frequency with which group A streptococci produce specific virulence factors (68). For example, M-1 and M-3 serotypes have predominated among patients with shock and organ involvement, but it is not clear whether these proteins are in some way responsible for TSLS or serve as markers for other virulence factors. Several studies have shown an association between production of pyrogenic exotoxin A (SpeA) or with the phage-associated *speA* gene, but many cases have been caused by strains that are clearly negative for this toxin. Necrotizing soft tissue infection may be attributable to production of proteases or other extracellular toxins. In fact, TSLS may represent multiple clinical entities that reflect both the virulence factors of the organism and specific and nonspecific immunity of the host.

Kawasaki Syndrome (KS) Also known as mucocutaneous lymph node syndrome, KS can be as difficult to differentiate from nonmenstrual TSS in a child as streptococcal TSS is in an adult. KS is an illness of young children, with 80% of patients being less than 4 years of age. As with TSS, KS is a clinical diagnosis that rests upon fulfillment of established criteria: fever lasting 5 days or more that is unresponsive to antibiotics, plus conjunctival injection, changes in oropharyngeal mucosae, erythema or edema of the hands and feet and/or periungual desquamation during convalescence, a polymorphous rash, and cervical lymphadenopathy (69). KS and nonmenstrual TSS differ in that KS is more of a subacute process and is not generally accompanied by hypotension and multiple organ dysfunction. (These differences may be more apparent than real, however, in that the working definition for TSS does not accommodate mild cases.) TSS is also accompanied by thrombocytopenia (vs. a normal or increased platelet count in KS), a sunburn-like erythroderm, and hypocalcemia, and a primary site of infection may be evident.

The striking similarity between the two diseases most likely represents similar pathogenic mechanisms, such as induction of cytokines by an infectious agent of some kind. A wide variety of agents, including viruses, fungi, bacteria, and toxins, has been touted as putative causes of KS. Most recently, it was reported that many children with KS are colonized with toxigenic staphylococci or streptococci (70), and there is reason to believe that some patients who fulfill the KS criteria are actually manifesting the effects of bacterial toxins. Subsequent studies have not confirmed, however, that the majority of KS cases are caused by gram-positive bacterial toxins. The similarity between KS and TSS (and, for that matter, a variety of streptococcal syndromes) mandates that patients with KS be evaluated meticulously for gram-positive pathogens, including cultures of throat, vagina, and rectum.

Other Entities A variety of other diagnoses merit consideration, if only because of the consequences of delayed initiation of therapy. Staphylococcal scalded skin syndrome (SSSS) is caused by exfoliation or epidermolytic toxin, which is produced by *S. aureus* during colonization or infection. SSSS differs from TSS in that the desquamation, which is bullous in nature, occurs during the acute illness as opposed to during convalescence. Furthermore, hypotension and multisystem failure are usually absent. This is generally a disease of young children, who are more likely to lack antibody to the toxin.

Rocky Mountain spotted fever and meningococcemia are acute febrile illnesses that are frequently accompanied by rash, hypotension, and multiple organ involvement. The rashes caused by these organisms are classically purpuric in nature, however, whereas that of TSS is only rarely so. Unfortunately, from a diagnostic standpoint, skin lesions may be subtle, evanescent, or absent in all three diseases, so it is unwise to base therapeutic decisions solely on the presence or character of a rash. A careful epidemiologic history, including history of travel, exposure to ticks, use of tampons or barrier contraceptives, and residence in a dormitory or other such facility, may suggest one or another of these diseases. Differentiation between them is obviously critical, as optimal therapy for infections due to *S. aureus* (such as nafcillin or clindamycin) will generally be inadequate for treatment of those due to *N. meningitidis* and *R. rickettsii*.

Patients with gram-negative bacillary bacteremia can certainly present with fever, hypotension, and multiple organ system dysfunction, but a diffuse rash would be uncharacteristic (unless from a drug reaction). Vomiting, diarrhea, and abdominal pain may be prominent features of pneumonia, intra-abdominal sepsis, and TSS, however; thus, it is not always possible to differentiate among these entities before the results of radiologic and microbiologic studies have returned. In such cases, use of broad spectrum antibiotics that would cover both *S. aureus* and common gram-negative bacilli and anaerobes may be warranted.

Most viral illnesses cause neither hypotension nor multiple organ system dysfunction in normal hosts, although severe measles has been confused with TSS (71). Infection with hantavirus may result in hypotension and multisystem disease (hantavirus pulmonary syndrome), but rash appears to be uncommon in this disease (72).

Finally, a careful history of drug ingestion must be taken to exclude the possibility of a severe adverse drug reaction. In the author's experience, adverse reactions to sulfa drugs, quinolones, β-lactam antibiotics, and quinidine have been confused with TSS; pseudoephedrine has also been reported to cause a TSS-like illness (73). Fever, rash, hypotension, myocardial dysfunction, rhabdomyolysis, renal failure, and peripheral vasoconstriction can also occur as a result of cocaine injection or inhalation (74,75); blood and urine toxicology screens should be performed under the appropriate circumstances.

Laboratory Evaluation

Because TSS may be complicated by dysfunction of multiple organ systems, patients require close monitoring for life-threatening and remediable physiologic abnormalities. Initial evaluation should include a complete blood count, platelet count, and prothrombin time; determination of electrolyte, calcium, magnesium, phosphate, and albumin concentrations; tests of renal and hepatic function; and a creatine phosphokinase (CPK level). A urinalysis should be performed, plus a urine culture if pyuria is present. A chest radiograph and an electrocardiogram should be performed. Additional studies may be required depending on the circumstances.

Although recovery of *S. aureus* is not officially part of the case definition of TSS, it is important to try to recover this organism from patients with a suggestive clinical illness. In the evaluation of nonmenstrual TSS, this would typically involve culturing any wound or other skin or soft tissue site. It is important to emphasize that in many cases of nonmenstrual TSS, the primary site of infection is not immediately apparent. Infected surgical or traumatic wounds are notoriously benign in appearance in TSS; surgeons may have to be pressured before they are willing to violate what appears to be a benign wound for the sake of obtaining deep wound cultures. Although bacteremia is uncommon in TSS, blood should be cultured, both to evaluate the patient for alternative diagnoses and for the possibility of disseminated staphylococcal infection. Some cases of nonmenstrual TSS occur in the setting of what would more properly be called colonization than infection. In the absence of a primary site of infection, cultures should be obtained from the throat, vagina, and rectum.

There are numerous pitfalls in trying to establish a diagnosis of TSS, as listed in Table 1.3. TSS is probably underrecognized in children, for reasons that are both biologic and related to physician awareness. Some cases of TSS are missed because of a persistent misconception that a foreign body is required for development of illness. Because TSS is caused by the release of toxins rather than by rapid bacterial multiplication and development of pyogenic infection, benign-appearing lesions are often overlooked as the source of illness. Confusion over the timing of desquamation continues to lead physicians away from considering this diagnosis. Physicians may fail to obtain appropriate cultures, especially of mucosal sites, or obtain cultures only after antibiotics have been administered. Finally, laboratories may fail to recognize *S. aureus* in cultures that have been appropriately obtained. TSS-associated strains of *S. aureus* are often minimally β-hemolytic and tend to be hypopigmented in comparison with other pathogenic strains (76–79). This may result in misidentification of *S. aureus* as a coagulase-negative staphylococcus.

The question often arises as to the utility of performing special studies for TSST-1 and other TSS toxins, as well as for antibody to same. Such studies are often useful, but more for the sake of long-term management than for diagnosis and more for menstrual than for nonmenstrual disease. Almost all cases of menstrual TSS are caused by TSST-1. Therefore, the finding of a TSST-1–producing strain of *S. aureus* in combination with an absence of antibody to TSST-1 is strongly supportive of the diagnosis. Development of a protective level of antibody during convalescence (seroconversion) will protect a patient from recurrent episodes of TSS, which is useful information in counseling patients as to the risks of using tampons and contraceptive devices. Unfortunately, many patients with definite menstrual TSS—probably on the order of two thirds—do not seroconvert, which makes the running of paired samples a test of low diagnostic sensitivity.

The utility of special studies for diagnosis of nonmenstrual TSS is made problematic by the fact that as many as 40% of cases are caused by staphylococcal toxins other than TSST-1. Therefore, it may be necessary to test recovered strains for production of multiple toxins (particularly if the strain is negative for

Table 1.3. Pitfalls in Establishing a Diagnosis of Toxic Shock Syndrome

- Failure to suspect TSS in the nonmenstrual setting, especially among children.
- Failure to suspect TSS in menstruating women who are not using tampons or who are using low absorbency or "natural fiber" tampons.
- Failure to suspect menstrual TSS because of an absence of vaginal discharge or inflammation, and nonmenstrual TSS because of the nonpurulent appearance of a wound (i.e., no obvious staphylococcal infection).
- Failure to suspect TSS because of the absence of a diffuse erythroderm at the time of presentation.
- Failure to diagnose TSS because desquamation is absent at the time of presentation.
- Failure to recognize the "flu-like" presentation of TSS.
- Failure to obtain appropriate cultures of wounds and mucous membranes.
- Failure of laboratory personnel to recognize hypopigmented or nonhemolytic strains of *S. aureus*, especially when present in mixed culture.

TSST-1) before antibody testing can be conducted. In addition, less is known about the rate of seroconversion after nonmenstrual TSS. Finally, nonmenstrual TSS is much less likely to recur than is menstrual TSS, which decreases the utility of determining a patient's serologic status.

For these reasons, a compelling case can be made for sending staphylococcal isolates plus acute and convalescent sera for toxin and antibody testing in the setting of menstrual TSS but not routinely for nonmenstrual disease. The author welcomes submission of staphylococcal isolates and sera for testing; samples can be sent to Dr. Jeffrey Parsonnet at Dartmouth-Hitchcock Medical Center, Lebanon, NH 03756. Several commercial laboratories in the United States also offer both toxin and antibody testing.

TREATMENT

General Management

The cornerstones of treatment of nonmenstrual TSS are intravascular volume repletion and removal or drainage of any focus of infection. Fluid requirements are often massive because of capillary leak, which may result in anasarca and pulmonary edema. Because TSST-1 is rapidly cleared from the bloodstream, drainage or removal of the primary site of infection may bring about prompt improvement, particularly if end-organ damage, such as tubular necrosis, ARDS, or rhabdomyolysis, has not yet occurred.

Treatment with vasopressors is indicated when intravenous fluids are inadequate to reverse hypotension or when pulmonary edema prevents further fluid administration. Cardiac dysfunction, in the form of ventricular hypokinesis, is common in severe cases of TSS and may also warrant and benefit from pharmacologic intervention (58,61). Dopamine is usually the most appropriate agent because of its diverse effects on renal perfusion, myocardial function, and vascular tone, but dobutamine and norepinephrine may be preferable or required under some circumstances. Ventilatory support is occasionally necessary, especially after large volumes of fluid have been administered in the setting of oliguria.

Certain physiologic parameters require close monitoring, even in mild and moderate cases of nonmenstrual TSS. Hypocalcemia can be severe and life threatening. To some extent this is related to hypoalbuminemia, but a decrease in ionized calcium is also present in most cases. Hypocalcemia may be most profound a few days after the onset of illness; for this reason the serum calcium should be monitored daily over this period of time. Hypomagnesemia is also quite common and may complicate efforts to correct serum calcium levels (80). Rhabdomyolysis is a common complication of TSS, with creatine phosphokinase (CPK) levels often rising into the tens of thousands on the second or third day of illness. This may result in myoglobinuria, further complicating efforts to restore renal function (81). Coagulopathy may be severe, with thrombocytopenia and other laboratory manifestations of disseminated intravascular coagulation; clinical bleeding is relatively uncommon, however. Azotemia is often rapidly corrected with administration of fluids, but dialysis is occasionally required for removal of fluid and progressive renal insufficiency.

Antimicrobial Therapy

Administration of an antistaphylococcal antibiotic is important in nonmenstrual TSS to arrest staphylococcal multiplication and toxin production. This is especially true when there is no drainable focus of infection or removable device. Most TSS-associated strains of *S. aureus* are resistant to penicillin but susceptible to β-lactamase–resistant penicillins and cephalosporins; reports of methicillin resistance have been few. Accordingly, empiric therapy with nafcillin (or oxacillin) or, in the setting of penicillin allergy, cefazolin is appropriate. Empiric therapy with vancomycin is indicated only when a patient is considered to be at higher than usual risk of infection with a methicillin-resistant strain or when there is a history of anaphylaxis to penicillin. Intravenous therapy is usually indicated, either because of gastrointestinal symptoms or the need for higher drug levels than could be achieved by oral agents. Some mild cases of TSS can be managed with oral agents alone, particularly when there is a removable device or easily drained superficial infection.

Anecdotal clinical reports and laboratory studies suggest that antibiotics that inhibit protein synthesis, such as clindamycin, may be more effective than the β-lactam antibiotics (including penicillins and cephalosporins), which interfere with cell-wall synthesis (82,83). β-Lactams exert their bactericidal effect only on dividing bacteria. When bacterial numbers are high, many bacteria may be in stationary phase and remain viable in the face of therapy with these agents; these bacteria may continue to produce exoproducts, including TSST-1. This phenomenon, which is known as the "Eagle effect," was first described by Eagle (84) in relation to group A streptococci and has recently been re-examined by Stevens et al (85).

We recently showed that clindamycin almost completely blocks production of TSST-1 by toxigenic strains of *S. aureus* at a concentration as low as 1/64 of the minimum inhibitory concentration (86). Other inhibitors of protein synthesis, such as clarithromycin and gentamicin, were also effective at subinhibitory concentrations. An unexpected finding was that all β-lactam antibiotics, to one extent or another, actually increased production of TSST-1 when incubated with bacteria at subinhibitory concentrations. These data suggest that when antibiotic levels are low, which might be the case at mucosal sites or within abscesses or devitalized tissue, clindamycin may be superior to β-lactam antibiotics for treatment of infection syndromes mediated principally by toxins, such as TSS. As most strains of *S. aureus* are susceptible to clindamycin, it is the author's practice to treat nonmenstrual TSS with clindamycin, either initially or after susceptibility tests have returned.

Other Therapeutic Measures

Absence of antibody to TSST-1 (or other TSS toxins) is a prerequisite for development of disease. We have found that all commercially available preparations of immune globulin have high levels of antibody to TSST-1, as expected (as they are prepared from sera of healthy adults) (Parsonnet, unpublished data, 1994). It is reasonable to expect, therefore, that administration of high-dose immune globulin (IVIG) would be a useful adjunctive measure for treatment of severe cases of TSS, and this expectation has been supported by the author's and others' clinical experience (54).

Most patients with TSS recover quickly once the diagnosis has been considered and therapy has been initiated. Some patients continue to deteriorate, however, particularly those with nonmenstrual disease who have a persistent nidus of infection. It is this group of patients that should be considered for treatment with IVIG. Although the frequency of adverse events associated with IVIG is low, the cost is high, with a single dose costing our institution $690 for an average-sized adult (with a higher cost to the patient). Therefore, IVIG should not be administered unless there is a reasonable degree of certainty that a patient has TSS and has failed to respond or has been intolerant of conventional therapies, including aggressive fluid administration, antibiotics, and surgical drainage. The author's practice is to administer IVIG only when a patient begins to develop pulmonary edema, thereby limiting his or her tolerance of fluids, or when vasopressor support is required beyond an initial period of several hours.

When the decision is made to treat with IVIG, the dose most often used has been 400 mg/kg, given as a single dose over a period of several hours. The response to treatment often appears to be quite dramatic, although the uncontrolled nature of these observations must be acknowledged. Treatment results in a serum antibody titer many times higher than that which seems to provide immunity to TSST-1. Figure 1.1 shows the results of a representative patient with TSS treated by the author with IVIG. The anti-TSST-1 titer rose from less than 1:4 before treatment to 1:512 after treatment, and the titer was still in the protective range almost 3 months later.

Of paramount importance in treating TSS is removal of any foreign body or drainage of any site of infection. Most cases of nonmenstrual TSS result from skin and soft tissue infections, but cases have been reported in association with endocarditis, osteomyelitis, endometritis, and other foci that are not easily amenable to drainage. The usual indications for surgical debridement should be applied to such patients. This group of patients stands to benefit the most from administration of IVIG.

Corticosteroids should not be a administered routinely to patients with nonmenstrual TSS. In a retrospective analysis, Todd et al (87) showed that patients treated with steroids had a shorter time until defervescence and clinical stability than patients not so treated, but there was no difference in mortality. In this author's opinion, it makes more sense to treat with IVIG than with steroids for patients with serious or refractory illness.

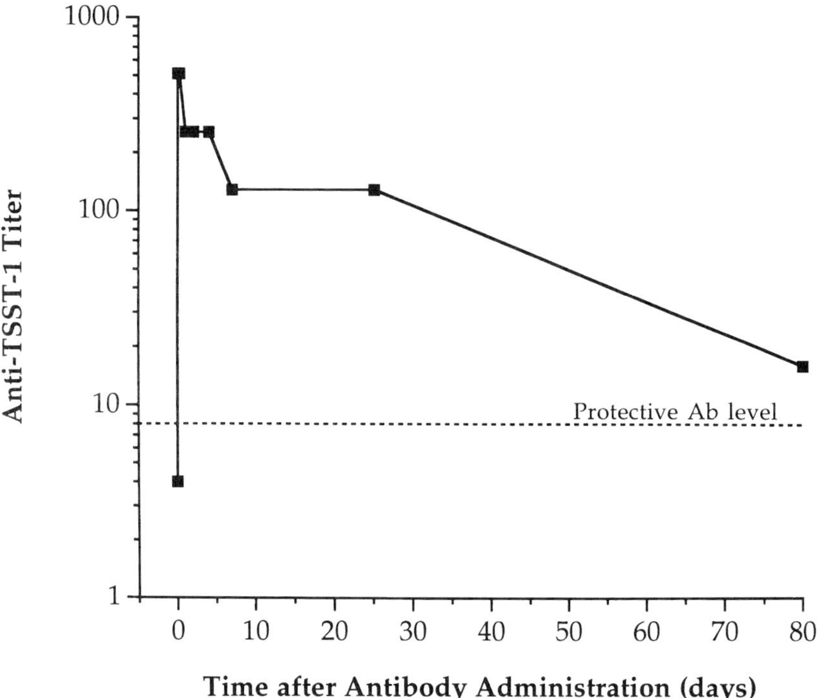

Figure 1.1. Serum antibody to TSST-1 before and after administration of high-dose immunoglobin. The patient, an 18-year old woman with menstrual TSS, was given 400 mg/kg of immunoglobulin over a period of 4 hours. Her antibody titer was 1:4 (plotted as 1:4) prior to treatment; immediately after the infusion, her antibody level was 1:512.

PROGNOSIS

The mortality rate of nonmenstrual TSS is low, probably on the order of 2–5%. Nonmenstrual TSS seems to carry a worse prognosis than menstrual disease, probably because of delayed diagnosis and the more serious nature of the primary infection. Most fatalities occur when there has been a long period of hypotension before initiation of therapy, which increases the likelihood of serious end-organ damage.

The major complications of TSS are ARDS, often requiring mechanical ventilation and occasionally resulting in chronic lung disease; cardiovascular collapse, with refractory hypotension; cardiac dysfunction, including refractory arrhythmias; acute renal insufficiency, requiring dialysis; peripheral vasoconstriction, resulting in gangrene; and rhabdomyolysis. Patients who develop renal failure may require dialysis for several weeks before renal function begins to improve. Less serious sequelae include alopecia and nail loss, which occur several months after acute illness and are reversible; a late rash, which occurs several weeks after illness; and persistent neuropsychological symptoms, such as fatigue, depression, and memory loss (88).

Recurrent nonmenstrual TSS does occur but much less frequently than does menstrual disease. We were recently involved in the care of three patients with recurrent nonmenstrual TSS—one with a breast abscess, one with postpartum TSS, and one with lower respiratory tract infection. In each case, the diagnosis was not suspected during the initial illness but only after the patient returned with recurrent symptoms and desquamation that had developed after the first episode. In none of the cases was the patient treated with a full course of antistaphylococcal antibiotics during the initial episode of illness.

For reasons that are unclear, most patients do not develop a protective level of antibody after an episode of menstrual TSS (89–91). Data on seroconversion after nonmenstrual TSS are scanty; in our experience with several dozen patients, however, approximately three quarters of patients with nonmenstrual TSS did not develop antibody, making them vulnerable to recurrent disease. The reason for the lower recurrence rate in nonmenstrual TSS could be that initial episodes tend to be more adequately treated or that the risk factor for disease is less likely to be periodic in nonmenstrual than in menstrual TSS.

Elimination of carriage of toxigenic strains of *S. aureus* would decrease what is already a low rate of recurrence. This is somewhat problematic, however, as patients may be colonized with more than one strain of *S. aureus* (requiring repeated testing of multiple strains) or may become recolonized with the original strain at a remote time. My usual recommendation, therefore, is that patients be treated for a total of 2 weeks with antistaphylococcal antibiotics, given intravenously until a patient has improved and can take oral medications. Staphylococcal carriage could probably be decreased further by use of combination regimens of antibiotics, but the incidence of recurrent nonmenstrual TSS is low enough as not to warrant this approach on a routine basis.

REFERENCES

1 **Todd J, Fishaut M, Kapral F, Welch T.** Toxic-shock syndrome associated with phage-group-I staphylococci. Lancet 1978;2: 1116–1118.

2 **Reingold AL, Hargrett NT, Shands KN, et al.** Toxic shock syndrome surveillance in the United States, 1980 to 1981. Ann Intern Med 1982;96(Part 2):875–880.

3 **Bergdoll MS, Crass BA, Reiser RF, et al.** A new staphylococcal enterotoxin, enterotoxin F, associated with toxic-shock-syndrome *Staphylococcus aureus* isolates. Lancet 1981;1: 1017–1021.

4 **Schlievert PM, Shands KN, Dan BB, et al.** Identification and characterization of an exotoxin from *Staphylococcus aureus* associated with toxic-shock syndrome. J Infect Dis 1981;143:509–516.

5 **Lee VT, Chang AH, Chow AW.** Detection of staphylococcal enterotoxin B among toxic shock syndrome (TSS)- and non-TSS-associated *Staphylococcus aureus* isolates. J Infect Dis 1992;166:911–915.

6 **Schlievert PM.** Staphylococcal enterotoxin B and toxic-shock syndrome toxin-1 are significantly associated with non-menstrual TSS. Lancet 1986;1:1149–1150. Letter.

7 **Crass BA, Bergdoll MS.** Involvement of staphylococcal enterotoxins in nonmenstrual toxic shock syndrome. J Clin Microbiol 1986;23:1138–1139.

8 **Reiser RF, Jacobson JA, Kasworm EM, Bergdoll MS.** Staphylococcal enterotoxin antibodies in pediatric patients from Utah. J Infect Dis 1988;158:1105–1108.

9 **Vergeront JM, Stolz SJ, Crass BA, et al.** Prevalence of serum antibody to staphylococcal enterotoxin F among Wisconsin residents: implications for toxic-shock syndrome. J Infect Dis 1983;148:692–698.

10 **Reingold AL, Hargrett NT, Dan BB, et al.** Nonmenstrual toxic shock syndrome: a review of 130 cases. Ann Intern Med 1982; 96(Part 2):871–874.

11 **Hirsch B, Stair T, Horowitz BZ, Brooks C.** Toxic shock syndrome from staphylococcal pharyngitis. Ear Nose Throat J 1984;63:494–497.

12 **Chow AW, Wong CK, MacFarlane AM, Bartlett KH.** Toxic shock syndrome: clinical and laboratory findings in 30 patients. Can Med Assoc J 1984;130:425–430.

13 **Reingold AL, Broome CV, Gaventa S, Hightower AW.** Risk factors for menstrual toxic shock syndrome: results of a multistate case-control study. Rev Infect Dis 1989; 11(suppl 1):S35–S41.

14 **Osterholm MT, Davis JP, Gibson RW, et al.** Tri-state toxic-shock syndrome study. I. Epidemiologic findings. J Infect Dis 1982; 145:431–440.

15 **Davis JP, Chesney PJ, Wand PJ, LaVenture M, and the Investigation and Laboratory Team.** Toxic-shock syndrome: epidemiologic features, recurrence, risk factors, and prevention. N Engl J Med 1980;303:1429–1435.

16 **Tofte RW, Williams DN.** Toxic shock syndrome: clinical and laboratory features in 15 patients. Ann Intern Med 1981;94:149–156.

17 **Faich G, Pearson K, Fleming D, et al.** Toxic shock syndrome and the vaginal contraceptive sponge. JAMA 1986;255:216–218.

18 **Schwartz B, Gaventa S, Broome CV, et al.** Nonmenstrual toxic shock syndrome associated with barrier contraceptives: report of a case-control study. Rev Infect Dis 1989; 11(suppl 1):S43–S49.

19 **Ferguson MA, Todd JK.** Toxic shock syndrome associated with *Staphylococcus aureus* sinusitis in children. J Infect Dis 1990;161: 953–955.

20 **Griffith JA, Perkin RM.** Toxic shock syndrome and sinusitis—a hidden site of infection. West J Med 1988;148:580–581.

21 **Wood SD, Ries K, White GLJ, et al.** Maxillary sinusitis—the focus of toxic shock syndrome in a male patient. West J Med 1987;147:467–469.

22 **Nahass RG, Gocke DJ.** Toxic shock syndrome associated with use of a nasal tampon. Am J Med 1988;8:4629–46231.

23 **Hull HF, Mann JM, Sands CJ, et al.** Toxic shock syndrome related to nasal packing. Arch Otolaryngol 1983;109:624–626.

24 **Allen ST, Liland JB, Nichols CG, Glew RH.** Toxic shock syndrome associated with use of latex nasal packing. Arch Intern Med 1990;150:2587–2588.

25 **Jacobson JA, Kasworm EM.** Toxic shock syndrome after nasal surgery. Case reports and analysis of risk factors. Arch Otolaryngol Head Neck Surg 1986;112:329–332.

26 **Thomas SW, Baird IM, Frazier RD.** Toxic shock syndrome following submucous resection and rhinoplasty. JAMA 1982;247: 2402–2403.

27 **Wilkins EG, Nye F, Roberts C, de Saxe M.** Probable toxic shock syndrome with

primary staphylococcal pneumonia. J Infect 1985;11:231–232.

28 **Dann EJ, Weinberger M, Gillis S, et al.** Bacterial laryngotracheitis associated with toxic shock syndrome in an adult. Clin Infect Dis 1994;18:437–439.

29 **Surh L, Read SE.** Staphylococcal tracheitis and toxic shock syndrome in a young child. J Pediatr 1984;105:585–587.

30 **Solomon R, Truman T, Murray DL.** Toxic shock syndrome as a complication of bacterial tracheitis. Pediatr Infect Dis 1985;4:298–299.

31 **Tolan RW Jr.** Toxic shock syndrome complicating influenze A in a child: case report and review. Clin Infect Dis 1993;17:43–45.

32 **Sperber SJ, Francis JB.** Toxic shock syndrome during an influenza outbreak. JAMA 1987;257:1086–1087.

33 **MacDonald KL, Osterholm MT, Hedberg CW, et al.** Toxic shock syndrome: a newly recognized complication of influenza and influenzalike illness. JAMA 1987;257:1053–1058.

34 **Kain KC, Schulzer M, Chow AW.** Clinical spectrum of nonmenstrual toxic shock syndrome (TSS): comparison with menstrual TSS by multivariate discriminant analyses. Clin Infect Dis 1993;16:100–106.

35 **Kreiswirth BN.** Genetics and expression of toxic shock syndrome toxin 1: overview. Rev Infect Dis 1989;11(suppl 1):S97–S100.

36 **Peng HL, Novick RP, Kreiswirth B, et al.** Cloning, characterization, and sequencing of an accessory gene regulator (agr) in *Staphylococcus aureus*. J Bacteriol 1988;170:4365–4372.

37 **Wong ACL, Bergdoll MS.** Effect of environmental conditions on production of toxic shock syndrome toxin 1 by *Staphylococcus aureus*. Infect Immun 1990;58:1026–1029.

38 **Todd JK, Todd BH, Franco BA, et al.** Influence of focal growth conditions on the pathogenesis of toxic shock syndrome. J Infect Dis 1987;155:673–681.

39 **Schlievert PM, Blomster DA.** Production of staphylococcal pyrogenic exotoxin type C: influence of physical and chemical factors. J Infect Dis 1983;147:236–242.

40 **Kass EH, Kendrick MI, Tsai YC, Parsonnet J.** Interaction of magnesium ion, oxygen tension, and temperature in the production of toxic shock syndrome toxin-1 by *Staphylococcus aureus*. J Infect Dis 1987;155:812–815.

41 **Salamon FT, Fayen JD, Leonard ML, et al.** Accessory function of human mononuclear phagocytes for lymphocyte responses to the superantigen staphylococcal enterotoxin B. Cell Immunol 1992;141:466–484.

42 **Scholl P, Diez A, Mourad W, et al.** Toxic shock syndrome toxin-1 binds to MHC class II molecules. Proc Natl Acad Sci USA 1989;86:4210–4214.

43 **Scholl PR, Diez A, Geha RS.** Staphylococcal enterotoxin B and toxic shock syndrome toxin-1 bind to distinct sites on HLA-DR and HLA-DQ molecules. J Immunol 1989;143:2583–2588.

44 **Parsonnet J.** Mediators in the pathogenesis of toxic shock syndrome: overview. Rev Infect Dis 1989;11(suppl 1):S263–S269.

45 **Ikejima T, Dinarello CA, Gill DM, Wolff SM.** Induction of human interleukin-1 by a product of *Staphylococcus aureus* associated with toxic shock syndrome. J Clin Invest 1984;73:1312–1320.

46 **Ikejima T, Okusawa S, van der Meer JW, Dinarello CA.** Induction by toxic-shock-syndrome toxin-1 of a circulating tumor necrosis factor-like substance in rabbits and of immunoreactive tumor necrosis factor and interleukin-1 from human mononuclear cells. J Infect Dis 1988;158:1017–1025.

47 **Micusan VV, Mercier G, Bhatti AR, et al.** Production of human and murine interleukin-2 by toxic shock syndrome toxin-1. Immunology 1986;58:203–208.

48 **Parsonnet J, Hickman RK, Eardley DD, Pier GB.** Induction of human interleukin-1 by toxic shock syndrome toxin-1. J Infect Dis 1985;151:514–522.

49 **Parsonnet J, Gillis ZA.** Production of tumor necrosis factor by human monocytes in response to toxic shock syndrome toxin-1. J Infect Dis 1988;158:1026–1033.

50 **Uchiyama T, Kamagata Y, Yan XJ, et al.** Relative strength of the mitogenic and interleukin-2-production-inducing activities of staphylococcal exotoxins presumed to be causative exotoxins of toxic shock syndrome: toxic shock syndrome toxin-1 and enterotoxins A, B and C to murine and human T cells. Clin Exp Immunol 1989;75:239–244.

51 **Dinarello CA, Gelfand JA, Wolff SM.** Anticytokine strategies in the treatment of the systemic inflammatory response syndrome. JAMA 1993;269:1829–1835.

52 **Melish ME, Murata S, Fukunaga C, et al.** Endotoxin is not an essential mediator in toxic shock syndrome. Rev Infect Dis 1989;11(suppl 1):S219–S228.

53 **Best GK, Scott DF, Kling JM, et al.** Protection of rabbits in an infection model of toxic

shock syndrome (TSS) by a TSS toxin-1-specific monoclonal antibody. Infect Immun 1988;56:998–999.

54 **Barry W, Hudgins L, Donta ST, Pesanti EL.** Intravenous immunoglobulin therapy for toxic shock syndrome. JAMA 1992;267: 3315–3316.

55 **Chesney RW, McCarron DM, Haddad JG, et al.** Pathogenic mechanisms of the hypocalcemia of the staphylococcal toxic-shock syndrome. J Lab Clin Med 1983;101: 576–585.

56 **Sperber SJ, Blevins DD, Francis JB.** Hypercalcitoninemia, hypocalcemia, and toxic shock syndrome. Rev Infect Dis 1990;12:736–739.

57 **Heimburger DC.** Hyperthyrocalcitoninemia in toxic shock syndrome. South Med J 1981;74:1265–1266.

58 **Olson RD, Stevens DL, Melish ME.** Direct effects of purified staphylococcal toxic shock syndrome toxin 1 on myocardial function of isolated rabbit atria. Rev Infect Dis 1989;11(suppl 1):S313–S315.

59 **Fitz JD, Weeks KDJ, Duff P.** Left ventricular dysfunction in a patient with toxic shock syndrome. Am J Obstet Gynecol 1983;146: 467–468.

60 **Burns JR, Menapace FJ.** Acute reversible cardiomyopathy complicating toxic shock syndrome. Arch Intern Med 1982;142:1032–1034.

61 **Crews JR, Harrison JK, Corey GR, et al.** Stunned myocardium in the toxic shock syndrome. Ann Intern Med 1992;117:912–913.

62 **Bartter T, Dascal A, Carroll K, Curley FJ.** "Toxic strep syndrome." A manifestation of group A streptococcal infection. Arch Intern Med 1988;148:1421–1424.

63 **Cone LA, Woodard DR, Schlievert PM, Tomory GS.** Clinical and bacteriologic observations of a toxic shock-like syndrome due to *Streptococcus pyogenes*. N Engl J Med 1987;317:146–149.

64 **Stevens DL, Tanner MH, Winship J, et al.** Severe group A streptococcal infections associated with a toxic shock-like syndrome and scarlet fever toxin A. N Engl J Med 1989;321:1–7.

65 **Working Group on Severe Streptococcal Infections.** Defining the group A streptococcal toxic shock syndrome. JAMA 1993;269: 390–391.

66 **Chapnick EK, Gradon JD, Lutwick LI, et al.** Streptococcal toxic shock syndrome due to noninvasive pharyngitis. Clin Infect Dis 1992;14:1074–1077.

67 **Stevens DL.** Invasive group A streptococcus infections. Clin Infect Dis 1992;14:2–13.

68 **Talkington DF, Schwartz B, Black CM, et al.** Association of phenotypic and genotypic characteristics of invasive *Streptococcus pyogenes* isolates with clinical components of streptococcal toxic shock syndrome. Infect Immun 1993;62:3369–3374.

69 **Rauch AM, Hurwitz ES.** Centers for Disease Control (CDC) case definition for Kawasaki syndrome. Pediatr Infect Dis 1985;4:702–703. Letter.

70 **Leung DY, Meissner HC, Fulton DR, et al.** Toxic shock syndrome toxin-secreting *Staphylococcus aureus* in Kawasaki syndrome. Lancet 1993;342:1385–1388.

71 **Makhene MK, Diaz PS.** Clinical presentations and complications of suspected measles in hospitalized children. Pediatr Infect Dis J 1993;12:836–840.

72 **Duchin JS, Koster FT, Peters CJ, et al.** Hantavirus pulmonary syndrome: a clinical description of 17 patients with a newly recognized disease. N Engl J Med 1994;330: 949–955.

73 **Cavanah DK, Ballas ZK.** Pseudoephedrine reaction presenting as recurrent toxic shock syndrome. Ann Intern Med 1993;119:302–303.

74 **Enriquez R, Palacios FO, Gonzalez CM, et al.** Skin vasculitis, hypokalemia and acute renal failure in rhabdomyolysis associated with cocaine. Nephron 1991;59:336–337.

75 **Brody SL, Wrenn KD, Wilber MM, Slovis CM.** Predicting the severity of cocaine-associated rhabdomyolysis. Ann Emerg Med 1990;19:1137–1143.

76 **Barbour AG.** Vaginal isolates of *Staphylococcus aureus* associated with toxic shock syndrome. Infect Immun 1981;33:442–449.

77 **Clyne M, De AJ, Carlson E, Arbuthnott J.** Production of gamma-hemolysin and lack of production of alpha-hemolysin by *Staphylococcus aureus* strains associated with toxic shock syndrome. J Clin Microbiol 1988;26: 535–539.

78 **Chow AW, Gribble MJ, Bartlett KH.** Characterization of the hemolytic activity of *Staphylococcus aureus* strains associated with toxic shock syndrome. J Clin Microbiol 1983;17:524–528.

79 **Todd JK, Franco BA, Lawellin DW, Vasil ML.** Phenotypic distinctiveness of *Staphylococcus aureus* strains associated with toxic shock syndrome. Infect Immun 1984;45:339–344.

80 **Rudick JH, Sheehan JP.** Hypomagnesemia,

hypocalcemia, and toxic-shock syndrome: a case report. Magnesium 1987;6:325–329.

81 **Bachhuber R, Parker RA, Bennett WM.** Acute renal failure in toxic shock syndrome owing to rhabdomyolysis. Ann Clin Lab Sci 1983;13:25–26.

82 **Dickgiesser N, Wallach U.** Toxic shock syndrome toxin-1 (TSST-1): influence of its production by subinhibitory antibiotic concentrations. Infection 1987;15:351–353.

83 **Schlievert PM, Kelly JA.** Clindamycin-induced suppression of toxic-shock syndrome-associated exotoxin production. J Infect Dis 1984;149:471.

84 **Eagle H.** Experimental approach to the problem of treatment failure with penicillin. I. Group A streptococcal infection in mice. Am J Med 1952;13:389–399.

85 **Stevens DL, Yan S, Bryant AE.** Penicillin-binding protein expression at different growth stages determines penicillin efficacy in vitro and in vivo: an explanation for the inoculum effect. J Infect Dis 1993;167:1401–1405.

86 **Parsonnet J, Modern PA, Giacobbe KD.** Effect of subinhibitory concentrations of antibiotics on production of toxic shock syndrome toxin-1 (TSST-1). Presented at the 32nd Annual Meeting of Infectious Diseases Society of America, Orlando, October 1994.

87 **Todd JK, Ressman M, Caston SA, et al.** Corticosteriod therapy for patients with toxic shock syndrome. JAMA 1984;252: 3399–3402.

88 **Rosene KA, Copass MK, Kastner LS, et al.** Persistent neuropsychological sequelae of toxic shock syndrome. Ann Intern Med 1982;96(Part 2):865–870.

89 **Bonventre PF, Linnemann C, Weckbach LS, et al.** Antibody responses to toxic-shock-syndrome (TSS) toxin by patients with TSS and by healthy staphylococcal carriers. J Infect Dis 1984;150:662–666.

90 **Davis JP, Osterholm MT, Helms CM, et al.** Tri-state toxic-shock syndrome study. II. Clinical and laboratory findings. J Infect Dis 1982;145:441–448.

91 **Stolz SJ, Davis JP, Vergeront JM, et al.** Development of serum antibody to toxic shock toxin among individuals with toxic shock syndrome in Wisconsin. J Infect Dis 1985;151:883–889.

Antibiotic Resistance in *Enterococcus* Species: An Update

GEORGE M. ELIOPOULOS

The relative resistance of enterococci to inhibition and killing by penicillin, leading to unacceptably low cure rates when this antibiotic was used alone in the treatment of infective endocarditis, has been recognized since the 1940s (1–3). Documentation of cures when penicillin was combined with streptomycin and demonstration of synergistic bactericidal activity of this combination in vitro led to the adoption of such combinations as routine treatment of enterococcal endocarditis (2–6). Over the ensuing decades, regimens consisting of a cell wall-active antibiotic in combination with an aminoglycoside yielded high rates of cure with relative consistency and remained the standard approach to such infections (7–9).

However, by the early 1990s, it became obvious that any complacency regarding treatment of serious enterococcal infections was unwarranted. This was a consequence of two factors that, to a large extent, are related. First, the spread of high-level resistance to streptomycin and gentamicin rendered traditional "synergistic" regimens ineffective, whereas the emergence of resistance to vancomycin and other antimicrobials rendered selection of even a single active agent problematic (10,11). In addition, enterococci were recognized as increasingly important nosocomial pathogens (12), with strains resistant to vancomycin especially worrisome in critical care settings (13). In 1994, the Centers for Disease Control and Prevention (CDC) (14) proposed guidelines to limit the spread of multiple drug-resistant enterococci, amply demonstrating the magnitude of concern regarding this ominous development.

This chapter is intended to provide an overview and update of mechanisms leading to antimicrobial resistance in enterococci, factors associated with the increasing prevalence of resistant strains, and options available for treatment of infections caused by these organisms. Additional details may be found in several recent reviews (10,11,15–17).

TRADITIONAL CONCERNS WITH ANTIBIOTIC RESISTANCE IN ENTEROCOCCI

Intrinsic Resistance to β-Lactam Antibiotics

Enterococci are, in general, substantially more resistant to penicillin than are streptococci. Strains of *Streptococcus bovis* are inhibited by penicillin at concentrations less than or equal to 0.12 μg/mL, whereas minimal inhibitory concentrations (MICs) against typical isolates of *Enterococcus faecalis* range from 2 to 4 μg/mL (18). *E. faecium* are even more resistant to penicillin with MICs 8 to 64 μg/mL against isolates recovered before 1980 (19). As will be discussed below, a shift toward even greater penicillin resistance in the latter species has occurred in recent years.

Activities of other penicillins and carbapenems parallel those of penicillin G against enterococci, with ampicillin and amoxicillin tending to be more active than penicillin, imipenem generally comparable with penicillin, and piperacillin somewhat less active (Table 2.1). Activities of antistaphylococcal penicillins and cephalosporins are not predictably adequate when tested in serum or in animals (34–36). A curious, and as yet unexplained, observation is that blood products enhance the activities in vitro of several aminothiazoyl oxime cephalosporins (e.g., cefotaxime) against some strains of *E. faecalis* (37). This is not known to have therapeutic relevance at present.

Mechanisms of intrinsic resistance to β-lactams in enterococci have been explored in naturally occurring strains and in more resistant or hypersusceptible laboratory mutants. In *Enterococcus hirae* ATCC 9790, a peni-

Table 2.1. Activity of β-Lactam Antibiotics Against Enterococci

Antibiotic	*Representative MIC_{90}s (μg/mL)*			
	E. faecalis	*E. faecium*	*E. avium*	*E. raffinosus*
Amoxicillin	1–2	⩽32	0.5	16
Ampicillin	1–4	4–16	0.5–2	16
Penicillin	2–4	32	1	128
Oxacillin	16–32	⩾128	32 to ⩾128	⩾128
Imipenem	2–4	⩾32	1–2	⩾128
Mezlocillin	2–16	64		
Piperacillin	4–8	64		
Ticarcillin	>16			
Cephalexin	⩾64	⩾64	⩾64	⩾64
Cefuroxime	⩾64	⩾64	⩾64	⩾64
Cefoperazone	32–64	⩾128		
Cefotaxime	⩾64	⩾64		
Ceftriaxone	⩾128	⩾128		

Derived from references 8 and 20–33.

cillin-binding protein (PBP5) of unusually low affinity for radiolabeled penicillin was identified after prolonged incubation of cell membranes with the antibiotic (38). Cells grew normally in concentrations of penicillin saturating other PBPs, and mutants of this strain demonstrating higher penicillin resistance produced greater amounts of this protein. Strains of *E. faecium* resistant to penicillin produce abundant quantities of a low-affinity PBP (PBP5, molecular weight 79.5 kDa); spontaneous penicillin-susceptible mutants demonstrated reduced amounts of PBP5, with the appearance of a higher affinity protein termed PBP5* (81 kDa) (39). Based on amino acid sequences of peptide fragments of a low-affinity PBP (PBP3^r) from a penicillin-resistant swine isolate *E. hirae* 5185, oligonucleotides were derived for use as polymerase chain reaction (PCR) primers to generate a 233-bp DNA sequence (40). Analysis of the corresponding amino acid sequence revealed considerable similarity with the low-affinity PBP2′ of methicillin-resistant staphylococci. PBP3^r was also found to be related to PBP5 of *E. hirae* ATCC 9790 (40).

Tolerance to Bactericidal Effects of Cell Wall-Active Agents

Penicillin may fail to completely sterilize cultures of enterococci at concentrations substantially above the MIC. Tolerance of enterococci to bactericidal effects of cell wall-active antimicrobials, including β-lactams, vancomycin, bacitracin, and cycloserine, is reflected by minimal bactericidal concentrations (MBCs) at least 32-fold higher than MICs (41). Incomplete killing is probably best detected by time-kill methods, however, because MBC testing can sometimes indicate a bactericidal effect by the generally accepted criterion of 99.9% killing even when a substantial fraction of the original inoculum survives.

Although tolerance to killing by cell wall-active antimicrobials is a common finding among enterococci, it is by no means a universal feature in this genus. As illustrated in Figure 2.1, the magnitude of killing by ampicillin is generally greater than that seen with vancomycin, but considerable heterogeneity in susceptibility of individual isolates to killing exists (42). Working with a nontolerant strain of *E. faecalis* isolated from an antibiotic-naive population on the Solomon Islands in the 1960s, Hodges and coworkers (43) found that repetitive exposure to pulses of penicillin facilitated selection of tolerant clones. By comparison, when the isolate was exposed to constant levels of penicillin above the MIC, surviving colonies retained the lytic nontolerant phenotype of the original isolate. This phenomenon may be relevant to treatment of infections. In an animal model of *E. faecalis* endocarditis, ampicillin was more effective in reducing bacterial densities in cardiac vegetations when administered by continuous intravenous infusion than when the same total daily dose was fractionated in three intramuscular injections (44). Although another study of endocarditis in animals found no advantage of continuous infusion therapy (45), the strains used appeared to be inherently more tolerant to ampicillin than the one used in the previously mentioned study. The potential significance of tolerance to β-lactams in treatment outcome is further illustrated by a study by

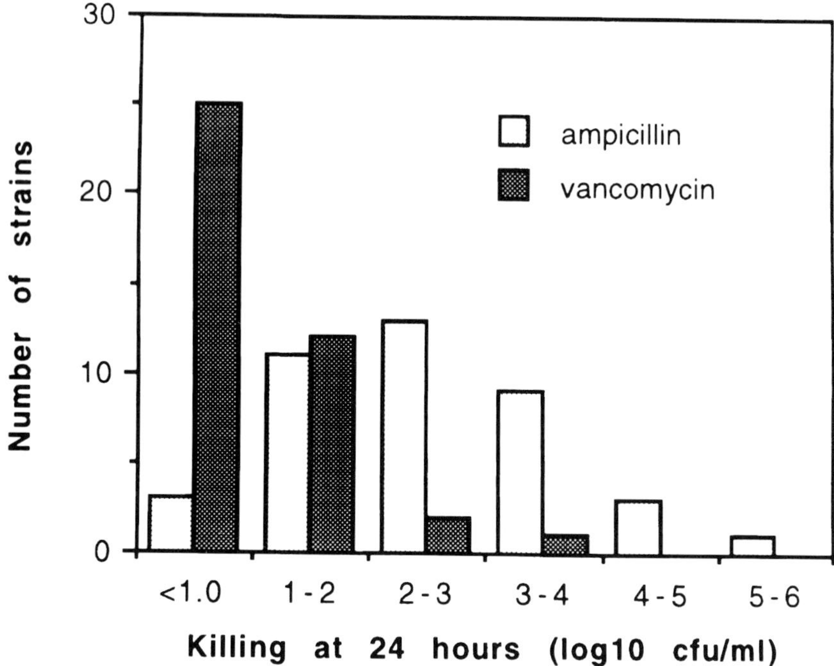

Figure 2.1. Magnitude of killing at 24 hr by ampicillin or vancomycin at 20 μg/mL against 40 strains of *E. faecalis*. (Adapted from data in reference 42.)

Kim and Bayer (46), who found procaine penicillin to be significantly more effective in experimental endocarditis created with a nontolerant enterococcus than with a tolerant isolate.

Mechanisms of tolerance to killing by cell wall-active antibiotics in enterococci are incompletely understood. Fontana and colleagues (47) reported that enterococci that produced only an autolytic enzyme that lysed heat-killed *Micrococcus luteus* cells demonstrated a paradoxical response to killing by penicillin (i.e., less killing as drug concentrations are increased), whereas strains that produced large amounts of a second enzyme that lysed heat-killed *E. faecalis* cells did not show this paradoxical response. Earlier work had shown that a lytic response on exposure of enterococcal isolates to β-lactams correlated with spontaneous cell lysis in antibiotic-free media (48,49). Such evidence suggests that susceptibility to lysis and killing is genetically determined. However, the fact that only a fraction of the cell population survives antibiotic exposure suggests that other factors influence phenotypic expression of tolerance or lysis in a single cell (47). In vitro, single colonies of a tolerant strain can give rise to both tolerant and nontolerant clones, with progeny of the latter yielding both tolerant and nontolerant clones at approximately the same frequency as in the preceding generation (50).

Synergism Between Cell Wall-Active Antimicrobials and Aminoglycosides

The Mayo Clinic experience in the treatment of enterococcal endocarditis from 1944 to 1953 was reported in 1954 (3). In that series, 4 of 10 patients who received penicillin alone at a daily dose of at least 6 million units were considered cured. However, excluding one patient who appeared to have a good response but was lost to follow-up and one who had a mixed infection, four of the remaining eight patients were cured with penicillin alone. Of those patients treated with penicillin combined with dihydrostreptomycin, 11 (78.6%) of 14 recovered, and one failure was successfully treated with a penicillin alone, for an overall response rate of 86%. This is not substantially different from results reported in series of β-lactam-aminoglycoside–treated patients published more recently (8).

Combinations of penicillin with streptomycin demonstrate bactericidal synergism against the vast majority of enterococci that do not exhibit high-level resistance (MIC > 2000 μg/mL) to the aminoglycoside. This occurs as a consequence of enhanced intracellular uptake of streptomycin in the presence of penicillin (51). High-level streptomycin resistance is usually due to acquisition of genes mediating streptomycin modifying (adenylylating) enzymes (52) but can arise from insensitivity of the ribosomal target (53). By 1973 to 1976, 54% of enterococcal blood culture isolates in Boston demonstrated high-level streptomycin resistance (54). When bactericidal activity was needed in the therapy of infections caused by such isolates, gentamicin was substituted for streptomycin. Until the emergence of high-level resistance to gentamicin (which is discussed below), bactericidal synergism and good clinical efficacy with penicillin-gentamicin combinations could be anticipated with reasonable likelihood (7,8).

The presence of various aminoglycoside-modifying enzymes limits the effectiveness of other 2-deoxystreptamine aminoglycosides in certain situations. Combinations of penicillin with kanamycin, tobramycin, or netilmicin, all of which are subject to acetylation at the 6′ position, fail to produce synergistic killing of *E. faecium* (19). This is due to production of a 6′-acetyltransferase mediated by a chromosomal gene *aac(6′)-Ii* specific to this species (55). Although amikacin is not effectively modified by this enzyme, it is rendered ineffective by a phosphorylating enzyme (APH(3′)-III) that is commonly found in *E. faecalis* as well as *E. faecium* and that is detected by screening for high-level kanamycin resistance (56). Penicillin-amikacin combinations actually can be antagonistic in vitro against strains producing this enzyme (57). A more recently described enzyme, 4′,4″-nucleotidyltransferase, produces high-level resistance to kanamycin and tobramycin and also prevents synergistic activity of amikacin (58). Originally described in an isolate of *E. faecium*, the genetic determinant was plasmid mediated and transferable to other enterococcal strains. Although gentamicin retains activity in the presence of the aforementioned enzymes, one isolate of *E. faecalis* resistant to penicillin-gentamicin synergism (in the absence of high-level gentamicin resistance) but susceptible to enhanced killing by penicillin combined with tobramycin has been found to have a specific defect in uptake of gentamicin in the presence of penicillin (59).

EMERGING RESISTANCE PROBLEMS

High-Level Resistance to Gentamicin

Discovery, Mechanisms, and Genetics In 1978, three strains of *E. faecalis* with plasmid-mediated high-level resistance to gentamicin (HLGR) were isolated in Paris hospitals (60). HLGR appeared in U.S. isolates of *E. faecalis* as early as 1981 (61). The latter also demonstrated high-level streptomycin resistance and were resistant to synergism by all penicillin-aminoglycoside combinations. HLGR was recognized in *E. faecium* in 1987 (62) and has since been found in several other enterococcal species (63).

HLGR in enterococci is due to the presence of a bifunctional enzyme with 6′-acetylating and 2″-phosphorylating activities. The gene specifying this activity was cloned from an *E. faecalis* plasmid into *Escherichia coli*, sequenced, and by subcloning experiments shown to consist of gene segments that specified each enzyme activity separately (64). HLGR was shown to be mediated by conjugative and nonconjugative plasmids ranging in size from 34 to 124 kb (65,66), and the gene was also localized to chromosomal DNA by hybridization with a probe for the bifunctional enzyme gene (67). Mobilization of the resistance determinant from plasmid pBEM10 (present in *E. faecalis* HH22 from Houston) into two sites of a tetracycline resistance plasmid further suggested that the HLGR determinant was on a transposon (68). This proposition was subsequently proven, and the transposon Tn*5281* was shown to be closely related to transposons specifying the bifunctional enzyme in Australian isolates of *Staphylococcus aureus* (Tn*4001*) and U.S. isolates of *Staphylococcus epidermidis* (Tn*4031*) (69). Plasmid DNA from two other strains of *E. faecalis* (from Texas and Chile) revealed gentamicin resistance transposons similar to Tn*5281*, whereas in two other isolates (from Texas and Pennsylvania), regions surrounding the resistance genes were more closely related to those of North American isolates of *S. aureus*. A third pattern was identified in an HLGR *E. faecalis* from Thailand (70). A large chromosome-borne HLGR transposable element (designated Tn*924*) has been identified in a strain of *E. faecalis* isolated in Winnipeg, Canada. The organization of this element resembles that of North American gentamicin-resistant *S. aureus* (71).

Although the presence of this bifunctional enzyme usually results in gentamicin MICs greater than 500 μg/mL, resistance to synergism can also occur in uncommonly encountered strains with moderate levels of gentamicin resistance (MIC = 500 μg/mL) (72). Rare strains of HLGR enterococci (MICs > 16,000 μg/mL) do not appear to contain DNA that hybridizes with *aph2″-aac6′*

gene probes, suggesting an alternative mechanism of resistance to gentamicin (63). Therefore, neither lack of HLGR by the standard criterion of MIC greater than 500 μg/mL nor failure to detect the bifunctional gene by DNA hybridization exclude with certainty the possibility of resistance to penicillin-gentamicin bactericidal synergism.

Epidemiology and Risk Factors for Acquisition The prevalence of HLGR among recent isolates of enterococci has reached significant levels worldwide (16). Resistance rates of 25% to 65% among *E. faecalis* isolates have been reported from laboratories in Europe (73–75). Eight (29%) of 28 patients hospitalized in a Zimbabwe hospital had stool colonization with HLGR *E. faecalis* (76). In the United States, HLGR was found in 15% of enterococci isolated at the University of Pennsylvania in 1985 (77), in 24% of *E. faecalis* at the VA Medical Center in Memphis in 1986 (78), and in 24% of enterococci in Youngstown, Ohio, in 1988 (79). Particularly high rates of HLGR among enterococci, from 52% to 55%, were identified in Brooklyn in 1990 (80), in Ann Arbor between 1985 and 1986 (81), and in Chicago between 1987 and 1990 (82). We found that approximately 60% of *E. faecium* isolated at two Boston hospitals between 1989 and 1990 exhibited HLGR (83).

A variable but important percentage of isolates demonstrating HLGR are also highly resistant to streptomycin. In the report from Pennsylvania (77), 67% of HLGR isolates were resistant to high levels of streptomycin. In Chicago, 54% were high-level streptomycin resistant (82).

Within any city, rates of patient colonization with HLGR enterococci can vary widely in different institutions, ranging in one case from 4.3% of patients in a private nursing home to 36% of patients in an acute care hospital, to 47% of patients in a nursing home affiliated with the latter (84). Within an institution, geographic clustering of cases has been described (84–86). Similarity of plasmid patterns among strains from individual patients provides evidence for both nosocomial acquisition of HLGR strains and interhospital spread of these organisms (81). Case-control studies have identified several potential risk factors for acquisition of HLGR strains by patients, including the following: prior exposure to antibiotics, including aminoglycosides and cephalosporins; longer duration of hospitalization; prior surgery; and need for intravenous lines, urinary catheters, and advanced nursing care (76,81,84–87). Resistant enterococci have been recovered both from environmental surfaces near colonized patients and from the hands of hospital personnel (81,84,85).

Resistance to β-Lactams

β-Lactamase Production The first β-lactamase–producing isolate of *E. faecalis* (strain HH22) was recovered in Houston, Texas, in 1981 (88). Constitutive production of low amounts of enzyme did not result in unusually elevated MICs of penicillin or ampicillin at standard inocula, but MICs exceeded 1000 μg/mL at higher inocula (10^7 CFU/mL). The enzyme was inhibited by clavulanic acid, sulbactam, and tazobactam, restoring susceptibility to penicillins (89). Almost all β-lactamase–producing isolates studied to date also demonstrate HLGR. The enzyme has also been detected in at least one strain of *E. faecium* (90).

Genetic determinants mediating β-lactamase production in the first few isolates identified were plasmid associated (88,91,92). A staphylococcal origin of the resistance gene was strongly suggested by demonstration of hybridization with an *S. aureus* penicillinase gene probe (91,93,94). The DNA sequence of the β-lactamase structural gene of *E. faecalis* HH22 was shown to be identical with those of staphylococcal penicillinase genes, but functional studies and analysis of adjacent sequences indicated the absence or truncation of sequences corresponding to regulatory genes of *S. aureus* (95–97). Hybridization of the staphylococcal penicillinase gene probe with chromosomal, but not plasmid, DNA from an isolate of *E. faecalis* (67) suggested the possibility of transposon-mediated resistance. Subsequent comparison of restriction maps of surrounding DNA sequences with those of recognized staphylococcal transposons provided further evidence in support of this hypothesis (98).

β-Lactamase–producing *E. faecalis* have been identified in several U.S. cities and other countries. Isolates from Texas, Delaware, Pennsylvania, Florida, and Virginia demonstrated similar restriction patterns of total DNA, suggesting they were derived from a single strain, whereas organisms from Argentina, Lebanon, Massachusetts, and Connecticut each had distinctly different patterns (99). Identical or nearly identical pulsed-field gel electrophoresis patterns of total DNA from several outbreak-related strains in Argentina and Virginia demonstrated the potential for intrahospital spread (100,101). In Argentina, 6 isolates were recovered over a 17-month period in a pediatric hospital; the latter outbreak of colonization and infection in adult patients included about 10% of enterococcal isolates from the Virginia hospital during the study period (100–103). A case of probable endocarditis due to a β-lactamase–producing *E. faecalis* has been reported (104), but most patients have had less serious infections or only colonization (102,105). Prolonged gastrointestinal carriage of such isolates has been reported in patients and hospital personnel (105,106).

In an outbreak of colonization on pediatric surgical ward, significant independent risk factors for acquisition of a β-lactamase–producing enterococcus included location in the nursery, need for mechanical and antibiotic bowel preparation, and exposure to one nurse who was persistently colonized (105). Two nurses had positive hand cultures, and eight of the employees tested had positive stool cultures during the outbreak. In the adult outbreak, multivariate analysis demonstrated significant risk for acquisition associated with an APACHE II score greater than 6 and antibiotic treatment (101). In the latter study, β-lactamase–producing strains were found on environmental surfaces but not on the hands of personnel.

Increasing Intrinsic β-Lactam Resistance Susceptibility to penicillin among current isolates of *E. faecalis* does not seem to be appreciably different from that encountered in the United States in the 1940s or on the Solomon Islands despite the fact that higher levels of resistance can be achieved by serial passage of strains through increasing concentrations of the antibiotic in vitro (3,43). Occasional β-lactamase–negative isolates with ampicillin MICs of 16 μg/mL have been encountered, however (107).

Isolates of the recently recognized species *Enterococcus raffinosus* are intrinsically more resistant to penicillin (MIC 4 to 64 μg/mL, MIC_{90} = 64 μg/mL) than are *Enterococcus avium* (MIC 0.5 to 2 μg/mL) with which they were once grouped and also differ from these in PBP patterns (108). *E. raffinosus* accounted for one third of the ampicillin-resistant enterococci isolated at the Martinez, California VA medical center (109). Nine *E. raffinosus* isolates were recovered in a Providence hospital between 1986 and 1988, four of which appeared to be identical and clustered by period of isolation and location, suggesting nosocomial spread (110).

Grayson and colleagues (83) documented a disturbing trend in increasing levels of resistance to penicillin and ampicillin among isolates of *E. faecium* recovered at one Boston hospital between 1969 and 1990. In the period to 1988, MIC_{90}s of penicillin and ampicillin were 64 and 32 μg/mL, respectively. For strains recovered in 1989 to 1990, these values had risen to 512 and 128 μg/mL. This was in marked contrast to isolates of *E. faecium* from the Solomon Islands, 90% of which were inhibited by ampicillin at 2 μg/mL. Strains with the highest levels of resistance produced a very low-affinity PBP, requiring incubation with 500 μg/mL of labeled penicillin for visualization by fluorography. Synthesis of low-affinity PBPs as an explanation for high levels of resistance to ampicillin in *E. faecium* was also suggested by studies of Klare et al (111) and documented in subsequent work by Fontana et al (112).

Highly penicillin- and ampicillin-resistant strains of *E. faecium* are now common. In London, 71% of *E. faecium* had penicillin MICs greater than 100 μg/mL (75). One third of those from Philadelphia hospitals had penicillin MICs at least 200 μg/mL (113), and the ampicillin MIC_{90} for *E. faecium* recovered in Rome was at least 128 μg/mL (74). In addition to the fact that many of these *E. faecium* isolates are also HLGR (83), very high-level penicillin resistance has further implications with respect to the possibility of achieving bactericidal synergism. Because demonstration of bactericidal synergism between penicillin and an aminoglycoside in vitro generally requires that the former be used at concentrations of at least one half of the MIC (114), it is likely that attaining high enough levels to accomplish this in vivo would be difficult if not impossible, as suggested by an animal model of infective endocarditis (113).

Boyce et al (110) noted a sevenfold increase in the incidence of ampicillin-resistant enterococci from 1986 to 1988 at their institution. Nineteen patients had acquired isolates of *E. faecium* that were identical or closely related by analysis of plasmid content and chromosomal DNA restriction digest patterns. Hospitalization for more than two weeks and exposure to one intern were risk factors for acquisition of this strain. Prolonged hospitalization and imipenem therapy were associated with acquisition of other ampicillin-resistant enterococci. A prospective study, which included routine culturing of rectal swabs and urine of patients admitted to a medical ward and intensive care unit, identified prior antibiotic therapy, presence of a urinary catheter, and a bedridden status as risk factors for acquisition of ampicillin-resistant enterococci. This study also demonstrated that gastrointestinal colonization usually preceded detection of the isolates elsewhere (115).

Glycopeptide Resistance

Vancomycin resistance in enterococci was described in several reports published in 1988 from the United Kingdom (116), Germany (117), France (118), and the United States (119). Vancomycin MICs of these isolates ranged from 16 µg/mL in an *Enterococcus gallinarum* to 2000 µg/mL in a strain of *E. faecium*; some of the latter were also resistant to the related glycopeptide teicoplanin (investigational drug in the United States) (118). Several of the patients described suffered from chronic renal disease or multiple organ dysfunction and had received treatment with vancomycin (119,120). Nosocomial transmission was suspected (120), and plasmid-mediated transfer of resistance to susceptible donor strains was demonstrated in vitro (118,120).

Description of Phenotypic Classes Several features of the vancomycin resistance phenotype were noted in early studies. Some isolates were highly resistant to vancomycin (MICs $\geqslant$ 128 µg/mL) and resistant to teicoplanin (MICs $\geqslant$ 16 µg/mL); others showed more moderate resistance to vancomycin (MICs 32 to 64 µg/mL) and remained susceptible to teicoplanin (121,122). In *E. faecium* and *E. faecalis*, vancomycin resistance was inducible by preincubation with low concentrations of vancomycin or teicoplanin and induction was associated with the appearance of a cytoplasmic membrane protein of approximately 39 kDa (121,123,124). Isolates of *E. gallinarum* and *Enterococcus casseliflavus* appeared, in contrast, to be intrinsically resistant to low levels of vancomycin with MICs of 4 to 32 µg/mL (125). In early reports, plasmid-mediated transfer of resistance to suitable recipients could be demonstrated in vitro from donors with the high-level resistance phenotypes but not from those showing moderate levels of resistance (although later studies showed transfer from some moderately resistant strains as well).

Based on these characteristics, vancomycin resistant strains were designated as class A (vancomycin MICs $\geqslant$ 64 µg/mL, teicoplanin resistant, usually inducible resistance), class B (teicoplanin susceptible, vancomycin MICs usually 32 to 64 µg/mL), and class C (*E. gallinarum* or *E. casseliflavus* with low-level resistance) (126,127). This classification scheme was initially useful in categorizing isolates, but its limitations were shown by subsequent genetic studies and investigation of additional isolates. For example, the class A phenotype (*vanA* genotype) has now appeared in *E. gallinarum* and *E. casseliflavus* (128), some class B phenotype strains develop resistance to teicoplanin during vancomycin exposure thus resembling class A strains phenotypically (129), and enormous heterogeneity in levels of vancomycin resistance (MICs 4 to greater than 1024 μg/mL) is now appreciated among class B isolates (*vanB* genotype). This trait is now known to be potentially transmissible (130).

Mechanisms and Genetics of Resistance ***Class A Resistance*** Plasmid localization of vancomycin resistance determinants facilitated genetic studies. The first gene related to vancomycin resistance to be cloned was termed *vanA* (131). A DNA probe from this gene hybridized with DNA from class A phenotype enterococci but not from those of classes B and C or from intrinsically vancomycin-resistant strains of *Leuconostoc* spp., *Pediococcus* spp., or lactobacilli (132). Comparison of the VanA sequence with those of known proteins revealed significant homology with D-alanine-D-alanine ligases of *E. coli* and *Salmonella typhimurium* (133). These enzymes are involved in peptidoglycan synthesis, producing a D-Ala-D-Ala dipeptide that is added to UDP-MurNAc-tripeptide to produce a pentapeptide involved in cross-linking of the cell wall. This was of great interest because the terminal D-Ala-D-Ala of the pentapeptide is the target of vancomycin inhibition of cell wall synthesis (134). The calculated molecular weight of the VanA protein was 37,400, comparable with that of the membrane protein induced in class A strains during incubation with vancomycin (133).

Bugg et al (135) purified the VanA protein and demonstrated ligase activity, but of altered substrate specificity, forming mixed dipeptides containing D-alanine. Sequencing upstream from *vanA* revealed an open reading frame (*vanH*) coding for a protein with extensive amino acid similarity with 2-hydroxycarboxylic acid dehydrogenase (136). VanH protein was subsequently purified and shown to produce D-hydroxy acids from a variety of substrates, which could then be condensed into D-Ala-D-hydroxy acid depsipeptides that demonstrated markedly reduced binding affinity for vancomycin as compared with D-Ala-D-Ala (137). Synthesis of UDP-MurNAc-depsipentapeptide terminating in D-lactate was demonstrated in vancomycin-resistant *E. faecium* (138). Addition of lactate to a culture of *E. faecium* in which *vanH* was inactivated was found to restore vancomycin resistance (139), indicating that vancomycin resistance was due to the formation of the altered peptidoglycan precursor terminating in D-Ala-D-lactate.

The genetic basis of vancomycin resistance in the class A phenotype strain of *E. faecium* originally studied has now been extensively characterized (17). This consists of a 10,851-bp transposon (Tn*1546*) containing seven genes involved in resistance and putative transposase and resolvase functions (140). In addition to *vanA* and *vanH*, it contains gene *vanY* determining a vancomycin-inducible D,D-carboxypeptidase, which can cleave D-Ala from preformed pentapeptide (and which also has carboxyesterase activity) but is not essential for vancomycin resistance (141–145), and *vanX*, which is essential and codes for a protein VanX that hydrolyzes D-Ala-D-Ala, reducing pools available for production of normal cell wall (142) (Figure 2.2). The element also contains genes *vanR* and *vanS*, which appear to constitute a two-component system regulating

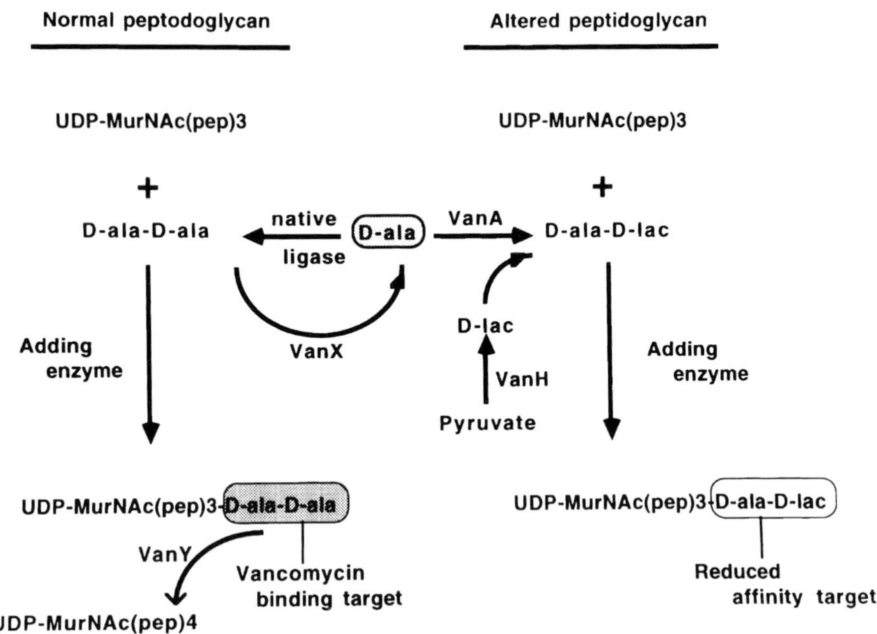

Figure 2.2. Schematic representation of peptidoglycan synthesis pathway alterations leading to class A vancomycin resistance in enterococci. (Adapted from references 135, 137, and 140–145.)

the synthesis of the aforementioned resistance genes (146,147). Presence of the transposon has been documented in three additional strains (17).

Plasmid-mediated vancomycin resistance genes of the class A type can be transferred into other species of gram-positive organisms with heterogeneous expression. Levels of vancomycin resistance conferred ranged from MICs of 16μg/mL in *Streptococcus pyogenes* and *S. sanguis* to 512μg/mL in *Listeria monocytogenes* (127). Conjugal transfer of vancomycin resistance from an enterococcus into *S. aureus* has been demonstrated in vitro and on the skin of mice, with resulting vancomycin MICs to 1000μg/mL (148).

Class B Resistance Availability of the *vanA* sequence and those of gram-negative bacterial ligases permitted design of degenerate primer systems to explore by PCR vancomycin resistance genes in other phenotypic classes. Sequences of genes analogous to *vanA* were determined in a typical class B phenotype *E. faecalis* (MIC 32 to 64μg/mL) (*vanB*) (149) and from a strain that was highly vancomycin resistant but teicoplanin susceptible (*vanB2*) (150). Deduced amino acid sequences of these two gene products revealed approximately 96% identity, and each shared approximately 76% homology with VanA (150–152). An adjacent sequence shows substantial similarity to *vanH* (151), and depsipentapeptide precursors from a *vanB* strain also terminated in D-Ala-D-lactate (153). *vanB* resistance genes are also transferable between enterococci, from chromosomal sites in donor strains to the chromosome of the resulting transconjugants (130,150,154).

Class C Resistance Gene probes specific for *vanA* or *vanB* do not hybridize with DNA of the low-level vancomycin-resistant species *E. gallinarum* and *E. casseliflavus*. A gene designated *vanC* (subsequently referred to as *vanC-1*) was identified in *E. gallinarum* and demonstrated to be specific to this species, with less than 40% deduced amino acid sequence homology with the VanA protein (155). In contrast to class A and B strains, which produce peptidoglycan precursors terminating in D-Ala-D-lactate, the VanC ligase in *E. gallinarum* results in D-Ala-D-serine termini (156,157). Fragments of the ligase gene in *E. casseliflavus* (designated *vanC-2*) have been identified and shown to specify amino acid sequences with approximately 73% identity after alignment with those of the *vanC-1* gene of *E. gallinarum* (158).

Epidemiology and Risk Factors for Acquisition Vancomycin-resistant enterococci (VRE) are now a significant problem in many U.S. hospitals. Data from the National Nocosomial Infections Surveillance system indicate that 7.9% of enterococci examined in 1993 demonstrated vancomycin resistance, up from 0.3% in 1989. Intensive care unit isolates were even more often resistant, 13.6% versus 0.4% in the same time periods (13). Recovery rates of VRE were highest in large hospitals and in teaching hospitals. Approximately two thirds were of the class A phenotype and one third of class B. Of 105 isolates from 1988 to 1992 examined at the CDC, approximately 70% were class A VRE, 25% class B, and the remainder class C phenotype (159). Phenotype and genotype did not correlate completely. One isolate of *E. raffinosus* was inhibited by vancomycin at 16 µg/mL and was susceptible to teicoplanin but was of the *vanA* genotype. Genotypic *vanB* strains that were teicoplanin resistant were also encountered. Another curious fact is the existence of apparently rare isolates of vancomycin-dependent VRE, reported from the United States and United Kingdom (160,161). These were detected by growth only around vancomycin discs during susceptibility testing and appear to reflect inactivity of the native enterococcal ligase (160). VRE have been isolated from general sewage samples in Spain (162) and from sewage and animal sources in the United Kingdom (163).

In two outbreaks of VRE among hospitalized children, colonization with apparently identical (164) as well as genetically distinct (165) strains has been reported. Among pediatric liver transplant patients in one center, stool colonization with several species of VRE was detected in 36 of 49 individuals monitored prospectively over a 2-year period (166). Other reports from general hospitals provide evidence both for clonal spread and for the coexistence of multiple clones, sometimes sharing a common vancomycin-resistance plasmid (167–170). Clonal outbreaks have involved both *vanA* and *vanB* resistance genes.

One report of an outbreak of infection with VRE (*E. faecium*) implicated contamination of rectal thermometer probe handles (171). VRE have been recovered from environmental surfaces near colonized patients in other outbreaks (169,172), with more extensive contamination when patients had diarrhea (169). In case-control studies, several risk factors for acquisition of VRE have been suggested. These include the need for prolonged intensive care unit stay (171), intense prior antibiotic exposure (168,171,173), and proximity to a case or exposure to a nurse who cared for a case (169). Exposure to vancomycin was reported as a risk factor for VRE acquisition in several studies (164,168,172). Intensive application of contact isolation procedures, sometimes with restriction of vancomycin use, appears to have been effective in curbing several outbreaks (164,169,171,172).

Emergence of Resistance to Multiple Antimicrobials

Because VRE are frequently *E. faecium*, it should be obvious from the preceding discussion of penicillin resistance and high-level aminoglycoside resistance in this species that many isolates will demonstrate resistance to all cell wall-active agents and combinations generally regarded as first-line therapy for enterococcal infections. This unfortunate situation is further aggravated by intrinsic and acquired resistance to other antimicrobials commonly encountered in enterococci. These additional resistance traits have been reviewed elsewhere (10,15).

Enterococci demonstrate low-level intrinsic resistance to clindamycin, and acquired resistance to higher levels is common (30). Erythromycin resistance is widespread; recently, only 6% of VRE from New Jersey were susceptible (174). Resistance to chloramphenicol is common (30), but some multiply resistant enterococci retain susceptibility to this agent that has been used in therapy (175). Although many enterococcal isolates appear susceptible to trimethoprim-sulfamethoxazole in vitro, these organisms can use exogenous products of the folate synthesis pathway, raising concerns about activity of this agent in vivo (10). In animal models of enterococcal endocarditis (176) and peritonitis (177), the drug was ineffective.

The effect of rifampin against enterococci is primarily inhibitory, and the drug can antagonize killing by ampicillin, at least when tested by time-kill methods (178,179). Moreover, resistance to this agent develops readily and is now common among VRE in some institutions (75,180). Resistance to fluoroquinolones has increased over recent years. Schaberg et al (181) noted that although no strain of HLGR enterococcus recovered in their institution between 1985 and 1986 was resistant to ciprofloxacin, 24% of isolates from 1989 to 1990 were resistant. Although several strain types contributed to the group of resistant isolates, 80% were of a single type, suggesting hospital spread. Boyle et al (168) noted that 52% of VRE collected in 1992 were susceptible to this agent, down from 70% in 1990. In the later period, 51% of isolates of VRE from the United Kingdom and 26% of VRE from a New York hospital demonstrated susceptibility to ciprofloxacin (75,180). Although tetracycline resistance determinants are common in enterococci (10), a variable proportion of isolates are susceptible to this agent (75,182). Minocycline inhibits some strains of VRE that are resistant to tetracycline (182).

CONSIDERATIONS IN TREATMENT

High-Level Aminoglycoside Resistance

High-level resistance to both streptomycin and gentamicin, which precludes synergism between cell wall-active agents and any aminoglycoside currently available, presents a problem when bactericidal activity is desirable, as in infective endocarditis. A few patients have apparently been cured with antibiotic treatment alone; others have required valve replacement (Table 2.2). At present, no combination regimen is known to be clearly and predictably superior to ampicillin alone based on such limited data. Any potential benefit of alternative combinations is likely to be strain dependent, as is the likelihood of success with a cell wall-active agent alone. It is worth recalling that in early experience, a small number of patients with enterococcal endocarditis were cured with penicillin alone (3). It is not known, however, whether current isolates are more likely to demonstrate tolerance to cell wall-active agents than those of the patients who were cured with penicillin alone decades ago.

Results from animal studies of experimental endocarditis provide conflicting data as to whether administration of ampicillin by continuous infusion over a

Table 2.2. Reports of Successful Therapy of High-Level Gentamicin Resistant Enterococcal Endocarditis

Case	*Antibiotic Regimen*	*Treatment Duration (wk)*	*Follow-Up (mo)*	*Surgery*	*Reference*
1	V(P) + SM[a]	5	6		183
2	V + GM[b]	6	12		104
3	Amp	6	2		184
4	Amp	4	8		185
5	Amp	8	6		186
6	Amp + SM[c]	4	6		186
7	P + GM	4	1	MVR	187
8	Amp	6	>14	AVR	188
9	Amp + Cip	6	3	AVR	189
10	Amp	5	>12	AVR	190
11	Vancomycin[d]	6		AVR	191

[a] Not high-level streptomycin resistant; rash on penicillin, switched to vancomycin for 36 days.
[b] Possible endocarditis; β-lactamase–producing strain.
[c] Possibly not high-level streptomycin resistant; details not given.
[d] Ampicillin-resistant *E. faecium* grown from valve culture.
V, vancomycin; P, penicillin; Amp, ampicillin; SM, streptomycin; GM, gentamicin; Cip, ciprofloxacin; AVR, aortic valve replacement; MVR, mitral valve replacement.

24-hour period offers any advantage over intermittent administration of the same daily dose (44,45). The former mode has been used satisfactorily in traditional combination regimens of penicillin with streptomycin or gentamicin (192), as has the latter. In view of in vitro data showing that pulse exposure to penicillin can select tolerant enterococcal clones (43), if intermittent dosage is selected, it seems reasonable to administer doses of ampicillin frequently enough that trough levels would not be expected to fall below inhibitory concentrations of the drug.

Presterl et al (193) have reported a cure of enterococcal endocarditis in five patients with teicoplanin alone. Although intriguing, this approach cannot be recommended in patients with infection due to high-level aminoglycoside-resistant infections because the drug is not licensed in the United States and because of the limited strain and case descriptions provided for this small number of patients. Although teicoplanin was effective in a rat endocarditis model (HLGR strain) (194), caution must be exercised in extrapolating from studies of glycopeptide efficacy in rats because of possible potentiation of drug activity by unknown factors in rat serum (195).

As discussed earlier, some (apparently rare) isolates are resistant to bactericidal effects of certain penicillin-aminoglycoside combinations even in the absence of high-level resistance. This point should be kept in mind when cases of endocarditis appear refractory to cure despite seemingly appropriate therapy. In such cases, formal study of the isolates by time-kill curve methods may provide an explanation for clinical failure and may point to alternative regimens.

Resistance to Cell Wall-Active Agents

Many enterococcal isolates exhibiting unusual levels of resistance to β-lactams or glycopeptides also demonstrate high-level aminoglycoside resistance, and the considerations discussed above apply. In the absence of high-level resistance to both streptomycin or gentamicin, efforts should be made to select a cell wall-active agent that is likely to contribute to a synergistic effect with the appropriate aminoglycoside if bactericidal activity is deemed necessary, as in the treatment of endocarditis.

β-Lactam Resistance β-Lactamase–producing enterococci have been rarely encountered except in a few outbreaks. Currently available β-lactamase inhibitors inhibit enzymes studied to date, restoring susceptibility in vitro to penicillins (89), but the possibility exists that enzymes resistant to inhibition may arise in the future. In animal studies, penicillin plus clavulanate and ampicillin plus sulbactam have been more effective than the penicillin alone against β-lactamase–producing strains (196,197). The only report to date of a clinical case of probable endocarditis due to a β-lactamase–producing *E. faecalis* described apparent cure with vancomycin (plus gentamicin, despite HLGR) (104). There is, of course, no reason why β-lactamase production *per se* would affect susceptibility to glycopeptides, and vancomycin has demonstrated some activity in experimental models with β-lactamase–producing strains (194,197,198). A case of bacteremia due to a β-lactamase–producing HLGR *E. faecalis* has been reported in which the patient failed to respond to treatment with vancomycin plus gentamicin, with subsequent response to vancomycin plus imipenem (106). The relative contribution of individual agents or the combination to response could not be precisely determined. In the outbreak of infections due to β-lactamase–producing enterococci described by Wells et al (101), some patients responded to "inappropriate" antibiotics, whereas others failed treatment with β-lactamase–stable antibiotics. Thus, at present, it is impossible to draw firm conclusions regarding optimal therapy of such infections.

β-Lactamase inhibitors have no recognized beneficial role against non-β-lactamase–producing enterococci that are intrinsically resistant to β-lactam antibiotics. High doses of penicillin combined with an aminoglycoside have been used in the treatment of endocarditis due to *E. faecium* with moderate levels of penicillin resistance (190). This approach is likely to be suboptimal for those isolates of *E. faecium* with substantially higher penicillin MICs. This concept is supported by in vitro and in vivo experiments with a highly penicillin-resistant *E. faecium* that showed lack of bactericidal synergism when penicillin 200 μg/mL was combined with gentamicin (despite synergism between vancomycin with gentamicin) and ineffectiveness of penicillin-gentamicin combination therapy in an animal model despite peak serum penicillin concentrations of 120 μg/mL (113). The alternative approach in such cases would be to use vancomycin plus gentamicin, assuming susceptibility to the former and lack of HLGR, as such regimens are considered acceptable for use in penicillin-allergic patients with enterococcal endocarditis (7). Vancomycin used alone resulted in cure of one patient with *E. faecium* endocarditis due to an ampicillin-resistant, HLGR, and high-level streptomycin-resistant strain (191). This case is atypical, however, because the diagnosis was only established after culture of a surgically excised aortic valve.

Vancomycin Resistance Isolated vancomycin resistance in enterococcal infections should not pose a problem when a penicillin can be used. The β-lactam–allergic patient who cannot undergo desensitization presents a greater problem. When bactericidal activity is nonessential, the standard antibiogram may be helpful in pointing out suitable alternatives. When bactericidal activity is needed and neither β-lactams nor vancomycin can be used, there is no currently approved or widely accepted alternative. For class B or C strains of VRE (i.e., susceptible to teicoplanin), the physician can inquire about the availability of this investigational antibiotic through U.S. Food and Drug Administration-approved experimental protocol. Teicoplanin, like vancomycin, provides enhanced killing of enterococci in experimental animals when combined with an appropriate aminoglycoside (199,200). As noted earlier, resistance to teicoplanin can emerge during treatment of infection due to *vanB* genotype VRE with vancomycin (129); therefore, physicians using teicoplanin for class B VRE infections should remain alert for this potential complication.

Resistance to Multiple Antimicrobials

A major problem likely to be encountered with increasing frequency is infection because of enterococci resistance to high levels of penicillin and ampicillin, glycopeptides, and multiple other antimicrobials of various classes. Many of these isolates exhibit high-level resistant to streptomycin, gentamicin, or to both aminoglycosides. When a suitable agent cannot be identified that is both active against the infecting organism and approved for use in enterococcal infections, approaches to therapy are highly empiric. The remainder of this section discusses observations from in vitro and in vivo studies and clinical reports possibly relevant to treatment of infections due to multiple drugresistant enterococci. However, because such regimens are neither widely accepted as optimal for treating enterococcal infections nor specifically approved for this purpose, these discussions must not be construed as recommendations for treatment.

Combinations of Cell Wall-Active Agents Several groups have observed bacteriostatic synergism with β-lactam–glycopeptide combinations in vitro against VRE, including strains resistant to ampicillin (201–204). It has been suggested that the modified peptidoglycan produced once glycopeptide resistance proteins have been induced might not be suitable substrates for cross-linking by the low-affinity PBP5, rendering the cells susceptible to the β-lactam at concentrations sufficient to saturate higher affinity PBPs (205). However, glycopeptide–β-lactam inhibitory synergism is not a consistent finding against VRE (206–208), and subpopulations resistant to synergism can be isolated from high inoculum cultures (202).

Caron et al (209), using a non-HLGR VRE (MIC of vancomycin = 1024 μg/mL, MIC of penicillin = 32, which dropped to 0.5 μg/mL after induction with vancomycin 10 μg/mL), showed an enhanced effect of penicillin plus vancomycin together with gentamicin in a rabbit model of endocarditis. However, high doses of penicillin combined with gentamicin were just as effective. In a second study using a VRE strain with higher level penicillin resistance (MIC = 128 μg/mL, reduced to 16 μg/mL with vancomycin 10 μg/mL), the triple drug combination was effective in reducing bacterial counts in cardiac vegetations, whereas neither penicillin-gentamicin nor vancomycin-gentamicin showed activity (210). Similar results were also noted with combinations of ceftriaxone (MIC > 512 μg/mL, reduced to 32 with vancomycin 10 μg/mL or to 2 μg/mL with teicoplanin 10 μg/mL), plus either vancomycin or teicoplanin, plus gentamicin (211). In both of these last two studies, subpopulations resistant to synergistic inhibition were encountered in some animals despite use of the triple combination.

Recent preliminary reports have called attention to potential synergistic interactions arising from double β-lactam combinations against VRE. One group demonstrated inhibitory synergism between amoxicillin and cefotaxime in vitro (212). Another paper reported enhanced effectiveness of ampicillin-imipenem combinations in a rabbit endocarditis model using a vancomycin-resistant *E. faecium* (213). The generality of these findings and their clinical applicability remains to be determined.

Combinations Involving Fluoroquinolones Landman et al (214) studied ampicillin-ciprofloxacin combinations against ampicillin-resistant *E. faecium* by time-kill methods and concluded that significant killing occurred if ciprofloxacin MICs did not exceed 8 μg/mL. Ampicillin concentrations at which this effect was seen (40 μg/mL) were relatively high. Ampicillin 20 μg/mL combined with the investigational drug clinafloxacin, which is more potent than ciprofloxacin against enterococci, resulted in a bactericidal effect against 12 strains of multidrug-resistant *E. faecium* that were susceptible to the fluoroquinine but not against resistant isolates (215). Ünal et al (216) reported inhibitory synergism between ciprofloxacin and vancomycin against enterococcal isolates resistant to both agents but generally at concentrations too high to be clinically relevant.

In vitro, two investigational fluoroquinolones, sparfloxacin and clinafloxacin, demonstrated a modest degree of killing activity against enterococci susceptible to these agents; for 12 of 15 non-HLGR isolates, killing was further enhanced by addition of gentamicin (217). Modest benefits of these combinations were observed in an animal model (218). In another endocarditis model using an ampicillin- and vancomycin-resistant *E. faecium*, addition of rifampin (MIC = 0.098 μg/mL) to a ciprofloxacin (MIC = 3.1 μg/mL) plus gentamicin (MIC = 12.5 μg/mL) combination resulted in significant reduction in bacterial densities in cardiac vegetations after 5 days of treatment (219). Rifampin resistance was detected among organisms that persisted after discontinuation of therapy.

Novobiocin, another DNA gyrase inhibitor that was introduced years ago as an antistaphylococcal agent, shows significant in vitro activity against *E. faecium*, including vancomycin-resistant isolates (MIC_{90} = 1.0 μg/mL) (220). Activity is less against *E. faecalis* (MIC_{90} = 16 μg/mL) or in media supplemented with 50% serum. Combinations of novobiocin with ciprofloxacin or ofloxacin resulted in additive bactericidal activity against multiresistant *E. faecium* (214, 220). In an animal model, treatment with the combination significantly decreased numbers of surviving organisms compared with those in untreated animals, but any advantage of the combination compared with novobiocin alone was less apparent (221). Novobiocin plus ciprofloxacin combinations demonstrating synergy by checkerboard testing have been used with favorable initial clinical response in 10 liver transplant patients with infections due to vancomycin-resistant *E. faecium* (222). In that study, novobiocin resistance emerged when one patient received this agent alone.

Other Antimicrobial Agents Among recent VRE, a number show susceptibility to chloramphenicol or tetracycline, or both (174,223). Tetracyclines have been among the most commonly used drugs in VRE bacteremia treatment

lin, and ticarcillin against gram-positive bacteria and *Haemophilus influenzae.* Antimicrob Agents Chemother 1981;20: 843–846.

32 **Sentochnik DE, Eliopoulos GM, Ferraro MJ, Moellering RC Jr.** Comparative in vitro activity of SM7338, a new carbapenem antimicrobial agent. Antimicrob Agents Chemother 1989;33:1232–1236.

33 **White GW, Malow JB, Zimelis VM, et al.** Comparative in vitro activity of azlocillin, ampicillin, mezlocillin, piperacillin, and ticarcillin, alone and in combination with an aminoglycoside. Antimicrob Agents Chemother 1979;15:540–543.

34 **Lincoln LJ, Weinstein AJ, Gallagher M, Abrutyn E.** Penicillinase-resistant penicillins plus gentamicin in experimental enterococcal endocarditis. Antimicrob Agents Chemother 1977;12:484–489.

35 **Glew RH, Moellering RC Jr.** Effect of protein binding on the activity of penicillins in combination with gentamicin against enterococci. Antimicrob Agents Chemother 1979;15:87–92.

36 **Weinstein AJ, Lentnek AL.** Cephalosporin-aminoglycoside synergism in experimental enterococcal endocarditis. Antimicrob Agents Chemother 1976;9:983–987.

37 **Eliopoulos GM, Reiszner E, Willey S, et al.** Effect of blood product medium supplements on the activity of cefotaxime and other cephalosporins against *Enterococcus faecalis.* Diagn Microbiol Infect Dis 1989:12:149–156.

38 **Fontana R, Cerini R, Longoni P, et al.** Identification of a streptococcal penicillin-binding protein that reacts very slowly with penicillin. J Bacteriol 1983;155:1343–1350.

39 **Williamson R, LeBouguénec C, Gutmann L, Horaud T.** One or two low af-finity penicillin-binding proteins may be responsible for the range of susceptibility of *Enterococcus faecium* to benzylpenicillin. J Gen Microbiol 1985;131:1933–1940.

40 **Piras G, El Kharroubi A, van Beeumen J, et al.** Characterization of an *Enterococcus hirae* penicillin-binding protein 3 with low penicillin affinity. J Bacteriol 1990;172: 6856–6862.

41 **Krogstad DJ, Parquette AR.** Defective killing of enterococci: a common property of antimicrobial agents acting on the cell wall. Antimicrob Agents Chemother 1980;17: 965–968.

42 **Cercenado E, Eliopoulos GM, Wennersten CB, Moellering RC Jr.** Influence of high-level gentamicin resistance and beta-hemolysis on susceptibility of enterococci to the bactericidal activities of ampicillin and vancomycin. Antimicrob Agent Chemother 1992;36:2526–2528.

43 **Hodges TL, Zighelboim-Daum S, Eliopoulos GM, et al.** Antimicrobial susceptibility changes in *Enterococcus faecalis* following various penicillin exposure regimens. Antimicrob Agents Chemother 1992; 36:121–125.

44 **Thauvin C, Eliopoulos GM, Willey S, et al.** Continuous-infusion ampicillin therapy of enterococcal endocarditis in rats. Antimicrob Agents Chemother 1987;31: 139–143.

45 **Hellinger WC, Rouse MS, Rabadan PM, et al.** Continuous intravenous versus intermittent ampicillin therapy of experimental endocarditis caused by aminoglycoside-resistant enterococci. Antimicrob Agents Chemother 1992;36:1272–1275.

46 **Kim KS, Bayer AB.** Significance of in-vitro penicillin tolerance in experimental enterococcal endocarditis. J Antimicrob Chemother 1987;19:475–485.

47 **Fontana R, Boaretti M, Grossato A, et al.** Paradoxical response of *Enterococcus faecalis* to the bactericidal activity of penicillin is associated with reduced activity of one autolysin. Antimicrob Agents Chemother 1990;34:314–320.

48 **Said I, Fletcher H, Volpe A, Daneo-Moore L.** Penicillin tolerance in *Streptococcus faecium* ATCC 9790. Antimicrob Agents Chemother 1987;31:1150–1152.

49 **Storch GA, Krogstad DJ.** Antibiotic-induced lysis of enterococci. J Clin Invest 1981;68:639–645.

50 **Daneo-Moore L, Volpe A, Said I.** Variation between penicillin-tolerant and penicillin-sensitive states in *Streptococcus faecium* ATCC9790. FEMS Microbiol Lett 1985;30:319–323.

51 **Moellering RC Jr, Weinberg AN.** Studies on antibiotic synergism against enterococci. II. Effect of various antibiotics on the uptake of ^{14}C-labeled streptomycin by enterococci. J Clin Invest 1971;50:2580–2584.

52 **Krogstad DJ, Korfhagen TR, Moellering RC Jr, et al.** Aminoglycoside-inactivating enzymes in clinical isolates of *Streptococcus faecalis.* An explanation for resistance to antibiotic synergism. J Clin Invest 1978;62: 480–486.

53 **Eliopoulos GM, Farber BF, Murray BE, et al.** Ribosomal resistance of clinical enterococcal isolates to streptomycin. Antimicrob Agents Chemother 1984;25:398–399.

54 **Calderwood SA, Wennersten C, Moellering RC Jr, et al.** Resistance to six aminoglycosidic aminocyclitol antibiotics among enterococci: prevalence, evolution, and relationship to synergism with penicillin. Antimicrob Agents Chemother 1977;12: 401–405.

55 **Costa Y, Galimand M, Leclercq R, et al.** Characterization of the chromosomal *aac(6')-Ii* gene specific for *Enterococcus faecium.* Antimicrob Agents Chemother 1993;37:1896–1903.

56 **Calderwood SB, Wennersten C, Moellering RC Jr.** Resistance to antibiotic synergism in *Streptococcus faecalis*: further studies with amikacin and with a new amikacin derivative, 4'-deoxy, 6'-*N*-methylamikacin. Antimicrob Agents Chemother 1981;19:549–555.

57 **Thauvin C, Eliopoulos GM, Wennersten C, Moellering RC Jr.** Antagonistic effect of penicillin-amikacin combinations against enterococci. Antimicrob Agents Chemother 1985;28:78–83.

58 **Carlier C, Courvalin C.** Emergence of 4',4''-aminoglycoside nucleotidyltransferase in enterococci. Antimicrob Agents Chemother 1990;34:1565–1569.

59 **Moellering RC Jr, Murray BE, Schoenbaum SC, et al.** A novel mechanism of resistance to penicillin-gentamicin synergism in *Streptococcus faecalis.* J Infect Dis 1980;141:81–86.

60 **Horodniceanu T, Bougueleret L, El-Solh N, et al.** High-level, plasmid-borne resistance to gentamicin in *Streptococcus faecalis* subsp. *zymogenes.* Antimicrob Agents Chemother 1979;16:686–689.

61 **Mederski-Samoraj BD, Murray BE.** High-level resistance to gentamicin in clinical isolates of enterococci. J Infect Dis 1983;147:751–757.

62 **Eliopoulos GM, Wennersten C, Zighelboim-Daum S, et al.** High-level resistance to gentamicin in clinical isolates of *Streptococcus (Enterococcus) faecium.* Antimicrob Agents Chemother 1988;32: 1528–1532.

63 **Sahm DF, Gilmore MS.** Transferability and genetic relatedness of high-level gentamicin resistance among enterococci. Antimicrob Agents Chemother 1994;38: 1194–1196.

64 **Ferretti JJ, Gilmore KS, Courvalin P.** Nucleotide sequence analysis of the gene specifying the bifunctional 6'-aminoglycoside acetyltransferase 2''-aminoglycoside phosphotransferase enzyme in *Streptococcus faecalis* and identification and cloning of gene regions specifying the two activities. J Bacteriol 1986;167:631–638.

65 **Zervos MJ, Mikesell TS, Schaberg DR.** Heterogeneity of plasmids determining high-level resistance to gentamicin in clinical isolates of *Streptococcus faecalis.* Antimicrob Agents Chemother 1986;30:78–81.

66 **Patterson JE, Masecar BL, Kauffman CA, et al.** Gentamicin resistance plasmids of enterococci from diverse geographic areas are heterogeneous. J Infect Dis 1988;158: 212–216.

67 **Rice LB, Eliopoulos GM, Wennersten C, et al.** Chromosomally mediated β-lactamase production and gentamicin resistance in *Enterococcus faecalis.* Antimicrob Agents Chemother 1991;35:272–276.

68 **Hodel-Christian SL, Murray BE.** Mobilization of the gentamicin resistance gene in *Enterococcus faecalis.* Antimicrob Agents Chemother 1990;34:1278–1280.

69 **Hodel-Christian SL, Murray BE.** Characterization of the gentamicin resistance transposon Tn*5281* from *Enterococcus faecalis* and comparison to staphylococcal transposons Tn*4001* and Tn*4031.* Antimicrob Agents Chemother 1991;35:1147–1152.

70 **Hodel-Christian SL, Murray BE.** Comparison of the gentamicin resistance transposon Tn*5281* with regions encoding gentamicin resistance in *Enterococcus faecalis* isolates from diverse geographic locations. Antimicrob Agents Chemother 1992;36:2259–2264.

71 **Thal LA, Chow JW, Clewell DB, Zervos MJ.** Tn*924,* a chromosome-borne transposon encoding high-level gentamicin resistance in *Enterococcus faecalis.* Antimicrob Agents Chemother 1994;38: 1152–1156.

72 **Bantar CE, Micucci M, Fernandez Canigia L, et al.** Synergy characterization for *Enterococcus faecalis* strains displaying moderately high-level gentamicin and streptomycin resistance. J Clin Microbiol 1993;31:1921–1923.

73 **Bartoloni A, Stefani S, Orsi A, et al.** High-level aminoglycoside resistance among enterococci isolated from blood cultures. J Antimicrob Chemother 1992;29:729–731.

74 **Venditti M, Tarasi A, Gelfusa V, et al.**

Antimicrobial susceptibilities of enterococci isolated from hospitalized patients. Antimicrob Agents Chemother 1993;37: 1190–1192.

75 **Woodford N, Morrison D, Johnson AP, George RC.** Antimicrobial resistance amongst enterococci isolated in the United Kingdom: a reference laboratory perspective. J Antimicrob Chemother 1993;32:344–346.

76 **Patterson JE, Barry M, Gallant J, et al.** Epidemiology of high-level gentamicin resistant enterococci isolates from Zimbabwe. Am J Trop Med Hyg 1990;43:397–399.

77 **Nachamkin I, Axelrod P, Talbot GH, et al.** Multiply high-level-aminoglycoside-resistant enterococci isolated from patients in a university hospital. J Clin Microbiol 1988; 26:1287–1291.

78 **Weems JJ Jr, Lowrance JH, Baddour LM, Simpson WA.** Molecular epidemiology of nosocomial, multiply aminoglycoside resistant *Enterococcus faecalis*. J Antimicrob Chemother 1989;24:121–130.

79 **Watanakunakorn C.** The prevalence of high-level aminoglycoside resistance among enterococci isolated from blood cultures during 1980–1988. J Antimicrob Chemother 1989;24:63–68.

80 **Gradon JR, Lutwick S, Lutwick LI, Levi MH.** *Enterococcus faecium* with high-level resistance to gentamicin. Lancet 1991;338: 762–763.

81 **Zervos MJ, Kauffman CA, Therasse PM, et al.** Nosocomial infection by gentamicin-resistant *Streptococcus faecalis*. Ann Intern Med 1987;106:687–691.

82 **Wurtz R, Sahm D, Flaherty J.** Gentamicin-resistant, streptomycin-susceptible *Enterococcus (Streptococcus) faecalis* bacteremia. J Infect Dis 1991;163:1393–1394.

83 **Grayson ML, Eliopoulos GM, Wennersten CB, et al.** Increasing resistance to β-lactam antibiotics among clinical isolates of *Enterococcus faecium*: a 22-year review at one institution. Antimicrob Agents Chemother 1991;35:2180–2184.

84 **Zervos MJ, Terpenning MS, Schaberg DR, et al.** High-level aminoglycoside-resistant enterococci. Colonization of nursing home and acute care hospital patients. Arch Intern Med 1987;147:1591–1594.

85 **Zervos MS, Dembinski S, Mikesell T, Schaberg DR.** High-level resistance to gentamicin in *Streptococcus faecalis*: risk factors and evidence for exogenous acquisition of infection. J Infect Dis 1986;153: 1075–1083.

86 **Axelrod P, Talbot GH.** Risk factors for acquisition of gentamicin-resistant enterococci. Arch Intern Med 1989;149:1397–1401.

87 **Noskin GA, Till M, Patterson BK, et al.** High-level gentamicin resistance in *Enterococcus faecalis* bacteremia. J Infect Dis 1991;164:1212–1215.

88 **Murray BE, Mederski-Samaroj B.** Transferable β-lactamase. A new mechanism for in vitro penicillin resistance in *Streptococcus faecalis*. J Clin Invest 1983;72:1168–1171.

89 **Murray BE.** β-Lactamase-producing enterococci. Antimicrob Agents Chemother 1992;36:2355–2359.

90 **Coudron PE, Markowitz SM, Wong ES.** Isolation of a β-lactamase-producing, aminoglycoside-resistant strain of *Enterococcus faecium*. Antimicrob Agents Chemother 1992;36:1125–1126.

91 **Murray BE, Church DA, Wanger A, et al.** Comparison of two β-lactamase-producing strains of *Streptococcus faecalis*. Antimicrob Agents Chemother 1986;30:861–864.

92 **Patterson JE, Masecar BL, Zervos MJ.** Characterization and comparison of two penicillinase-producing strains of *Streptococcus (Enterococcus) faecalis*. Antimicrob Agents Chemother 1988;32:122–124.

93 **Murray BE, Mederski-Samoraj B, Foster SK, et al**. In vitro studies of plasmid-mediated penicillinase from *Streptococcus faecalis* suggest a staphylococcal origin. J Clin Invest 1986;77:289–293.

94 **Zscheck KK, Hull R, Murray BE.** Restriction mapping and hybridization studies of a β-lactamase-encoding fragment from *Streptococcus (Enterococcus) faecalis*. Antimicrob Agents Chemother 1988;32:768–769.

95 **Zscheck KK, Murray BE.** Nucleotide sequence of the β-lactamase gene from *Enterococcus faecalis* HH22 and its similarity to staphylococcal β-lactamase genes. Antimicrob Agents Chemother 1991;35: 1736–1740.

96 **Zscheck KK, Murray BE**. Genes involved in the regulation of β-lactamase production in enterococci and staphylococci. Antimicrob Agents Chemother 1993;37:1966–1970.

97 **Smith MC, Murray BE.** Sequence analysis of the β-lactamase repressor from *Staphylococcus aureus* and hybridization studies with two β-lactamase-producing isolates of *Enterococcus faecalis*. Antimicrob Agents Chemother 1992;36:2265–2269.

98 **Rice LB, Marshall SH.** Evidence of incorporation of the chromosomal β-lactamase gene of *Enterococcus faecalis* CH19 into a transposon derived from staphylococci.

Antimicrob Agents Chemother 1992;36: 1843–1846.

99 **Murray BE, Singh KV, Markowitz SM, et al.** Evidence for clonal spread of a single strain of β-lactamase-producing *Enterococcus (Streptococcus) faecalis* to six hospitals in five states. J Infect Dis 1991;163:780–785.

100 **Murray BE, Lopardo HA, Rubeglio EA, et al.** Intrahospital spread of a single gentamicin-resistant, β-lactamase-producing strain of *Enterococcus faecalis* in Argentina. Antimicrob Agents Chemother 1992;36: 230–232.

101 **Wells VD, Wong ES, Murray BE, et al.** Infections due to beta-lactamase-producing, high-level gentamicin-resistant *Enterococcus faecalis*. Ann Intern Med 1992; 116:285–292.

102 **Markowitz SM, Wells VD, Williams DS, et al.** Antimicrobial susceptibility and molecular epidemiology of β-lactamase-producing, aminoglycoside-resistant isolates of *Enterococcus faecalis*. Antimicrob Agents Chemother 1991;35:1075–1080.

103 **Lopardo H, Casimir L, Hernández C, Rubeglio EA.** Isolation of three strains of beta-lactamase-producing *Enterococcus faecalis* in Argentina. Eur J Clin Microbiol Infect Dis 1990;9:402–405.

104 **Patterson JE, Colodny SM, Zervos MJ.** Serious infection due to β-lactamase-producing *Streptococcus faecalis* with high-level resistance to gentamicin. J Infect Dis 1988;158:1144–1145.

105 **Rhinehart E, Smith NE, Wennersten C, et al.** Rapid dissemination of β-lactamase-producing, aminoglycoside-resistant *Enterococcus faecalis* among patients and staff on an infant-toddler surgical ward. N Engl J Med 1990;323:1814–1818.

106 **Mazzulli T, King SM, Richardson SE.** Bacteremia due to β-lactamase-producing *Enterococcus faecalis* with high-level resistance to gentamicin in a child with Wiskott-Aldrich syndrome. Clin Infect Dis 1992; 14:780–781.

107 **Cercenado E, Garcia-Leoni ME, Rodeño P, Rodriguez-Créixems M.** Ampicillin-resistant enterococci. J Clin Microbiol 1990; 28:829.

108 **Grayson ML, Eliopoulos GM, Wennersten CB, et al.** Comparison of *Enterococcus raffinosus* with *Enterococcus avium* on the basis of penicillin susceptibility, penicillin-binding protein analysis, and high-level aminoglycoside resistance. Antimicrob Agents Chemother 1991;35:1408–1412.

109 **Oster SE, Chirurgi VA, Goldberg AA, et al.** Ampicillin-resistant enterococcal sepsis in an acute-care hospital. Antimicrob Agents Chemother 1990;34:1821–1823.

110 **Boyce JM, Opal SM, Potter-Bynoe G, et al.** Emergence and nosocomial transmission of ampicillin-resistant enterococci. Antimicrob Agents Chemother 1992;36:1032–1039.

111 **Klare I, Rodloff AC, Wagner J, et al.** Overproduction of a penicillin-binding protein is not the only mechanism of penicillin resistance in *Enterococcus faecium*. Antimicrob Agents Chemother 1992;36:783–787.

112 **Fontana R, Aldegheri M, Ligozzi M, et al.** Overproduction of a low-affinity penicillin-binding protein and high-level ampicillin resistance in *Enterococcus faecium*. Antimicrob Agents Chemother 1994;38: 1980–1983.

113 **Bush LM, Calmon J, Cherney CL, et al.** High-level penicillin resistance among isolates of enterococci. Implications for treatment of enterococcal infections. Ann Intern Med 1989;110:515–520.

114 **Torres C, Tenorio C, Lantero M, et al.** High-level penicillin resistance and penicillin-gentamicin synergy in *Enterococcus faecium*. Antimicrob Agents Chemother 1993;37:2427–2431.

115 **Chirurgi VA, Oster SE, Goldberg AA, McCabe RE.** Nosocomial acquisition of β-lactamase-negative, ampicillin-resistant enterococcus. Arch Intern Med 1992;152: 1457–1461.

116 **Uttley AH, Collins CH, Naidoo J, George RC.** Vancomycin-resistant enterococci. Lancet 1988;1:57–58.

117 **Lütticken R, Kunstmann G.** Vancomycin-resistant streptococcaceae from clinical material. Zentralbl Bakt Hyg 1988;267: 379–382.

118 **Leclercq R, Derlot E, Duval J, Courvalin P.** Plasmid-mediated resistance to vancomycin and teicoplanin in *Enterococcus faecium*. N Engl J Med 1988;319:157–161.

119 **Kaplan AH, Gilligan PH, Facklam RR.** Recovery of resistant enterococci during vancomycin prophylaxis. J Clin Microbiol 1988;26:1216–1218.

120 **Uttley AHC, George RC, Naidoo J, et al.** High-level vancomycin-resistant enterococci causing hospital infections. Epidemiol Infect 1989;103:173–181.

121 **Williamson R, Al-Obeid S, Shlaes JH, et al.** Inducible resistance to vancomycin in *Enterococcus faecium* D366. J Infect Dis 1989;159:1095–1104.

122 **Sahm DF, Kissinger J, Gilmore MS, et al.** In vitro susceptibility studies of

vancomycin-resistant *Enterococcus faecalis*. Antimicrob Agents Chemother 1989;33: 1588–1591.

123 **Shlaes DM, Bouvet A, Devine C, et al.** Inducible, transferable resistance to vancomycin in *Enterococcus faecalis* A256. Antimicrob Agents Chemother 1989;33: 198–203.

124 **Nicas TI, Wu CYE, Hobbs JN Jr, et al.** Characterization of vancomycin resistance in *Enterococcus faecium* and *Enterococcus faecalis*. Antimicrob Agents Chemother 1989;33:1121–1124.

125 **Vincent S, Knight RG, Green M, et al.** Vancomycin susceptibility and identification of motile enterococci. J Clin Microbiol 1991;29:2335–2337.

126 **Shlaes DM.** Vancomycin-resistant bacteria. Infect Control Hosp Epidemiol 1992;13:193–194.

127 **Courvalin P.** Resistance of enterococci to glycopeptides. Antimicrob Agent Chemother 1990;34:2291–2296.

128 **Dutka-Malen S, Blaimont B, Wauters G, Courvalin P.** Emergence of high-level resistance to glycopeptides in *Enterococcus gallinarum* and *Enterococcus casseliflavus*. Antimicrob Agents Chemother 1994;38: 1675–1677.

129 **Hayden MK, Trenholme GM, Schultz JE, Sahm DF.** In vivo development of teicoplanin resistance in a VanB *Enterococcus faecium* isolate. J Infect Dis 1993;167: 1224–1227.

130 **Quintiliani R Jr, Evers S, Courvalin P.** The *vanB* gene confers various levels of self-transferable resistance to vancomycin in enterococci. J Infect Dis 1993;167:1220–1223.

131 **Brisson-Noël A, Dutka-Malen S, Molinas C, et al.** Cloning and heterospecific expression of the resistance determinant *vanA* encoding high-level resistance to glycopeptides in *Enterococcus faecium* BM4147. Antimicrob Agents Chemother 1990;34:924–927.

132 **Dutka-Malen S, Leclercq R, Coutant V, et al.** Phenotypic and genotypic heterogeneity of glycopeptide resistance determinants in gram-positive bacteria. Antimicrob Agents Chemother 1990;34:1875–1879.

133 **Dutka-Malen S, Molinas C, Arthur M, Courvalin P.** The VANA glycopeptide resistance protein is related to D-alanyl-D-alanine ligase cell wall biosynthesis enzymes. Mol Gen Genet 1990;224:364–372.

134 **Walsh CT.** Vancomycin resistance: decoding the molecular logic. Science 1993;261: 308–309.

135 **Bugg TDH, Dutka-Malen S, Arthur M, et al.** Identification of vancomycin resistance protein VanA as a D-alanine:D-alanine ligase of altered substrate specificity. Biochemistry 1991;30:2017–2021.

136 **Arthur M, Molinas C, Dutka-Malen S, Courvalin P.** Structural relationship between the vancomycin resistance protein VanH and 2-hydroxycarboxylic acid dehydrogenases. Gene 1991;103:133–134.

137 **Bugg TDH, Wright GD, Dutka-Malen S, et al.** Molecular basis for vancomycin resistance in *Enterococcus faecium* BM4147: biosynthesis of a depsipeptide peptidoglycan precursor by vancomycin resistance proteins VanH and VanA. Biochemistry 1991;30:10408–10415.

138 **Allen NE, Hobbs JN Jr, Richardson JM, Riggin RM.** Biosynthesis of modified peptidoglycan precursors by vancomycin-resistant *Enterococcus faecium*. FEMS Microbiol Lett 1992;98:109–116.

139 **Arthur M, Molinas C, Bugg TDH, et al.** Evidence for in vivo incorporation of D-lactate into peptidoglycan precursors of vancomycin-resistant enterococci. Antimicrob Agents Chemother 1992;36:867–869.

140 **Arthur M, Molinas C, Depardieu F, Courvalin P.** Characterization of Tn*1546*, a Tn*3*-related transposon conferring glycopeptide resistance by synthesis of depsipeptide peptidoglycan precursors in *Enterococcus faecium* BM4147. J Bacteriol 1993;175:117–127.

141 **Arthur M, Molinas C, Courvalin P.** Sequence of the *vanY* gene required for production of a vancomycin-inducible, D,D-carboxypeptidase in *Enterococcus faecium* BM4147. Gene 1992;120:111–114.

142 **Arthur M, Depardieu F, Snaith HA, et al.** Contribution of VanY D,D-carboxypeptidase to glycopeptide resistance in *Enterococcus faecalis* by hydrolysis of peptidoglycan precursors. Antimicrob Agents Chemother 1994;38:1899–1903.

143 **Gutmann L, Billot-Klein D, Al-Obeid S, et al.** Inducible carboxypeptidase activity in vancomycin-resistant enterococci. Antimicrob Agents Chemother 1992;36:77–80.

144 **Handwerger S.** Alterations in peptidoglycan precursors and vancomycin susceptibility in Tn*917* insertion mutants of *Enterococcus faecalis* 221. Antimicrob Agents Chemother 1994;38:473–475.

145 **Wright GD, Molinas C, Arthur M, et al.**

Characterization of VanY, a D,D-carboxypeptidase from vancomycin-resistant *Enterococcus faecium* BM4147. Antimicrob Agents Chemother 1992;36:1514–1518.

146 **Arthur M, Molinas C, Courvalin P.** The VanS-VanR two-component regulatory system controls synthesis of depsipeptide peptidoglycan precursors in *Enterococcus faecium* BM4147. J Bacteriol 1992;174:2582–2591.

147 **Holman TR, Wu Z, Wanner BL, Walsh CT.** Identification of the DNA-binding site for the phosphorylated VanR protein required for vancomycin resistance in *Enterococcus faecium*. Biochemistry 1994;33:4625–4631.

148 **Noble WC, Virani Z, Cree RGA.** Co-transfer of vancomycin and other resistance genes from *Enterococcus faecalis* NCTC 12201 to *Staphylococcus aureus*. FEMS Microbiol Lett 1992;93:195–198.

149 **Evers S, Sahm DF, Courvalin P.** The *vanB* gene of vancomycin-resistant *Enterococcus faecalis* V583 is structurally related to genes encoding D-Ala:D-Ala ligases and glycopeptide-resistance proteins VanA and VanC. Gene 1993;124:143–144.

150 **Gold HS, Ünal S, Cercenado E, et al.** A gene conferring resistance to vancomycin but not teicoplanin in isolates of *Enterococcus faecalis* and *Enterococcus faecium* demonstrates homology with vanB, vanA, and vanC genes of enterococci. Antimicrob Agents Chemother 1993;37:1604–1609.

151 **Gold HS, Moellering RC Jr, Eliopoulos GM.** Sequence of *vanB2* gene and flanking DNA of vancomycin-resistant *Enterococcus faecalis* SF300. Presented at the 34th Interscience Conference Antimicrobial Agents Chemotherapy 1994.

152 **Evers S, Reynolds PE, Courvalin P.** Sequence of the *vanB* and *ddl* genes encoding D-alanine:D-lactate and D-alanine:D-alanine ligases in vancomycin-resistant *Enterococcus faecalis* V583. Gene 1994;140:97–102.

153 **Billot-Klein D, Gutmann L, Sablé S, et al.** Modification of peptidoglycan precursors is a common feature of the low-level vancomycin-resistant VANB-type Enterococcus D366 and of the naturally glycopeptide-resistant species *Lactobacillus casei, Pediococcus pentosaceus, Leuconostoc mesenteroides*, and *Enterococcus gallinarum*. J Bacteriol 1994;176:2398–2405.

154 **Quintiliani R Jr, Courvalin P.** Conjugal transfer of the vancomycin resistance determinant *vanB* between enterococci involves the movement of large genetic elements from chromosome to chromosome. FEMS Microbiol Lett 1994;119:359–364.

155 **Dutka-Malen S, Molinas C, Arthur M, Courvalin P.** Sequence of the *vanC* gene of *Enterococcus gallinarum* BM4174 encoding a D-alanine:D-alanine ligase-related protein necessary for vancomycin resistance. Gene 1992;112:53–58.

156 **Leclercq R, Dutka-Malen S, Duval J, Courvalin P.** Vancomycin resistance gene *vanC* is specific to *Enterococcus gallinarum*. Antimicrob Agents Chemother 1992;36:2005–2008.

157 **Reynolds PE, Snaith HA, Maguire AJ, et al.** Analysis of peptidoglycan precursors in vancomycin-resistant *Enterococcus gallinarum* BM4174. Biochem J 1994;301:5–8.

158 **Navarro F, Courvalin P.** Analysis of genes encoding D-alanine-D alanine ligase-related enzymes in *Enterococcus casseliflavus* and *Enterococcus flavescens*. Antimicrob Agents Chemother 1994;38:1788–1793.

159 **Clark NC, Cooksey RC, Hill BC, et al.** Characterization of glycopeptide-resistant enterococci from U.S. hospitals. Antimicrob Agents Chemother 1993;37:2311–2317.

160 **Fraimow HS, Jungkind DL, Lander DW, et al.** Urinary tract infection with an *Enterococcus faecalis* isolate that requires vancomycin for growth. Ann Intern Med 1994;121:22–26.

161 **Woodford N, Johnson AP, Morrison D, et al.** Vancomycin-dependent enterococci in the United Kingdom. J Antimicrob Chemother 1994;33:1066.

162 **Torres C, Reguera JA, Sanmartin MJ, et al.** *vanA*-Mediated vancomycin-resistant Enterococcus spp. in sewage. J Antimicrob Chemother 1994;33:553–561.

163 **Bates J, Jordens JZ, Griffiths DT.** Farm animals as a putative reservoir for vancomycin-resistant enterococcal infection in man. J Antimicrob Chemother 1994;34:507–516.

164 **Rubin LG, Tucci V, Cercenado E, et al.** Vancomycin-resistant *Enterococcus faecium* in hospitalized children. Infect Control Hosp Epidemiol 1992;13:700–705.

165 **Bingen EH, Denamur E, Lambert-Zechovsky NY, Elion J.** Evidence for the genetic unrelatedness of nosocomial vancomycin-resistant *Enterococcus faecium* strains in a pediatric hospital. J Clin Microbiol 1991;29:1888–1892.

166 **Green M, Barbadora K, Michaels M.** Re-

covery of vancomycin-resistant gram-positive cocci from pediatric liver transplant recipients. J Clin Microbiol 1991;29:2503–2506.

167 **Chow JW, Kuritza A, Shlaes DM, et al.** Clonal spread of vancomycin-resistant *Enterococcus faecium* between patients in three hospitals in two states. J Clin Microbiol 1993;31:1609–1611.

168 **Boyle JF, Soumakis SA, Rendo A, et al.** Epidemiologic analysis and genotypic characterization of nosocomial outbreak of vancomycin-resistant enterococci. J Clin Microbiol 1993;31:1280–1285.

169 **Boyce JM, Opal SM, Chow JW, et al.** Outbreak of multidrug-resistant *Enterococcus faecium* with transferable *vanB* class vancomycin resistance. J Clin Microbiol 1994;32:1148–1153.

170 **Woodford N, Morrison D, Johnson AP, et al.** Application of DNA probes for rRNA and *vanA* genes to investigation of a nosocomial cluster of vancomycin-resistant enterococci. J Clin Microbiol 1993;31:653–658.

171 **Livornese LL Jr, Dias S, Samel C, et al.** Hospital-acquired infection with vancomycin-resistant *Enterococcus faecium* transmitted by electronic thermometers. Ann Intern Med 1992;117:112–116.

172 **Karanfil LV, Murphy M, Josephson A, et al.** A cluster of vancomycin-resistant *Enterococcus faecium* in an intensive care unit. Infect Control Hosp Epidemiol 1992;13: 195–200.

173 **Montecalvo MA, Horowitz H, Gedris C, et al.** Outbreak of vancomycin-, ampicillin- and aminoglycoside-resistant *Enterococcus faecium* bacteremia in an adult oncology unit. Antimicrob Agents Chemother 1994; 38:1363–1367.

174 **Silber JL, Patel M, Paul SM, Kostman JR.** Statewide surveillance of isolates of vancomycin-resistant gram-positive cocci: genotyping of vancomycin resistance and activity of quinupristin/dalfopristin (RP 59500) and other antimicrobials. Presented at the 34th Intersci Conf Antimicrob Agents Chemother Orlando, Florida, October 4–7, 1994.

175 **Hardalo C, Rigsby M, Chen L, et al.** Chloramphenicol treatment of resistant *Enterococcus faecium* infections. Presented at the Infectious Diseases Society of America Annual Meeting, 1993.

176 **Grayson ML, Thauvin-Eliopoulos C, Eliopoulos GM, et al.** Failure of trimethoprim-sulfamethoxazole therapy in experimental enterococcal endocarditis. Antimicrob Agents Chemother 1990;34: 1792–1794.

177 **Chenoweth CE, Robinson KA, Schaberg DR.** Efficacy of ampicillin versus trimethoprim-sulfamethoxazole in a mouse model of lethal enterococcal peritonitis. Antimicrob Agents Chemother 1990;34: 1800–1802.

178 **Iannini PB, Ehret J, Eickhoff TC.** Effects of ampicillin-amikacin an ampicillin-rifampin on enterococci. Antimicrob Agents Chemother 1976;9:448–451.

179 **Moellering RC Jr, Wennersten C.** Therapeutic potential of rifampin in enterococcal infections. Rev Infect Dis 1983;5(suppl 3): S528–S532.

180 **Gedris G, van Horn K, Aguero-Rosenfeld M, Carbonaro C.** Incidence and susceptibility of vancomycin-resistant Enterococcus sp. blood isolates in a tertiary care hospital. Presented at the 93rd American Society of Microbiology General Meeting, 1993.

181 **Schaberg DR, Dillon WI, Terpenning MS, et al.** Increasing resistance of enterococci to ciprofloxacin. Antimicrob Agents Chemother 1992;36:2533–2535.

182 **Eliopoulos GM, Wennersten CB, Cole G, Moellering RC Jr.** In vitro activities of two glycylcyclines against gram-positive bacteria. Antimicrob Agents Chemother 1994;38:534–541.

183 **Spiegel CA, Huycke M.** Endocarditis due to streptomycin-susceptible *Enterococcus faecalis* with high-level gentamicin resistance. Arch Intern Med 1989;149;1873–1875.

184 **Lipman ML, Silva J Jr.** Endocarditis due to *Streptococcus faecalis* with high-level resistance to gentamicin. Rev Infect Dis 1989;11:325–328.

185 **Jones BL, Ludlam HA, Brown DFJ.** High dose ampicillin for the treatment of high-level aminoglycoside resistant enterococcal endocarditis. J Antimicrob Chemother 1994;33:891–892.

186 **Almirante B, Tornos MP, Gurgui M, et al.** Prognosis of enterococcal endocarditis. Rev Infect Dis 1991;13:1248–1249.

187 **Libertin CR, McKinley KM.** Gentamicin-resistant enterococcal endocarditis: the need for routine screening for high-level resistance to aminoglycosides. South Med J 1990;83:458–460.

188 **Fernández-Guerrero ML, Barros C, Rodriguez Tudela JL, et al.** Aortic endocarditis caused by gentamicin-resis-

tant *Enterococcus faecalis*. Eur J Clin Microbiol Infect Dis 1988;7:525–527.

189 **Holliman R, Smyth E.** Gentamicin-resistant enterococci and endocarditis. Postgrad Med J 1989;65:390–393.

190 **Rice LB, Calderwood SB, Eliopoulos GM, et al.** Enterococcal endocarditis: a comparison of prosthetic and native valve disease. Rev Infect Dis 1991;13:1–7.

191 **Das SS, Anderson JR, Macdonald AA, Somerville KW.** Endocarditis due to high level gentamicin resistant *Enterococcus faecium*. J Infect 1994;28:185–191.

192 **Wilson WR, Wilkowske CJ, Wright AJ, et al.** Treatment of streptomycin-susceptible and streptomycin-resistant enterococcal endocarditis. Ann Intern Med 1984;100: 816–823.

193 **Presterl E, Graninger W, Georgopoulos A.** The efficacy of teicoplanin in the treatment of endocarditis caused by gram-positive bacteria. J Antimicrob Chemother 1993; 31:755–766.

194 **Yao JDC, Thauvin-Eliopoulos C, Eliopoulos GM, Moellering RC Jr.** Efficacy of teicoplanin in two dosage regimens for experimental endocarditis caused by a β-lactamase-producing strain of *Enterococcus faecalis* with high-level resistance to gentamicin. Antimicrob Agents Chemother 1990;34:827–830.

195 **Gold MJ, Calmon J, Wendeler M, et al.** Synergistic bactericidal activity of rat serum with vancomycin against enterococci. J Infect Dis 1991;163:1358–1361.

196 **Hindes RG, Willey SH, Eliopoulos GM, et al.** Treatment of experimental endocarditis caused by a β-lactamase-producing strain of *Enterococcus faecalis* with high-level resistance to gentamicin. Antimicrob Agents Chemother 1989;33:1019–1022.

197 **Ingerman M, Pitsakis PG, Rosenberg A, et al.** β-Lactamase production in experimental endocarditis due to aminoglycoside-resistant *Streptococcus faecalis*. J Infect Dis 1987;155:1226–1232.

198 **Lavoie SR, Wong ES, Coudron PE, et al.** Comparison of ampicillin-sulbactam with vancomycin for treatment of experimental endocarditis due to a β-lactamase-producing, highly gentamicin-resistant isolate of *Enterococcus faecalis*. Antimicrob Agents Chemother 1993;37:1447–1451.

199 **Sullam PM, Täuber MG, Hackbarth CJ, Sande MA.** Therapeutic efficacy of teicoplanin in experimental enterococcal endocarditis. Antimicrob Agents Chemother 1985;27:135–136.

200 **Fantin B, Leclercq R, Arthur M, et al.** Influence of low-level resistance to vancomycin on efficacy of teicoplanin and vancomycin for treatment of experimental endocarditis due to *Enterococcus faecium*. Antimicrob Agents Chemother 1991;35: 1570–1575.

201 **Bingen E, Lambert-Zechovsky N, Leclercq R, et al.** Bactericidal activity of vancomycin, daptomycin, ampicillin and aminoglycosides against vancomycin-resistant *Enterococcus faecium*. J Antimiciob Chemother 1990;26:619–626.

202 **Gutmann L, Al-Obeid S, Billot-Klein D, et al.** Synergy and resistance to synergy between β-lactam antibiotics and glycopeptides against glycopeptide-resistant strains of *Enterococcus faecium*. Antimicrob Agents Chemother 1994;38:824–829.

203 **Hayden MK, Koenig GI, Trenholme GM.** Bactericidal activities of antibiotics against vancomycin-resistant *Enterococcus faecium* blood isolates and synergistic activities of combinations. Antimicrob Agents Chemother 1994;38:1225–1229.

204 **Leclercq R, Bingen E, Su QH, et al.** Effects of combinations of β-lactams, daptomycin, gentamicin, and glycopeptides against glycopeptide-resistant enterococci. Antimicrob Agents Chemother 1991;35:92–98.

205 **Al-Obeid S, Billot-Klein D, van Heijenoort J, et al.** Replacement of the essential penicillin-binding protein 5 by high-molecular mass PBPs may explain vancomycin-β-lactam synergy in low-level vancomycin-resistant *Enterococcus faecium* D366. FEMS Microbiol Lett 1992;91:79–84.

206 **Cercenado E, Eliopoulos GM, Wennersten CB, Moellering RC Jr.** Absence of synergistic activity between ampicillin and vancomycin against highly vancomycin-resistant enterococci. Antimicrob Agents Chemother 1992;36:2201–2203.

207 **Fraimow HS, Venuti E.** Inconsistent bactericidal activity of triple-combination therapy with vancomycin, ampicillin, and gentamicin against vancomycin-resistant, highly ampicillin-resistant *Enterococcus faecium*. Antimicrob Agents Chemother 1992;36:1563–1566.

208 **Handwerger S, Perlman DC, Altarac D, McAuliffe V.** Concomitant high-level vancomycin and penicillin resistance in clinical isolates of enterococci. Clin Infect Dis 1992;14:655–661.

209 **Caron F, Carbon C, Gutmann L.** Triple-combination penicillin-vancomycin-

gentamicin for experimental endocarditis caused by a moderately penicillin- and highly glycopeptide-resistant isolate of *Enterococcus faecium*. J Infect Dis 1991;164: 888–893.

210 **Caron F, Lemeland J-F, Humbert G, et al.** Triple combination penicillin-vancomycin-gentamicin for experimental endocarditis caused by a highly penicillin- and glycopeptide-resistant isolate of *Enterococcus faecium*. J Infect Dis 1993;168:681–686.

211 **Caron F, Pestel M, Kitzis M-D, et al.** Comparison of different β-lactam-glycopeptide-gentamicin combinations for an experimental endocarditis caused by a highly β-lactam-resistant and highly glycopeptide-resistant isolate of *Enterococcus faecium*. J Infect Dis 1995;171:106–112.

212 **Mainardi JL, Gutman L, Acar JF, Goldstein FW.** Synergistic effect of amoxicillin and cefotaxime against *Enterococcus faecalis*. Antimicrob Agents Chemother 1995;39:1984–1987.

213 **Brandt CM, Rouse MS, Tallan BM, et al.** Effective treatment of multidrug resistant enterococcal experimental endocarditis with combinations of cell-wall active agents. Presented at the 34th Intersci Conf Antimicrob Agents Chemother, 1994.

214 **Landman D, Mobarakai NK, Quale JM.** Novel antibiotic regimens against *Enterococcus faecium* resistant to ampicillin, vancomycin, and gentamicin. Antimicrob Agents Chemother 1993;37:1904–1908.

215 **Burney S, Landman D, Quale JM.** Activity of ciprofloxacin against multidrug resistant *Enterococcus faecium*. Antimicrob Agents Chemother 1994;38:1668–1670.

216 **Ünal S, Flokowitsch J, Mullen DL, et al.** In-vitro synergy and mechanism of interaction between vancomycin and ciprofloxacin against enterococcal isolates. J Antimicrob Chemother 1993;31:711–723.

217 **Perri MB, Chow JW, Zervos MJ.** In vitro activity of sparfloxacin and clinafloxacin against multidrug-resistant enterococci. Diagn Microbiol Infect Dis 1993;17:151–155.

218 **Vazquez J, Perri MB, Thal LA, et al.** Sparfloxacin and clinafloxacin alone or in combination with gentamicin for therapy for experimental ampicillin-resistant enterococcal endocarditis in rabbits. J Antimicrob Chemother 1993;32:715–721.

219 **Whitman MS, Pitsakis PG, Zausner A, et al.** Antibiotic treatment of experimental endocarditis due to vancomycin- and ampicillin-resistant *Enterococcus faecium*. Antimicrob Agents Chemother 1993;37: 2069–2073.

220 **French P, Venuti E, Fraimow HS.** In vitro activity of novobiocin against multiresistant strains of *Enterococcus faecium*. Antimicrob Agents Chemother 1993;37: 2736–2739.

221 **Quale JM, Landman D, Mobarakai N.** Treatment of experimental endocarditis due to multidrug resistant *Enterococcus faecium* with ciprofloxacin and novobiocin. J Antimicrob Chemother 1994;34:797–802.

222 **Linden P, Pasculle AW, Manez R, et al.** Utilization of novobiocin and ciprofloxacin for the treatment of serious infections due to vancomycin resistant *Enterococcus faecium*. Presented at the 33rd Intersci Conf Antimicrob Agents Chemother, 1993.

223 **Feldman RJ, Paul S, Cody R, et al.** Analysis of treatment for patients with vancomycin-resistant enterococcal bacteremia. Presented at the 34th Intersci Conf Antimicrob Agents Chemother Orlando, Florida, October 4–7, 1994.

224 **Montecalvo MA, Horowitz H, Carbonaro C, et al.** Effect of novobiocin-containing antimicrobial regimens on infection and colonization with vancomycin and ampicillin-resistant *Enterococcus faecium*. Presented at the 34th Intersci Conf Antimicrob Agents Chemother Orlando, Florida, October 4–7, 1994.

225 **Collins LA, Malanoski GJ, Eliopoulos GM, et al.** In vitro activity of RP59500, an injectable streptogramin antibiotic, against vancomycin-resistant gram-positive organisms. Antimicrob Agents Chemother 1993;37:598–601.

226 **Berthaud N, Gouin AM, Rousseau J, Desnottes JF.** RP59500: killing kinetics against gram-positive cocci in an *in vitro* pharmacokinetic model. Presented at the 33rd Intersci Conf Antimicrob Agents Chemother, 1993.

227 **Johnson CC, Slavoski L, Schwartz M, et al.** In vitro bactericidal activity of RP59500 (Synercid) against antibiotic resistant strains of *Streptococcus pneumoniae* and *Enterococcus* spp. Presented at the 34th Intersci Conf Antimicrob Agents Chemother Orlando, Florida, October 4–7, 1994.

228 **Pasculle AW, Linden PK, McDevitt DA, et al.** Susceptibility of vancomycin-resistant

Enterococcus faecium to alternative antimicrobial agents singly and in combination. Presented at the 33rd Intersci Conf Antimicrob Agents Chemother, 1993.

229 **Linden P, Pasculle AW, Riddler S, et al.** Quinupristin/dalfopristin (RP59500) for treatment of serious infection due to high-level vancomycin resistant *Enterococcus faecium*. Presented at the 34th Intersci Conf Antimicrob Agents Chemother Orlando, Florida, October 4–7, 1994.

230 **Lynn W, Wont S, Lacey S, et al.** Treatment of peritoneal dialysis-associated peritonitis due to vancomycin-resistant *Enterococcus faecium* with RP 59500 (quinupristin/dalfopristin). Presented at the 34th Intersci Conf Antimicrob Agents Chemother Orlando, Florida, October 4–7, 1994.

231 **Furlong WB, Bompart F.** Therapy for enterococci with vanA/vanB resistance patterns using RP59500 (quinupristin/dalfopristin). Presented at the 34th Intersci Conf Antimicrob Agents Chemother Orlando, Florida, October 4–7, 1994.

Resistant Nosocomial Gram-Negative Bacillary Pathogens: *Acinetobacter baumannii*, *Xanthomonas maltophilia*, and *Pseudomonas cepacia*

FERRIC C. FANG
NANCY E. MADINGER

> *"The microbial diseases which account for the greatest morbidity in our communities today are completely different in their origin and manifestations from those which are so effectively dealt with by modern techniques. . . . In an ever-changing world each period and each type of civilization will continue to have its burden of disease (1)."*

Acinetobacter baumannii (*calcoaceticus* var. *anitratus*), *Xanthomonas* (*Stenotrophomonas*) *maltophilia*, and *Pseudomonas* (*Burkholderia*) *cepacia* have emerged as important nosocomial pathogens, largely as a consequence of medical progress. Although these bacteria are only distantly related taxonomically, they share several significant characteristics: low intrinsic virulence, resistance to many commonly used antimicrobial or disinfectant agents, and an ability to grow in a wide range of microenvironments frequently found in the hospital setting. These characteristics have given *A. baumannii*, *X. maltophilia*, and *P. cepacia* particular prominence in the intensive care unit, where many of the patients are compromised hosts receiving broad-spectrum antibiotics and invasive procedures. *A. baumannii* alone accounted for 2.6% of bacterial blood culture isolates at the University of Colorado Health Sciences Center in 1994 (Fang, unpublished data, 1995), compared with less than 1% a decade earlier (2). This review focusec on the microbiologic, epidemiologic, clinical, therapeutic, and preventive aspects of infections caused by these ubiquitous organisms.

ACINETOBACTER BAUMANNII

Microbiology

Acinetobacter are nonfermentative gram-negative coccobacilli belonging to the family Neisseriaceae. *A. baumannii* (DNA group 2) is the most frequent clinical isolate and the species most often associated with nosocomial outbreaks (3,4). Previous names for this organism have included *Acinetobacter calcoaceticus* var.

anitratus, Diplococcus mucosus, Bacterium anitratum, Herellea vaginicola, Achromobacter anitratus, B5W, *Micrococcus calco-aceticus,* and *Moraxella glucidolytica* var. *nonliquefaciens* (5). Although the genus *Acinetobacter* is now well established, there are 17 genospecies that are definable only by DNA hybridization (3,6,7). Frequent name changes, use of differing phenotypic classifications (8), use of identical DNA group numbers, and clinical literature confounding different species and their historical counterparts have resulted in great confusion regarding species nomenclature (9,10). For clinical purposes, it is sufficient to perform a few phenotypic tests to identify the *A. baumannii-A. calcoaceticus* complex presumptively. However, epidemiologic investigations requiring more precise definitions must generally resort to molecular techniques.

Because nosocomial isolates of *Acinetobacter* may be highly drug resistant, prompt and accurate identification is essential. Clinicians should be aware of the characteristic Gram stain appearance and growth characteristics of this organism, because definitive identification of nonfermentative bacteria may require 72 to 96 hours. *Acinetobacter* are readily confused with other common bacteria on primary Gram stains from clinical material. *Acinetobacter* appear as gram-negative coccobacilli or short rods. Thus, they may be mistaken for *Neisseria gonorrhoeae, Haemophilus influenzae, Moraxella catarrhalis, Neisseria meningitidis,* or Enterobacteriaceae (11). Moreover, *Acinetobacter* tend to retain crystal violet more than other gram-negative bacteria and sometimes have been misidentified as gram-positive diplococci resembling *Streptococcus pneumoniae* (12).

As a genus, *Acinetobacter* have versatile metabolic characteristics, which probably accounts for their ubiquity in nature. Strictly aerobic, they will readily grow on conventional media used in clinical laboratories for primary isolation, such as blood agar, chocolate agar, MacConkey agar, broths, and blood culture media. Colonies are convex and opaque on blood agar and have a cornflower blue color on eosin-methylene blue agar. On MacConkey agar, a purple-pink pigment may be seen that can be mistaken for lactose fermentation. This appearance along with a negative cytochrome oxidase might lead to initial confusion with the Enterobacteriaceae. Presumptive identification of *Acinetobacter* species is made on the basis of a lack of carbohydrate fermentation, lack of cytochrome oxidase activity, absence of motility, and resistance to penicillin. Other characteristics include a positive catalase and negative indole reaction. The *A. baumannii-A. calcoaceticus* complex is further distinguished from other *Acinetobacter* spp. by rapid use and acid production from glucose, inability to reduce nitrate, and oxidative utilization of 10% lactose.

Acinetobacter have few identified virulence factors. Potential pathogenic factors include cell wall lipopolysaccharide (LPS), a capsule that inhibits phagocytosis, and bacteriocin production. Antibodies to outer membrane proteins and LPS O-polysaccharide have been detected in patients with either systemic or localized infections (13). Clinical isolates appear to be serum resistant relative to environmental strains (14), which may facilitate bloodstream invasion. In mice, slime-producing *Acinetobacter* strains were noted to enhance the virulence of other gram-negative bacteria present in mixed infections (15). This characteristic is clinically relevant since *A. baumannii* is frequently found in mixed cultures, particularly from respiratory specimens and wounds (16,17).

Epidemiology

Acinetobacter species are widespread in the environment, with their principle habitats probably water and soil (18). *Acinetobacter* isolates have been recovered from numerous sources, including milk and dairy products, poultry, and frozen food, as well as from the skin, conjunctiva, rectum, vagina, nasopharynx, human milk, throat, and urethra of healthy humans (18–20). However, food *Acinetobacter* isolates are typically *Acinetobacter* spp. other than *A. baumannii*, whereas hospital isolates are usually *A. baumannii* (21). With regard to culture specimens, *Acinetobacter* have been recovered from virtually every type of culture submitted from hospitalized patients. Colonized skin, respiratory tract, and gastrointestinal tract are believed to represent major reservoirs of infection (22–24).

Within the hospital environment, sources identified in association with infectious outbreaks have included gloves, distilled water, tap water, intravenous fluids and medications, needles, urinals, charts, monitors, intravenous poles, tables, washcloths, mattresses, ventilators or other respiratory equipment, water baths, humidifiers, and the hands of personnel (23,25–41). In one outbreak, *A. baumannii* was also detected in air samples obtained in the vicinity of colonized patients, raising the possibility of airborne spread (42). The ubiquity of *A. baumannii* in the environment frequently makes identification of a point source difficult and complicates control of infection in the hospital setting. Although transient and chronic skin carriage on the hands of hospital personnel has consistently been implicated in the transmission of *A. baumannii* (43–45), the reservoir of organisms colonizing inanimate objects and/or patients probably contributes to continued recolonization (46).

Despite the ubiquitous presence of *Acinetobacter* in the environment, there is evidence that endemic nosocomial isolates in an individual hospital represent clonal expansion of one or only a few strains (47–49). It is believed that pressures within the hospital select for a few prevailing strains which are then disseminated through the institution. It is also possible that some strains are more transmissible than others. Endemic (and epidemic) strains isolated from different institutions usually arise independently, although interhospital spread may occur when hospitals share staff or patients (50,51). Sporadic isolates, probably from endogenous sources, occur in the background of endemic and epidemic strains.

A. baumannii isolates are frequently recovered from patients in intensive care units, particularly burn units (48,52–54). Risk factors for *Acinetobacter* infection include major surgery, burns, instrumentation, diabetes, steroid use, chronic lung disease, alcohol abuse, underlying malignancy, and prolonged hospitalization. Patients with nosocomial *Acinetobacter* infections have been hospitalized for a mean of 15 days before the development of infection (range 5 to 35 days) (16,55–59). However, the single most significant risk factor is prior antibiotic use. Nearly 80% of patients have received antimicrobials before the development of serious *Acinetobacter* infections (16,50,60). In particular, prior use of cephalosporins is noted to significantly increase the risk of infection (50,61). Imipenem-resistant strains have arisen after increased use of this antimicrobial agent (26).

Seasonal variation in the frequency of cases has been noted in several reviews (17,58,60). Cases predominate during the late summer (July to September), a phenomenon independent of geographic location or type of hospital (teaching vs. private). The basis for this seasonal variation is not understood, although the possibility of increased transmission during periods of high humidity has been suggested (58).

Clinical Manifestations

Although community-acquired infections are common in some geographic locations (62), *A. baumannii* is particularly associated with nosocomial infections (63). *A. baumanii* has been implicated in infections of virtually any organ system (16,17,55,56,64). In several retrospective reviews, over half of isolates were part of mixed infections (17,56,57).

The most common site of colonization and infection is the respiratory tract (4,16,65). Moreover, respiratory tract infection is the leading identifiable source in cases of *Acinetobacter* bacteremia (43,58,61). Nosocomial *A. baumannii* pneumonia most often occurs in patients with endotracheal intubation or tracheostomy. Radiographic findings are frequently multilobar, and cavitation, empyema, and bronchopleural fistula have been reported (16). Mortality estimates vary with an overall reported mortality of about 40% (16,66). Although many fatalities have occurred in patients receiving suboptimal antimicrobial therapy, the reported experience with community-acquired *Acinetobacter* pneumonia confirms the considerable mortality rate associated with this illness (62).

Urine is the second most common site for recovery of *Acinetobacter* (16,67). Cystitis, acute and chronic pyelonephritis, and secondary bacteremia have been reported (64,65,67). Underlying renal or urologic disease is a common predisposing factor (65). Urinary isolates are frequently found in mixed cultures from patients with urinary catheters (64). Elston et al (67) reviewed urinary isolates and noted a predominance of infections associated with urinary tract obstruction.

Acinetobacter bacteremia usually occurs in association with a known localized infection, such as pneumonia, urinary tract infection, wound infection, or an infected intravascular catheter (16,58,68–70). Outbreaks of bacteremia have occurred in association with contaminated reusable pressure transducers (37). Clinical manifestations vary from septic shock to a well-tolerated febrile syndrome (71). Mortality may be considerable but is usually not a direct result of *Acinetobacter* bacteremia (72). Case series clearly document self-limited transient bacteremias that did not require aggressive therapy, and pseudobacteremia has also occurred (69,71). Both native valve and prosthetic valve endocarditis have been reported (73–75). Glew et al (16) reported prosthetic valve endocarditis, septic thrombophlebitis, and subhepatic abscess as complications of intravascular catheter infections.

Acinetobacter is an unusual cause of meningitis. However, patients with a breach in anatomic barriers (e.g., basilar skull fracture, neurosurgical procedure, or central nervous system [CNS] instrumentation) are at significant risk (11,36,76–78). In fact, *A. baumannii* is the second leading cause of postneurosurgical gram-negative meningitis (79). Occasional outbreaks have occurred in neonatal intensive care units (80). The clinical presentation is indistinguishable from that of other causes of bacterial meningitis, but many reports note that improper interpretation of Gram stains can lead to inappropriate therapy (11,76). A petechial rash and shock simulating meningococcemia have been reported in association with *Acinetobacter* spp. infections (30,64). In the largest reported series of *Acinetobacter* meningitis, one half of cases were polymicrobial (77). The mortality of *A. baumannii* meningitis is reported to be about 20%, comparing favorably with an overall 50% mortality for gram-negative meningitis in adults (77).

A. baumannii peritonitis has been reported in patients undergoing continuous ambulatory peritoneal dialysis (CAPD) (28,81–83). The source of infection is presumably colonized skin, with infection occurring at the time of insertion or during catheter maintenance. Infected patients have been noted to have mild illness.

Skin and wound infections are commonly associated with drains, catheters, or other foreign bodies (16). Other unusual forms of *Acinetobacter* infection include mediastinitis (84), endophthalmitis (85), corneal ulcer (86,87), osteomyelitis (88), septic arthritis (89), necrotizing fasciitis (90), thrombophlebitis (16), and intra-abdominal abscess (16,30). There is a single report of a saline infusion contaminated with killed *A. baumannii*, which caused an endotoxin reaction (27).

Therapy

Nosocomial *Acinetobacter* isolates tend to be highly drug resistant (26,50,91). *A. baumannii* may produce inducible and constitutive broad-spectrum β-lactamases, numerous aminoglycoside-modifying enzymes, altered penicillin-binding proteins, and altered outer membrane porin proteins (92–95). Resistance determinants may be plasmid borne, transposon associated, or chromosomal (96–98).

Although empiric therapy should take into account the usual susceptibility patterns of locally endemic strain(s), it is imperative that antibiotic selection be guided by susceptibility testing of specific isolates. Most of the older β-lactams are now ineffective and have been replaced by imipenem as the most effective agent, with a minimal inhibitory concentration $(MIC)_{90}$ of 0.5 μg/ml (92,99–102). Gentamicin resistance has been widely reported, and gentamicin-resistant strains may have elevated MICs for other aminoglycosides, although still within an achievable range (103). Although amikacin is currently the most active aminoglycoside (55,104), amikacin-resistant strains have been reported with increasing frequency (54,105). Ceftazidime, ceftriaxone, cefotaxime, piperacillin, ticarcillin, ciprofloxacin, sulfonamides, and doxycycline have in vitro activity against some isolates (99,101,104,106,107). However, it is now recognized that *Acinetobacter* possess broad-spectrum inducible β-lactamases that may not be detectable by routine methods in microbiology laboratories, leading some authorities to recommend against the use of cephalosporins in *Acinetobacter* infections irrespective of in vitro susceptibility determinations (108). Synergy has been demonstrated for β-lactams and aminoglycosides (16) or fluoroquinolones with aminoglycosides or β-lactams (102), and there is in vitro evidence suggesting that enhanced killing of aminoglycoside-resistant isolates is achieved with imipenem-aminoglycoside combinations (109). However, the clinical relevance of these observations has not been established.

Therapy for infections caused by *Acinetobacter* strains resistant to imipenem and/or amikacin is often problematic. Imipenem resistance appears to be associated with decreased expression of a specific outer membrane protein (110), and amikacin resistance can be mediated by an aminoglycoside-modifying enzyme (97). Sulbactam has activity against many isolates in vitro (111) and has been used with some success (112). However, a significant percentage of isolates are resistant (107,113,114), and sulbactam resistance may also arise rapidly on therapy (Fang, unpublished data, 1995). Piperacillin-tazobactam appears to be similarly active in vitro (115), but published clinical data are lacking. Although polymyxin B and colistimethate are active against *Acinetobacter* in vitro (113,116), the relative ineffectiveness of these agents in systemic infections (117) may limit their therapeutic role. Problems with polymyxin resistance have also been reported recently (54). Nevertheless, the use of such second-line agents must be considered when highly resistant strains are encountered (113).

There are no published trials to guide therapy of specific *Acinetobacter* syndromes. Recovery of *Acinetobacter* from contaminated sites or mixed cultures should first prompt clinical assessment of the need for therapy. Similarly, localized infections in normal hosts may respond to removal of foreign bodies and debridement without the use of antimicrobial agents. Monotherapy is appropriate for moderately severe infections when a brief course of treatment is anticipated, when high concentrations of the antimicrobial will be achieved, or when combination therapy is limited by drug penetration. The rationale for combination therapy of serious infections is based on anecdotal clinical experience, in vitro studies of synergy (16,102), and reports of resistance emerging during therapy (5,59,91,108,118). Empiric management often consists of a carbapenem and an aminoglycoside.

Despite reports describing spontaneous resolution of *Acinetobacter* bacteremia without specific therapy, it is prudent to consider nearly all *Acinetobacter* blood isolates as significant and to manage them accordingly (119). Infected intravascular devices such as catheters should be removed (56), and antibiotic selection should be guided by in vitro susceptibility tests. The recommended duration of therapy is similar to that for other gram-negative bacillary bacteremias, typically 10 to 14 days.

Successful therapy of *Acinetobacter* meningitis has usually consisted of β-lactam plus aminoglycoside combinations, selected according to susceptibility testing. Several authors have emphasized the use of intrathecal aminoglycosides for optimal results (76,120). Imipenem/cilastatin and fluoroquinolones have also been used successfully (121–123) and may be preferable to β-lactam agents for the reasons discussed above. Polymyxin B may be unsuitable as an intraventricular agent in the management of postneurosurgical ventriculitis because of its potential to cause chemical meningitis (124).

Catheter removal is usually unnecessary in the management of *A. baumannii* peritonitis complicating CAPD. Again, treatment regimens are guided by antimicrobial susceptibility testing, and successful eradication can been achieved with an oral fluoroquinolone, intraperitoneal aminoglycoside, or a combination of these agents (81–83). Because many patients receiving CAPD have positive cultures without signs of peritonitis, the decision to institute treatment must be individualized. Abrutyn et al (28) reported an outbreak of *Acinetobacter* peritonitis resulting from environmental contamination in which only 3 of 13 patients received short-course antimicrobial therapy. Although one of these patients developed *Acinetobacter* bacteremia, the authors believed that true peritonitis was not present in the majority of patients.

Prevention

Investigation of *A. baumannii* in the hospital environment requires surveillance of varied culture specimens, including potential sources of colonization (125). Analysis of frequency and rate of isolation data may underestimate nosocomial spread of a predominant strain (126). The *A. baumannii-A. calcoaceticus* complex is so homogeneous that biotype and antibiogram information are unlikely to assist in outbreak investigations (126,127). In addition to biotyping, numerous other methods have been used to delineate strains, including serotyping (128), restriction endonuclease analysis (26), pulsed-field gel electrophoresis (129), plasmid fingerprinting (126), polymerase chain reaction (PCR) fingerprinting (130,131), cell envelope protein electrophoresis (132), esterase electrophoresis (133), and ribotyping (134). Many investigators have used a combination of methods to achieve better discrimination (135).

Despite detailed epidemiologic investigation, environmental sources of *Acinetobacter* may remain obscure (50,91). When an environmental source is successfully identified, as in one outbreak resulting from contaminated ventilator circuits and resuscitation bags (136), a modification of sterilization protocols can result in prompt termination of the outbreak. Some outbreaks have been controlled with standard infection control practices, such as cohorting patients, improving handwashing technique, and increasing attention to universal precautions (34,50,137). Attempts to reduce inappropriate antibiotic use have also appeared to be beneficial (77,105). Topical application of polymyxin B may help to reduce skin and wound colonization (26). Selective decontamination of the gastrointestinal tract has been proposed (22), but the possible emergence of resistant bacteria is a concern (138). In the most drastic cases, some institutions have had to resort to bed closure, extensive decontamination procedures, and structural redesign of intensive care units to eradicate outbreak strains (43,91).

XANTHOMONAS (STENOTROPHOMONAS) MALTOPHILIA

Microbiology

Xanthomonas maltophilia is a motile nonfermentative gram-negative bacillus with multitrichous polar flagella. This organism was originally designated *Pseudomonas maltophilia* (139). However, distinguishing phenotypic features from other pseudomonads, including DNAse production, lysine decarboxylase activity, and the absence of an indophenol oxidase reaction, led to its transfer to the genus *Xanthomonas* in the 1980s (140,141). In 1993, reclassification to the new genus *Stenotrophomonas* was proposed (142), in recognition of yet other distinguishing features. Unlike *X. maltophilia*, other *Xanthomonas* sp. have a single polar flagellum, are unable to reduce nitrate, produce aryl polyene pigments (called "xanthomonadins"), and are primarily associated with plants. Although this recent proposed taxonomic change appears to be well justified, this review refers to *X. maltophilia*, in recognition of the nomenclature currently in widest use.

X. maltophilia colonies are flat and opaque with an irregular surface, typically appearing lavender-green or pale yellow. An ammonia-like odor is useful in preliminary identification. The oxidase reaction is generally negative but occasionally is positive. *X. maltophilia* produces extracellular DNAse, which may be detected on special media. As suggested by its name, *X. maltophilia* gives a vigorous acid reaction in oxidation-fermentation (OF) maltose medium, with weaker reactions in OF glucose or lactose. Like other Xanthomonas sp., *X. maltophilia* can hydrolyze esculin and (usually) orthonitrophenyl-β-D-galactopyranoside (ONPG) and produces catalase. Most strains require methionine for growth. A recent report has emphasized that *X. maltophilia* can occasionally be mistaken for *Pseudomonas* (*Burkholderia*) *cepacia*, particularly if oxidase and DNAse reactions are not performed carefully (143). This can be a clinically crucial distinction, because the isolation of *P. cepacia* has particular implications in the setting of cystic fibrosis.

Apart from intrinsic resistance to many antimicrobial agents, the virulence determinants of *X. maltophilia* have not been well characterized. Exoenzymes including elastase, esterase, lipase, mucinase, hyaluronidase, DNAse, RNAse, gelatinase, and hemolysin have been proposed as possible virulence factors (144). *X. maltophilia* adheres well to plastic materials (145), facilitating its role in infections of various medical devices.

Epidemiology

The normal environmental reservoir of *X. maltophilia* is not established, but the organism has been isolated from soil, fresh water, raw sewage, milk, and various animal and human sources (139,146). Notably, *X. maltophilia* has been isolated from water samples, water faucets, sink drains, vascular transducers, disinfectant solution, shaving brushes, anticoagulant solution in blood collection tubes, cardiopulmonary bypass pumps, and respiratory equipment in the hospital setting (147–153). In some cases, *X. maltophilia* transmission has been directly traced to contaminated solutions or equipment (150,154,155,156). However, in many instances, modes of transmission are unclear. Attempts to isolate *X. maltophilia* from the hands or throats of hospital personnel were unsuccessful in one outbreak setting (147), but colonization of nursing and respiratory therapy personnel was documented in another study (157).

X. maltophilia is an opportunistic pathogen that principally afflicts debilitated or immunocompromised hosts receiving broad-spectrum antimicrobial therapy. Nearly all *X. maltophilia* infections occur in the hospital setting; in one series, only 3% of isolates were community acquired (65). Patients with malignancies appear to be particularly predisposed to *X. maltophilia* infections (158,159), especially in the setting of granulocytopenia (147,160). Instrumentation is also an important risk factor. At one cancer hospital, *X. maltophilia* sepsis was associated with indwelling central venous or arterial catheters in 79% of cases (160). Infection with this organism has also complicated endotracheal intubation or tracheostomy (157,161), genitourinary catheterization (147), prosthetic valve implantation (153,159,162,163), continuous ambulatory peritoneal dialysis (164), and placement of an Ommaya reservoir or ventriculoperitoneal shunt (165–167). Broad-spectrum antimicrobial therapy provides a strong selection pressure favoring the emergence of these multiply resistant organisms, and the majority of patients infected with *X. maltophilia* has received antecedent antibiotics (147,168–171), particularly aminoglycosides, cephalosporins, antipseudomonal penicillins, and imipenem. Several centers have reported an increase in the incidence of *X. maltophilia* during the past decade (147,160,161,168), and increasing broad-spectrum antimicrobial use in the hospital setting is believed to be largely responsible for this trend.

Clinical Manifestations

X. maltophilia has been isolated from various clinical specimens, including respiratory secretions, throat swabs, lung tissue, wounds or skin lesions, blood, cerebrospinal fluid, urine, pericardial fluid, peritoneal fluid, amniotic fluid, ear drainage, eye drainage, and catheters (147,161,168,172). Not infrequently, *X. maltophilia* is isolated in mixed culture with other bacteria, making its clinical significance uncertain.

The respiratory tract is the most common site of *X. maltophilia* isolation overall, but the majority of isolates represents colonization rather than infection (147). Nevertheless, when pneumonia occurs, it is often complicated by bacteremia and a high mortality rate (160,161,173). Infiltrates are typically diffuse and bilateral (160). The overall crude mortality rate associated with respiratory isolation of *X. maltophilia* was 59% over a four year period at the University of Virginia (161). This may principally reflect the debilitated condition of patients predisposed to *X. maltophilia* infections rather than the intrinsic virulence of the pathogen. Other factors associated with *X. maltophilia* mortality include age greater than 40 years and hospitalization in an intensive care unit (161). The infrequent respiratory isolation of *X. maltophilia* in the outpatient setting appears to carry a less immediately ominous prognosis. It has been isolated in the setting of cystic fibrosis with increasing frequency (174,175) and was reported to cause pneumonia of mild severity in a patient with bronchiectasis (176).

X. maltophilia is occasionally isolated from postsurgical, posttraumatic, or burn wounds (146,161,177–179). Most of these infections appear to respond well to conventional measures of drainage and antimicrobial therapy. More serious *X. maltophilia* skin infections have been described in patients with cancer, particularly in those with granulocytopenia. Primary or metastatic cellulitis, mucocutaneous ulcers, purpura fulminans, or ecthyma gangrenosum have been reported (144,159,165,172,180–182). Primary cellulitis occurs mostly in the vicinity of a catheter site and responds to catheter removal. Metastatic nodular skin lesions may be mistaken for evidence of disseminated fungal infection (172), underscoring the importance of skin biopsy in this situation. Ecthyma gangrenosum may develop from metastatic cutaneous foci, mimicking skin lesions caused by *Pseudomonas aeruginosa*. Not surprisingly, metastatic skin lesions and mucocutaneous lesions of the oral cavity associated with *X. maltophilia* carry a poor prognosis unless resolution of neutropenia occurs.

The clinical spectrum of *X. maltophilia* bacteremia may range from nearly asymptomatic to fulminant septic shock. In one recent series from a cancer hospital, 43% of patients with *X. maltophilia* bacteremia were in shock upon presentation (160). Although *X. maltophilia* sepsis may be cryptogenic in immunocompromised hosts, indwelling central venous catheters are the most frequently identified portals of entry (160,183). Other associated sources of bacteremia include pneumonia, urinary tract infections, and intra-abdominal infections. No specific fever pattern is characteristic, and some patients have only low-grade temperature elevation (160). Because *X. maltophilia* readily colonizes a variety of microenvironments in the hospital setting, culture contamination or pseudobacteremia must always be considered when evaluating the significance of a positive blood culture. In one series, approximately one third of positive blood cultures were believed not to represent true infection (160). *X. maltophilia* contamination of the EDTA anticoagulant in blood collection tubes led to an outbreak of "pseudobacteremia" in one hospital (152). Concomitant procurement of blood samples for coagulation studies and culture resulted in blood culture cross-contamination. Contamination of devices or solutions can also result in true *X. maltophilia* bacteremia (150–152). Occasionally, *X. maltophilia* bacteremia signifies the presence of endocarditis, most often in the setting of intravenous drug abuse (165,184) or a prosthetic heart valve (153,159,162,163).

CNS infection with *X. maltophilia* is very uncommon, but seven cases of meningitis have been reported (165–167,185). Three of these patients had indwelling foreign bodies (Ommaya reservoir, ventricular drain, ventriculoperitoneal shunt) after neurosurgical procedures. Three of the four nonsurgical cases involved infants ranging from 7 days to 13 months of age (186,187). A neutrophilic pleocytosis was invariably noted in the cerebrospinal fluid, and those patients who received appropriate antimicrobial therapy and foreign body removal survived.

Urinary tract infection with *X. maltophilia* is usually associated with urinary tract catheterization or instrumentation (146,147). One cluster of cases was traced to contaminated chlorhexidine-cetramide disinfectant (150). Other unusual reported *X. maltophilia* infections include epididymitis (188), mastoiditis (189), cholangitis (173), dialysis-associated peritonitis (164), and eye infections (155,187,188,190).

Therapy

Antimicrobial therapy of infections with *X. maltophilia* is complicated by the intrinsic resistance of the organism to many commonly used broad-spectrum antimicrobial agents, including aminoglycosides, cephalosporins, antipseudomonal penicillins, aztreonam, and imipenem. Relative outer membrane impermeability (191) and several inducible β-lactamases are primarily responsible for the resistance to β-lactam agents (192–196). The L1 β-lactamase is a zinc metalloenzyme carbapenemase that is not inhibited by clavulanic acid (197), and the L2 β-lactamase is an unusual cephalosporinase that also hydrolyzes aztreonam and is inhibited by clavulanic acid or sulbactam. Recently, additional β-lactamases have been described in *X. maltophilia,* including a penicillinase that does not hydrolyze aztreonam (198). Taken together, the β-lactamases of *X. maltophilia* can inactivate nearly the entire spectrum of β-lactam antimicrobial agents (199). At least some of these β-lactam resistance determinants appear to be transmissible (200). Aminoglycoside resistance appears to involve a plasmid-mediated mechanism that has been incompletely characterized (184,201).

The most useful antimicrobial agent for *X. maltophilia* infections has been trimethoprim-sulfamethoxazole, which has demonstrated in vitro activity against 89% to 100% of tested strains in several series (160,161,202,203). Unfortunately, the prevalence of resistance to this agent may be increasing (204). Moreover, trimethoprim-sulfamethoxazole is only bacteriostatic for *X. maltophilia.* Other useful antimicrobial agents for susceptible strains include minocycline and ticarcillin-clavulanic acid (202,204–206). The use of a combination of active agents has been recently advocated to avoid the emergence of resistance (204) and because of disappointing results reported with trimethoprim-sulfamethoxazole monotherapy (207). Susceptibility to third-generation cephalosporins and antipseudomonal penicillins is highly variable

(160,161), and resistance to imipenem and aztreonam appears to be uniformly present. Moxalactam and chloramphenicol possess reasonable in vitro activity against many isolates (159) but are not widely used because of potential adverse hematologic effects. The susceptibility of *X. maltophilia* to available fluoroquinolones is variable (203,208,209), and resistant mutants appear to arise readily (210). Reduced susceptibility to these agents may result from reduced outer membrane permeability. Disk diffusion susceptibility testing (211) may fail to recognize the presence of quinolone resistance in *X. maltophilia* (206); agar dilution may be a preferable susceptibility testing method with regard to these agents. Newer quinolones such as clinafloxacin, sparfloxacin, or PD131628 may eventually prove to be more useful (212–215).

With such limited selection of active antimicrobial agents, the importance of the removal of infected catheters or other foreign bodies cannot be overemphasized in *X. maltophilia* infections (160,167). In a recent study of *X. maltophilia* bacteremia associated with intravascular catheters, catheter removal was much more significant with regard to ultimate survival than the selection of appropriate antimicrobial therapy.

Prevention

Because patients receiving broad-spectrum antimicrobial therapy (especially imipenem, antipseudomonal penicillins, cephalosporins, and aminoglycosides) or instrumentation (e.g., intravascular catheters) are at greatest risk for nosocomial *X. maltophilia* colonization, avoidance of inappropriate antibiotic use or prolonged implantation of foreign devices will help to minimize the incidence of infection. Assiduous handwashing, aseptic technique, and careful maintenance of the sterility of solutions used in the hospital setting are the most important measures for the prevention of both pseudoinfection and genuine infection (216). Personnel caring for patients with *X. maltophilia* infection should implement secretion and drainage precautions (157). High-level disinfection of devices, including respiratory equipment (157), bypass pumps, vascular transducers, and dialyzers (156), is also important.

Although strain typing of *X. maltophilia* has not been as actively investigated as for *A. baumannii*, serotyping (217), multilocus enzyme electrophoresis (218), restriction endonuclease analysis (219), contour-clamped homogeneous electric field gel electrophoresis (171,220), PCR-based genomic analysis (221), and pyrolysis mass spectroscopy (222) have been reported to be helpful methods in the recognition and analysis of nosocomial outbreaks.

PSEUDOMONAS (BURKHOLDERIA) CEPACIA

Microbiology

Pseudomonas (*Burkholderia*) *cepacia* was first identified by Burkholder (223) in 1950 as the causative agent of "sour skin," a disease of onions. Previous names used to describe this organism include Eugonic Oxidizer-group I, *Pseudomonas multivorans*, and *Pseudomonas kingii*. Nucleic acid analyses have placed *P. cepacia* in RNA group II of the family Pseudomonadaceae, along with *P. pseudomallei*, *P. mallei*, *P. gladioli*, and *P. pickettii* (224). Transfer of *P. cepacia* to a new genus, Burkholderia, has been proposed recently on the basis of nucleic acid, fatty acid, and phenotypic analyses (225). Although this review uses the older designation *P. cepacia*, increasing acceptance of the designation *B. cepacia* is anticipated in the near future.

Like *X. maltophilia*, *P. cepacia* is a motile nonfermentative gram-negative bacillus with multitrichous polar flagella. Colonies may appear yellow, green-yellow, brown, red, purple, or nonpigmented, depending on the individual strain and culture medium used. On blood agar, *P. cepacia* colonies appear opaque and convex with a rough surface and irregular border. Acid is produced from many carbohydrate substrates, including glucose, maltose, lactose, mannitol, sucrose (86% of strains), and xylose. Most strains give positive oxidase, lysine, ornithine, ONPG, gelatin, and esculin reactions. Intrinsic resistance to polymyxin B is also a useful diagnostic characteristic (226). Because *P. cepacia* may phenotypically resemble the closely related species *P. gladioli*, clinical isolates of *P. gladioli* should not automatically be dismissed as contaminants (227).

Growth on MacConkey agar is poor. A number of specialized media have been developed to facilitate the isolation of *P. cepacia* from sputum. These include *P. cepacia* (PCM), oxidative-fermentative base-polymyxin B-bacitracin-lactose (OFPBL), and trypan blue-tetracycline (TB-T) medium. A comparative study using PCM, OFPBL, and MacConkey agar demonstrated the superior sensitivity of the more selective media, particularly when mucoid *P. aeruginosa* is also present in the sputum specimen (228). However, even culture with selective media may be an insensitive test of *P. cepacia* colonization (229). A PCR-based test amplifying 16S ribosomal sequences from primary specimens may ultimately provide a rapid, specific, and highly sensitive method for the detection of *P. cepacia* in sputum (230).

Although the intrinsic pathogenicity of *P. cepacia* is quite low, a number of putative virulence factors have been identified (231). A majority of strains produces protease/gelatinase (232) and lipase (233). Lecithinase (phospholipase) (234), hemolysin, esterase, exopolysaccharide, and various siderophores have also been detected (231). The presence of rough lipopolysaccharide was suggested to be associated with virulence in one report (227). Nevertheless, *P. cepacia* has been found to possess very low virulence in guinea pig (235), mouse (236), or rat (237) models, and culture supernatants do not exhibit toxicity for eukaryotic cells in vitro (238). Resistance to nonoxidative neutrophil killing (239) and the ability to bind respiratory mucin (240) have been suggested as factors facilitating *P. cepacia* persistence in patients with chronic granulomatous disease and cystic fibrosis.

Epidemiology

P. cepacia is found widely in the environment and can use an astonishing array of metabolic substrates. It has been isolated from a variety of plants, soil, water, animal sources, and decaying organic matter (241), although the ability of such environmental isolates to infect humans has not been established (242). *P. cepacia* is able to grow in simple salt solutions, dye solutions (243), disinfectants (244), and even distilled or tap water (245). It can use penicillin G as a nutrient (246), a sobering observation for users of antimicrobial agents. The ability of *P. cepacia* to degrade complex molecules such as agent orange (2,3,4-trichlorophenoxyacetic acid) had led to investigation of its use in bioremediation.

It is therefore not surprising that *P. cepacia* has demonstrated an ability to colonize many niches in the hospital environment. Outbreaks of true infection and "pseudoinfection" have resulted from *P. cepacia* colonization of drug solutions, antiseptics (e.g., chlorhexidine, povidone-iodine, benzalkonium chloride), skin lotions, intravenous fluids, respiratory equipment, water baths, pressure transducers, catheters, blood gas analyzers, and dialysis machines (241,247–257). The resistance of *P. cepacia* to many antimicrobial agents has allowed transmission of the organism via contaminated prophylactic aerosolized antibiotics delivered via respiratory nebulizers (258). It is fortunate that this widely distributed and versatile organism has virtually no virulence for normal human hosts. However, *P. cepacia* can be a formidable pathogen in patients with impaired host defenses or instrumentation. Patients with cystic fibrosis (237), burns (259), chronic granulomatous disease (239,260–262), intravenous drug abuse (263), and sickle-cell hemoglobinopathies (264) are included among those at increased risk. In fact, *P. cepacia* pneumonia may be the presenting manifestation of an underlying immunodeficiency (261).

Although transmission by infected solutions or devices has been well described (241,249), compelling evidence of person-to-person spread has been documented over the past several years in the setting of cystic fibrosis (229,265). Initially, it was observed that the *P. cepacia* isolation rate had increased markedly at several cystic fibrosis centers (266–268). Studies at one cystic fibrosis center found that the *P. cepacia* colonization risk was increased if a sibling with cystic fibrosis was also colonized, suggesting the possibility of person-to-person spread (269). Cohorting of colonized patients appeared to result in a decline in the rate of colonization, further supporting this notion (270). In some cases, colonization was associated with subacute or acute clinical deterioration (267,268,271), making the issue of transmissibility a more urgent one. Moreover, fulminant courses of *P. cepacia* infection after lung transplantation led to the suggestion that colonized patients be excluded as transplant recipients (272–274).

Ultimately, molecular strain typing methods provided convincing evidence that *P. cepacia* can be spread on occasion from person-to-person in social settings, such as conferences (275) or cystic fibrosis camps (265,276,277). Moreover, analyses of *P. cepacia*-colonized patients at some cystic fibrosis centers have demonstrated the presence of predominant strains within centers (278–280). These findings have had an unfortunate detrimental impact on the social isolation of cystic fibrosis patients.

One recent case-control study of five *P. cepacia*-colonized patients with cystic fibrosis implicated respiratory equipment rather than person-to-person spread (281), and another recent study failed to demonstrate evidence of person-to-person spread over an 8-year period at a North Carolina cystic fibrosis center with 22 *P. cepacia*-colonized patients (282). Such observations suggest that *P. cepacia* transmission occurs via multiple routes and that individual strains may differ with regard to their transmissibility (265,283,284).

Clinical Manifestations

The lung is the most common site of *P. cepacia* infection (285). Nosocomial pneumonia caused by *P. cepacia* is clinically indistinguishable from nosocomial pneumonia of other causes (286). Lobular infiltrates are most frequently seen (258), and cavitation (258,287) or pleural effusions (258) occur in a significant minority of cases. In one outbreak, nearly half of patients with respiratory *P. cepacia* colonization developed pneumonia, usually within 2 weeks of initial isolation of the organism (258). Mortality specifically attributable to *P. cepacia* pneumonia is difficult to ascertain because infected patients frequently have serious underlying comorbidity, but fatal cases clearly occur.

The clinical course of *P. cepacia* respiratory infection in the setting of cystic fibrosis is highly variable. Some colonized patients have no apparent alteration in their clinical status (268,288), whereas others experience a respiratory deterioration (268,289) that may be abrupt or even fulminant (267). In the most severe cases, leukocytosis, an elevated erythrocyte sedimentation rate, high fever, and even bacteremia (290) occur. Lung pathology in fatal cases has demonstrated necrotizing pneumonia. Similarly, aggressive *P. cepacia* pulmonary disease, sometimes complicated by bacteremia or death, has also been reported in patients with chronic granulomatous disease (239,260–262,291–295). Some *P. cepacia*-colonized patients undergoing lung transplantation for cystic fibrosis have developed rapidly progressive postoperative pulmonary infection, sepsis, and death (268,272,296,297). This had led to the suggestion that it may be necessary to exclude *P. cepacia*-colonized patients from consideration for transplantation (272–274), although not all transplanted patients with *P. cepacia* colonization have fared poorly (280,298,299).

Skin and soft tissue infections with *P. cepacia* are principally related to the ability of this organism to contaminate water, saline solutions, disinfectants, and other solutions used in the hospital setting. Infected burns (259) and surgical wounds (300,301) are seen most frequently. Ecthyma gangrenosum has also been described as an unusual cutaneous complication of *P. cepacia* bacteremia (302). "Foot rot" related to *P. cepacia* has been reported in normal hosts subjected to prolonged immersion in swamp water during military exercises (303).

P. cepacia bacteremia may be seen as a complication of local infection (e.g., pulmonary, urinary tract) or in association with an intravenous catheter (160,304,305). Bacteremia resulting from contaminated intravenous anesthetic preparations (251,306,307), heparin intravenous flush solutions (305), serum albumin (308), arteriovenous hemodialysis access grafts (309), pressure transducers (310), or intraaortic balloon pumps (311) has also been described. Endocarditis occurs rarely (312–314) but should particularly be considered in intravenous drug abusers (63,302) or patients with prosthetic heart valves (315). Clinical interpretation of a positive blood culture for *P. cepacia* must also take the possibility of "pseudobacteremia" into account. False-positive blood cultures yielding *P. cepacia* have been traced to contaminated antiseptic solution (e.g., povidone-iodine) used to disinfect the skin before venipuncture (257,316–319) or to a contaminated blood-gas analyzer (253,256). However, true bacteremia may also result from such contamination (253).

Unusual types of *P. cepacia* infection include meningitis (320,321), ventriculoatrial shunt infection (322), osteomyelitis (310), dialysis-associated peritonitis (257,309,323), septic arthritis after intra-articular corticosteroid injection (324,325), and urinary tract infection associated with urethral instrumentation (300,309,326,327) or transrectal prostate biopsy (328).

Therapy

Treatment of *P. cepacia* infections is complicated by the resistance of this organism to many antimicrobial agents. In fact, some strains are resistant to all currently available drugs. The majority of isolates is resistant to many β-lactam agents, aminoglycosides, and polymyxins (226,329–332). An inducible chromosomal β-lactamase is partly responsible for the resistance to β-lactams (332); derepressed mutants may arise that possess high level resistance to both readily and poorly hydrolyzable substrates. Reduced outer membrane permeability appears to be another factor. Clinical isolates have diminished porin content (332,333) and fail to demonstrate aminoglycoside uptake (330). *P. cepacia* may also carry a gene conferring nonenzymatic resistance to multiple antimicrobial agents, possibly resulting from active drug efflux (334).

Trimethoprim-sulfamethoxazole has been used successfully in the treatment of *P. cepacia* infections (263,313,320), but some strains are resistant to this combination agent (335,336), especially in patients with cystic fibrosis (237). *P. cepacia* isolates may be susceptible in vitro to mezlocillin, piperacillin, ceftazidime, cefotaxime, imipenem, aztreonam, chloramphenicol, minocycline, sulbactam, or ciprofloxacin (174,329,337–339). However, ceftazidime has been reported to be ineffective in the setting of cystic fibrosis in some cases (340), and there is little published clinical experience concerning most of the other alternative agents. Meropenem, an investigational carbapenem, is of some interest because imipenem-resistant *P. cepacia* isolates appear to retain susceptibility to meropenem (341). Cystic fibrosis patients colonized or infected with *P. cepacia* pose a particularly difficult problem, because resistance to antimicrobial agents emerges readily during the course of treatment (237). Multidrug regimens involving ticarcillin, tobramycin, amikacin, piperacillin, aztreonam, imipenem, rifampin, or ciprofloxacin in various combinations have been reported to demonstrate synergistic activity against some resistant *P. cepacia* isolates in vitro

(337,342–344), but the clinical significance of these observations has not been established.

In light of the propensity of *P. cepacia* to develop increasing resistance to antimicrobial agents under selection pressure, it is important to withhold the use of antibiotics in instances of colonization or pseudoinfection. In addition, removal of the focus of infection in cases involving catheters or other foreign bodies is strongly recommended.

Prevention

As for the other pathogens discussed in this review, minimizing the use of broad-spectrum antimicrobial agents or prolonged implantation of foreign bodies will help to reduce the risk of *P. cepacia* infection in the hospital setting. Aggressive infection control practices to maintain the sterility of solutions (328,345,346) and devices (255,347,348) have been effective in preventing or curtailing nosocomial outbreaks.

Prevention of person-to-person transmission among patients with cystic fibrosis is a more complicated issue. Cohorting or isolation of colonized individuals (349) has been associated with a reduction in the increase of *P. cepacia* in cystic fibrosis centers (270), but the economic costs of these interventions and the adverse social impact on colonized patients have been significant. However, despite the apparent rarity of person-to-person transmission in some centers (282), there presently appears to be a consensus that aggressive measures to segregate *P. cepacia*-colonized patients with cystic fibrosis in both hospital and social settings are warranted (279,283,284,350).

In the investigation of possible nosocomial outbreaks or person-to-person transmission of *P. cepacia*, strain typing has become an indispensable tool. Phenotypic methods such as serotyping (351,352), biotyping (353), multilocus enzyme electrophoresis (354,355), or bacteriocin susceptibility (356,357) have generally given way to genotypic methods such as ribotyping (257,278,280,282,305,348,355,358–362), arbitrarily primed PCR (AP-PCR) (359), pulse-field electrophoresis (280,282,358,359), or plasmid analysis (257,311). As typing methods, pulse-field electrophoresis or AP-PCR generally possess greater discriminatory ability than ribotyping (363), and this also appears to be the case when applied to *P. cepacia* (280,282). Such methods have allowed epidemiologists to establish the clonality of multiple *P. cepacia* isolates with a high degree of certainty.

CONCLUSIONS

The gram-negative bacilli *A. baumannii* (*calcoaceticus* var. *anitratus*), *X.* (*Stenotrophomonas*) *maltophilia*, and *P.* (*Burkholderia*) *cepacia* have been isolated with increasing frequency as causes of nosocomial pneumonia, cutaneous infection, bacteremia, urinary tract infection, meningitis, and miscellaneous other infections. Pseudoinfection resulting from contamination of disinfectant agents or collection tubes can also occur. Resistance to multiple antimicrobial or antiseptic agents and an ability to colonize diverse microenvironments within the hospital setting are among the principal factors responsible for this trend. Patients with recent surgery, burn wounds, instrumentation, broad-spectrum antimicrobial therapy, prolonged hospitalization, and chronic underlying illness are at greatest risk. Patients with cystic fibrosis may have particularly severe problems associated with *P. cepacia* infection.

The most widely used antimicrobial agents are imipenem and amikacin in the case of *A. baumannii* and trimethoprim-sulfamethoxazole for infections caused by *X. maltophilia* or *P. cepacia*. However, resistance to each of these agents has been reported, and it is important to obtain in vitro susceptibility testing to guide antimicrobial therapy. Combination therapy may help to minimize the likelihood of resistance emerging during therapy.

Prevention of environmental or person-to-person transmission may best be accomplished by avoiding inappropriate antibiotic use, minimizing the implantation of foreign devices, maintaining the sterility of equipment and solutions used in the hospital setting, isolating infected patients, and carefully attending to aseptic technique and handwashing. Molecular strain typing methods such as ribotyping, restriction endonuclease analysis of plasmids, AP-PCR, and pulse-field electrophoresis have been demonstrated to be useful in the analysis of outbreaks in the hospital setting.

REFERENCES

1 **Dubos R.** Man adapting. New Haven: Yale University press, 1965.

2 **Weinstein MP, Reller LB, Murphy JR, Lichtenstein KA.** The clinical significance of positive blood cultures: a comprehensive analysis of 500 episodes of bacteremia and fungemia in adults. I. Laboratory and epidemiologic observations. Rev Infect Dis 1983;5:54–70.

3 **Bouvet PJM, Grimont PAD.** Taxonomy of the genus *Acinetobacter* with the recognition of *Acinetobacter baumannii* sp. nov., *Acinetobacter haemolyticus* sp. nov., *Acintobacter johnsonii* sp. nov., and *Acinetobacter junii* sp. nov. and emended descriptions of *Acinetobacter calcoaceticus* and *Acinetobacter iwoffii*. Int J Syst Bacteriol 1986; 36:228–240.

4 **Seifert H, Baginski R, Schulze A, Pulverer G.** The distribution of *Acinetobacter* species in clinical culture materials. Int J Med Microbiol Virol Parasitol Infect Dis 1993; 279:544–552.

5 **Allen DM, Hartman BJ.** *Acinetobacter* species. In: Mandell GL, Bennett JE, Dolin R, eds. Principles and practices of infectious diseases, 4th ed. New York: Churchill Livingstone, 1995:2009–2013.

6 **Bouvet PJM, Jeanjean S.** Delineation of new proteolytic genomic species in the genus *Acinetobacter*. Res Microbiol 1989; 140:291–299.

7 **Tjernberg I, Ursing J.** Clinical strains of *Acinetobacter* classified by DNA-DNA hybridization. APMIS 1989;97:595–605.

8 **Gerner-Smidt P, Tjernberg I, Ursing J.** Reliability of phenotypic tests for identification of *Acinetobacter* species. J Clin Microbiol 1991;29:277–282.

9 **Dijkshoorn L, van der Toorn J.** *Acinetobacter* species: which do we mean? Clin Infect Dis 1992;15:748–749.

10 **Weaver RE, Actis LA.** Identification of *Acinetobacter* species. J Clin Microbiol 1994;32:1833.

11 **Berkowitz FE.** *Acinetobacter* meningitis—a diagnostic pitfall. S Afr Med J 1982;61: 448–449.

12 **Hammett JB.** Death from pneumonia with bacteremia due to Mimeae tribe bacterium. JAMA 1968;206:641–642.

13 **Smith AW, Alpar KE.** Immune response to *Acinetobacter calcoaceticus* infection in man. J Med Microbiol 1991;34:83–88.

14 **Lian CJ, Jaszczak LJ, Palchaudhuri S, Prasad JK.** Resistance of *Acinetobacter calcoaceticus* isolates from burn patients to serum mediated killing. In: Abstracts of the 94th General Meeting of the American Society for Microbiology. Washington, D.C.: American Society for Microbiology, 1994.

15 **Obana Y.** Pathogenic significance of *Acinetobacter calcoaceticus*: analysis of experimental infection in mice. Microbiol Immunol 1986;30:645–657.

16 **Glew RH, Moellering RC, Kunz LJ.** Infection with *Acinetobacter calcoaceticus* (*Herellea vaginicola*): clinical and laboratory studies. Medicine (Baltimore) 1977;56:79–97.

17 **Retailliau HF, Hightower AW, Dixon RE, Allen JR.** *Acinetobacter calcoaceticus*: a nosocomial pathogen with an unusual seasonal pattern. J Infect Dis 1979;139: 371–375.

18 **Baumann P.** Isolation of *Acinetobacter* from soil and water. J Bacteriol 1968;96:39–42.

19 **Rosenthal SL.** Sources of *Pseudomonas* and *Acinetobacter* species found in human culture materials. Am J Clin Pathol 1974; 62:807–811.

20 **el-Mohandes AE, Schatz V, Keiser JF, Jackson BJ.** Bacterial contaminants of collected and frozen human milk used in an intensive care nursery. Am J Infect Control 1993;21:226–230.

21 **Gennari M, Lombardi P.** Comparative characterization of *Acinetobacter* strains isolated from different foods and clinical sources. Int J Med Microbiol Virol Parasitol Infect Dis 1993;279:553–564.

22 **Timsit J-F, Garrait V, Misset B, et al.** The digestive tract is a major site for *Acinetobacter baumannii* colonization in intensive care unit patients. J Infect Dis 1993;168: 1336–1337.

23 **Al-Khoja MS, Darrell JH.** The skin as the source of *Acinetobacter* and *Moraxella* species occurring in blood cultures. J Clin Microbiol 1979;32:497–499.

24 **Bergogne-Berezin E, Joly-Guillou ML, Vieu JF.** Epidemiology of nosocomial infections due to *Acinetobacter calcoaceticus*. J Hosp Infect 1987;10:105–113.

25 **Sherertz RJ, Sullivan ML.** An outbreak of infections with *Acinetobacter calcoaceticus* in burn patients: contamination of patients' mattresses. J Infect Dis 1985;151:252–258.

26 **Go ES, Urban C, Burns J, et al.** Clinical and molecular epidemiology of *Acinetobacter* infections sensitive only to polymyxin B and sulbactam. Lancet 1994;344:1329–1332.

27 **Reyes MP, Ganguly S, Fowler M, et al.** Pyrogenic reactions after inadvertent infusion of endotoxin during cardiac catheterizations. Ann Intern Med 1980;93: 32–35.

28 **Abrutyn E, Goodhart GL, Roos K, et al.** *Acinetobacter calcoaceticus* outbreak associated with peritoneal dialysis. Am J Epidemiol 1978;107:328–335.

29 **Schloesser RL, Laufkoetter EA, Lehners T, Mietens C.** An outbreak of *Acinetobacter calcoaceticus* infection in a neonatal care unit. Infection 1990;18:230–233.

30 **Henricksen SD.** Moraxella, *Acinetobacter*, and the Mimeae. Bacteriol Rev 1973;37: 522–561.

31 **Lowes JA, Smith J, Tabaqchali S, et al.** Outbreak of infection in a urological ward. Br Med J 1980;280:722.

32 **Buxton AE, Anderson RL, Werdegar D, et al.** Nosocomial respiratory tract infection and colonization with *Acinetobacter calcoaceticus*. Epidemiologic characteristics. Am J Med 1978;65:507–513.

33 **Irwin RS, Demers RR, Pratter MR, et al.** An outbreak of *Acinetobacter* infection associated with the use of a ventilator spirometer. Respir Care 1980;25:232–237.

34 **Patterson JE, Vecchio J, Pantelink EL, et al.** Association of contaminated gloves with transmission of *Acinetobacter calcoaceticus* var. *anitratus* in an intensive care unit. Am J Med 1991;91:479–483.

35 **Cefai C, Richards J, Gould FK, McPeake P.** An outbreak of *Acinetobacter* respiratory tract infection resulting from incomplete disinfection of ventilatory equipment. J Hosp Infect 1990;15:177–182.

36 **Kelkar R, Gordon SM, Giri N, et al.** Epidemic iatrogenic *Acinetobacter* spp. meningitis following administration of intrathecal methotrexate. J Hosp Infect 1989;14:233–243.

37 **Beck-Sague CM, Jarvis WR, Brook JH, et al.** Epidemic bacteremia due to *Acinetobacter baumannii* in five intensive care units. Am J Epidemiol 1990;132:723–733.

38 **Castle M, Tenney JH, Weinstein MP,**

Eickhoff TC. Outbreak of a multiply resistant *Acinetobacter* in a surgical care unit: epidemiology and control. Heart Lung 1978;7:641–644.

39 **Vandenbroucke-Grauls CM, Kerver AJ, Rommes JH, et al.** Endemic *Acinetobacter anitratus* in a surgical intensive care unit: mechanical ventilators as reservoir. Eur J Clin Microbiol Infect Dis 1988;7:485–489.

40 **Daschner FD, Habel H.** Hospital outbreak of multi-resistant *Acinetobacter anitratus*: an airborne mode of spread? J Hosp Infect 1987;10:211–212.

41 **Musa EK, Desai N, Casewell MW.** The survival of *Acinetobacter calcoaceticus* inoculated on fingertips and on formica. J Hosp Infect 1990;15:219–227.

42 **Allen KD, Green HT.** Hospital outbreak of multi-resistant *Acinetobacter anitratus*: an airborne mode of spread? J Hosp Infect 1987;9:110–119.

43 **Larson E.** A decade of nosocomial *Acinetobacter*. Am J Infect Control 1984;12:14–18.

44 **French GL, Casewell MW, Roncoroni AJ, et al.** A hospital outbreak of antibiotic-resistant *Acinetobacter anitratus*: epidemiology and control. J Hosp Infect 1980;1: 125–131.

45 **Guenthner SH, Hendley JO, Wenzel RP.** Gram-negative bacilli as nontransient flora on the hands of hospital personnel. J Clin Microbiol 1987;25:488–490.

46 **Getchell-White SI, Donowitz LG, Groschel DH.** The inanimate environment of an intensive care unit as a potential source of nosocomial bacteria: evidence for long survival of *Acinetobacter calcoaceticus*. Infect Control Hosp Epidemiol 1989;10: 402–407.

47 **Dijkshoorn L, Wubbels JL, Beunders AJ, et al.** Use of protein profiles to identify *Acinetobacter calcoaceticus* in a respiratory care unit. J Clin Pathol 1989;42:853–857.

48 **Dijkshoorn L, van Dalen R, van Ooyen A, et al.** Endemic *Acinetobacter* in intensive care units: epidemiology and clinical impact. J Clin Pathol 1993;46:533–536.

49 **Vila J, Almela M, Jimenez de Anta MT.** Laboratory investigation of hospital outbreak caused by two different multiresistant *Acinetobacter calcoaceticus* subsp. *anitratus*. J Clin Microbiol 1989;27:1086–1090.

50 **Scerpella EG, Wanger AR, Armitige L, et al.** Nosocomial outbreak caused by a multiresistant clone of *Acinetobacter baumannii*: results of the case-control and molecular epidemiologic investigations. Infect Control Hosp Epidemiol 1995;16:92–97.

51 **Struelens MJ, Carlier E, Maes N, et al.** Nosocomial colonization and infection with multiresistant *Acinetobacter baumannii*: outbreak delination using DNA macrorestriction analysis and PCR-fingerprinting. J Hosp Infect 1993;25:15–32.

52 **Green AR, Milling MA.** Infection with *Acinetobacter* in a burns unit. Burns Incl Therm Inj 1983;9:292–294.

53 **Frame JD, Kangesu L, Malik WM.** Changing flora in burn and trauma units: experience in the United Kingdom. J Burn Care Rehabil 1992;13:281–286.

54 **Ang SW, Lee ST.** Emergence of a multiply-resistant strain of *Acinetobacter* in a burns unit. Ann Acad Med Singapore 1992;21: 660–663.

55 **Thong ML.** *Acinetobacter anitratus* infections in man. Aust N Z J Med 1975;5:435–439.

56 **Rolston K, Guan S, Bodey GP, Elting L.** *Acinetobacter calcoaceticus* septicemia in patients with cancer. South Med J 1985;78:647–651.

57 **Green GS, Johnson RH, Shively JA.** Mimeae: opportunistic pathogens. A review of infections in a cancer hospital. JAMA 1965;194:163–166.

58 **Smego RA.** Endemic nosocomial *Acinetobacter calcoaceticus* bacteremia. Clinical significance, treatment and prognosis. Arch Intern Med 1985;145:2174–2179.

59 **Carlquist JF, Conti M, Burke JP.** Progressive resistance in a single strain of *Acinetobacter calcoaceticus* recovered during a nosocomial outbreak. Am J Infect Control 1982;10:43–48.

60 **Ramphal R, Kluge RM.** *Acinetobacter calcoaceticus* variety *anitratus*: an increasing nosocomial problem. Am J Med Sci 1979; 277:57–65.

61 **Peacock JE, Sorrell L, Sottile FD.** Nosocomial respiratory tract colonization and infection with aminoglycoside-resistant *Acinetobacter calcoaceticus* var *anitratus*: epidemiologic characteristics and clinical significance. Infect Control Hosp Epidemiol 1988;9:302–308.

62 **Anstey NM.** Community-acquired *Acinetobacter* pneumonia in the northern territory of Australia. Clin Infect Dis 1992;14:83–91.

63 **Mayer KH, Zinner SH.** Bacterial pathogens of increasing significance in hospital-acquired infections. Rev Infect Dis 1985; 7(suppl 3):S371–S379.

64 **O'Connell CJ, Hamilton R.** Gram-negative rod infections. II. *Acinetobacter* infections in general hospital. N Y State J Med 1981;81: 750–753.

65 **Gardner P, Griffin WB, Swartz MN, Kunz LJ.** Nonfermentative Gram-negative bacilli of nosocomial interest. Am J Med 1970; 48:735–749.

66 **Fagon J-Y, Chastre J, Hance AJ, et al.** Nosocomial pneumonia in ventilated patients: a cohort study evaluating attributable mortality and hospital stay. Am J Med 1993;94:281–288.

67 **Elston H, Hoffman KC.** Identification and clinical significance of *Achromobacter* (*Herellea*) *anitratus* in urinary tract infections. Am J Med Sci 1966;251:75–80.

68 **Tumbarello M, Tacconelli E, Del Forna A, et al.** Central venous catheter-related sepsis in HIV infected patients. Int Conf AIDS 1993;9:315.

69 **Snydman DR, Maloy MF, Brock SM, et al.** Pseudobacteremia: false positive blood cultures from mist tent contamination. Am J Epidemiol 1977:106:154–159.

70 **Tilley PAG, Roberts FJ.** Bacteremia with *Acinetobacter* species: risk factors and prognosis in different clinical settings. Clin Infect Dis 1994;18:896–900.

71 **Raz R, Alroy G, Solbel JD.** Nosocomial bacteremia due to *Acinetobacter calcoaceticus*. Infection 1982;10:168–171.

72 **Chen YC, Chang SC, Hsieh WC, Luh KT.** *Acinetobacter calcoaceticus* bacteremia: analysis of 48 cases. J Formos Med Assoc 1991;90:958–963.

73 **Cumberland NS, Jones KP.** Hospital acquired native valve endocarditis caused by *Acinetobacter calcoaceticus* and treated with imipenem/cilastatin. J R Army Med Corps 1987;133:156–158.

74 **Stein PD, Harken DE, Dexter L.** The nature and prevention of prosthetic valve endocarditis. Am Heart J 1966;71:393–407.

75 **Gradon JD, Chapnick EK, Lutwick LI.** Infective endocarditis of a native valve due to *Acinetobacter*: Case report and review. Clin Infect Dis 1992;14:1145–1148.

76 **Berk SL.** Meningitis caused by *Acinetobacter calcoaceticus* var. *anitratus*. A specific hazard in neurosurgical patients. Arch Neurol 1981;38:95–98.

77 **Siegman-Igra Y, Bar-Yosef S, Gorea A, Avram J.** Nosocomial *Acinetobacter* meningitis secondary to invasive procedure: report of 25 cases and review. Clin Infect Dis 1993;17:843–849.

78 **Nguyen MH, Harris SP, Muder RR, Pasculle AW.** Antibiotic-resistant *Acinetobacter* meningitis in neurosurgical patients. Neurosurgery 1994;35:851–885.

79 **Berk SL, McCabe WR.** Meningitis caused by Gram-negative bacilli. Ann Intern Med 1980;93:253–260.

80 **Morgan MEI, Hart CA.** *Acinetobacter* meningitis: acquired infection in a neonatal intensive care unit. Arch Dis Child 1982;57: 557–559.

81 **Said R, Krumlovsky FA, del Greco F.** Symptomatic *Acinetobacter calcoaceticus* peritonitis. A complication of peritoneal dialysis. J Dial 1980;4:101–107.

82 **Valdez JM, Asperilla MO, Smego RA.** *Acinetobacter* peritonitis in patients receiving continuous ambulatory peritoneal dialysis. South Med J 1991;84:607–610.

83 **Chan MK, Chau PY, Chan WWN, Cheng IKP.** Randomized controlled trial of oral oflaxacin vs. intraperitoneal tobramycin for the treatment of peritonitis in patients on continuous ambulatory peritoneal dialysis. Rev Infect Dis 1989;11(suppl 5):S1292.

84 **Stoutenbeek CP, van Saene HK, Miranda DR, van der Waaij D.** *Acinetobacter* mediastinitis and pneumonia in a thorotrastoma patient. The oropharyngeal flora as source of infection. Intensive Care Med 1983;9: 139–141.

85 **Peyman GA, Vastine DW, Diamond JG.** Vitrectomy and intraocular gentamicin management of *Herellea* endophthalmitis after incomplete phacoemulsification. Am J Ophthalmol 1975;80:764–765.

86 **Zabel RW, Winegarder T, Holland EJ, Doughman DJ.** *Acinetobacter* corneal ulcer after penetrating keratoplasty. Am J Ophthalmol 1989;107:677–678.

87 **Herbet RW.** *Herellea* corneal ulcer association with the use of soft contact lenses. Br J Ophthalmol 1972;56:848–850.

88 **Volpin G, Krivoy N, Stein H.** *Acinetobacter* spp. osteomyelitis of the femur: a late sequel of unrecognized foreign body implantation. Injury 1993;24:345–346.

89 **Haley S, Paul J, Crook DW, White SH.** *Acinetobacter* spp L-form infection of a cemented Charnley total hip replacement. J Clin Pathol 1990;43:781.

90 **Amsel MB, Horrilleno E.** Synergistic necrotizing fasciitis: a case of polymicrobic infection with *Acinetobacter calcoaceticus*. Curr Surg 1985;42:370–372.

91 **Tankovic J, Legrand P, De Gatinas G, et al.** Characterization of a hospital outbreak

of imipenem-resistant *Acinetobacter baumannii* by phenotypic and genotypic typing methods. J Clin Microbiol 1994;32:2677–2681.

92 **Joly-Guillou ML, Vallee E, Bergogne-Berezin E, Philippon A.** Distribution of β-lactamases and phenotype analysis in clinical strains of *Acinetobacter calcoaceticus*. J Antimicrob Chemother 1988;22: 597–604.

93 **Murray BE, Moellering RCJ.** Evidence of plasmid-mediated production of aminoglycoside-modifying enzymes not previously described in *Acinetobacter*. Antimicrob Agents Chemother 1990;17:30–36.

94 **Obara M, Nakae T.** Mechanisms of resistance to β-lactam antibiotics in *Acinetobacter calcoaceticus*. J Antimicrob Chemother 1991;28:791–800.

95 **Gerhlein M, Leying H, Cullmann W, et al.** Imipenem resistance in *Acinetobacter baumannii* is due to altered penicillin-binding proteins. Chemotherapy 1991;37:405–412.

96 **Goldstein FW, Labigne-Roussel A, Gerbaud G, et al.** Transferable plasmid-mediated antibiotic resistance in *Acinetobacter*. Plasmid 1983;10:138–147.

97 **Lambert T, Gerbaud G, Bouvet P, et al.** Dissemination of amikacin resistance gene *aph*A6 in *Acinetobacter* spp. Antimicrob Agents Chemother 1990;34:1244–1248.

98 **Devaud M, Kayser FH, Bachi B.** Transposon-mediated multiple antibiotic resistance in *Acinetobacter* strains. Antimicrob Agents Chemother 1982;22:323–329.

99 **Garcia I, Fainstein V, LeBlanc B, Bodey GP.** In vitro activities of new β-lactam antibiotics against *Acinetobacter* spp. Antimicrob Agents Chemother 1982;24:297–299.

100 **Cullmann W, Opferkuch W, Stieglitz M, Werkmeister U.** A comparison of the antibacterial activities of *N*-formimidoyl thienamycin (MK0787) with those of other recently developed β-lactam derivatives. Antimicrob Agents Chemother 1982;22:302–307.

101 **Rolston KVI, Bodey GP.** In vitro susceptibility of *Acinetobacter* species to various antimicrobial agents. Antimicrob Agents Chemother 1986;30:769–770.

102 **Chow AW, Wong J, Bartlett KH.** Synergistic interactions of ciprofloxacin and extended spectrum β-lactams or aminoglycosides against *Acintoebacter calcoaceticus* ss. *anitratus*. Diagn Microbiol Infect Dis 1988;9:213–217.

103 **Stiver HG, Bartlett KH, Chow AW.** Comparison of susceptibility of gentamicin-resistant and -susceptible *Acinetobacter anitratus* to 15 alternative antibiotics. Antimicrob Agents Chemother 1986;30:624–625.

104 **Seifert H, Baginski R, Schulze A, Pulverer G.** Antimicrobial susceptiblity of *Acinetobacter* species. Antimicrob Agents Chemother 1993;37:750–753.

105 **Buisson Y, Tran Van Nhieu G, Ginot L, et al.** Nosocomial outbreaks due to amikacin-resistant tobramycin sensitive *Acinetobacter* species: correlation with amikacin usage. J Hosp Infect 1990;15:83–93.

106 **Leonov Y, Schlaeffe RF, Karpuch J, et al.** Ciprofloxacin in the treatment of nosocomial multiply resistant *Acinetobacter calcoaceticus* bacteremia. Infection 1990;18: 234–236.

107 **Vila J, Marcos A, Marco F, et al.** In vitro antimicrobial production of β-lactamases, aminoglycoside-modifying enzymes, and chloramphenicol acetyltrasferase by and susceptibility of clinical isolates of *Acinetobacter baumannii*. Antimicrob Agents Chemother 1993;37:138–141.

108 **Anstey NM.** Use of cefotaxime for treatment of *Acinetobacter* infections. Clin Infect Dis 1992;15:374.

109 **Xirouchaki E, Giamarellou H.** In vitro interactions of aminoglycosides with imipenem or ciprofloxacin against aminoglycoside resistant *Acinetobacter baumannii*. J Chemother 1992;4:263–267.

110 **Clark RB.** Imipenem resistance among *Acinetobacter baumannii*: association with decreased expression of a 33–36 kDa outer membrane protein. In: Abstracts of the 94th General Meeting of the American Society for Microbiology. Washington, D.C.: American Society for Microbiology, 1994.

111 **Obana Y, Nishino T.** In-vitro and in-vivo activities of sulbactam and YTR830H against *Acinetobacter calcoaceticus*. J Antimicrob Chemother 1990;26:677–682.

112 **Urban C, Go E, Mariano B, et al.** Effect of sulbactam on infections caused by imipenem-resistant *Acinetobacter calcoaceticus* biotype *anitratus* strains. J Infect Dis 1993;167:448–451.

113 **Wood CA, Reboli AC.** Infections caused by imipenem-resistant *Acinetobacter calcoaceticus* biotype *anitratus*. J Infect Dis 1993;168: 1602–1603.

114 **Traub WH, Spohr M.** Antimicrobial drug susceptibility of clinical isolates of *Acinetobacter* species (*A. baumannii, A. haemolyticus*, genospecies 3 and genospecies 6). Antimicrob Agents Chemother 1989;33:1617–1619.

115 **Louie L, Lijnklater A, Mandarino E, et al.** Comparative in vitro activities of biapenem (CL186815) and piperacillin-tazobactam against multiresistant *Acinetobacter baumannii*. In: Abstracts of the 94th General Meeting of the American Society for Microbiology. Washington, D.C.: American Society for Microbiology, 1994.

116 **Obana Y, Nishino T, Tanino T.** In-vitro and in-vivo activities of antimicrobial agents against *Acinetobacter calcoaceticus*. J Antimicrob Chemother 1985;15:441–448.

117 **Tunkel AR.** Topical antibacterials. In: Mandell GL, Bennett JE, Dolin R, eds. Principles and practices of infectious diseases, 4th ed. New York: Churchill Livingstone, 1995:381–389.

118 **Kosmidis J, Koratzania G.** Emergence of resistant bacterial strains during treatment of infections in the respiratory tract. Scand J Infect Dis Suppl 1986;49:135–139.

119 **Seifert H, Baginski R.** The clinical significance of *Acinetobacter baumannii* in blood cultures. Int J Med Microbiol Virol Parasitol Infect Dis 1992;277:210–218.

120 **Rahal JJ, Simberkoff MS.** Host defense and antimicrobial therapy in adult gram-negative bacillary meningitis. Ann Intern Med 1982;96:468–474.

121 **Schonwald S, Beus I, Lisic M, et al.** Brief report: ciprofloxacin in the treatment of gram-negative bacillary meningitis. Am J Med 1989;87(suppl 5A):248S–249S.

122 **Segev S, Rosen N, Joseph G, et al.** Pefloxacin efficacy in gram-negative bacillary meningitis. J Antimicrob Chemother 1990;26:187–192.

123 **Rodriguez K, Dickinson GM, Greenman RL.** Successful treatment of gram-negative bacillary meningitis with imipenem/cilastatin. South Med J 1985;78:731–732.

124 **Simon C, Lang F, Holzman RS.** Successful treatment of *Acinetobacter calcoaceticus* ventriculitis and development of subsequent chemical meningitis following intraventricular polymyxin B. Clin Infect Dis 1994;19:598. Abstract.

125 **Johnson DR, Love-Dixon MA, Brown WJ.** Delayed detection of an increase in resistant *Acinetobacter* at a Detroit hospital. Infect Control Hosp Epidemiol 1992;13: 394–398.

126 **Hartstein AI, Morthland VH, Rourke JWJ, et al.** Plasmid DNA fingerprinting of *Acinetobacter calcoaceticus* subspecies *anitratus* from intubated and mechanically ventilated patients. Infect Control Hosp Epidemiol 1990;11:531–538.

127 **Dijkshoorn L, Aucken HM, Gerner-Smidt P, et al.** Correlation of typing methods for *Acinetobacter* isolates from hospital outbreaks. J Clin Microbiol 1993;31:702–705.

128 **Traub WH.** *Acinetobacter baumannii* serotyping for delineation of outbreaks of nosocomial cross-infection. J Clin Microbiol 1989;27:2713–2716.

129 **Gouby A, Carles-Nurit MJ, Bouziges N, et al.** Use of pulsed-field gel electrophoresis for investigation of hospital outbreaks of *Acinetobacter baumannii*. J Clin Microbiol 1992;30:1588–1591.

130 **Graser Y, Klare I, Halle E, et al.** Epidemiological study of an *Acinetobacter baumannii* outbreak by using polymerase chain reaction fingerprinting. J Clin Microbiol 1993; 31:2417–2420.

131 **Reboli AC, Houston ED, Monteforte JS, et al.** Discrimination of epidemic and sporadic isolates of *Acinetobacter baumannii* by repetitive element PCR-mediated DNA fingerprinting. J Clin Microbiol 1994;32: 2635–2640.

132 **Bouvet PJM, Jeanjean S, Vieu J-F, Dijkshoorn L.** Species, biotype and bacteriophage type determination compared with cell envelope protein profile for typing *Acinetobacter* strains. J Clin Microbiol 1990;28:170–176.

133 **Pouedras P, Gras S, Sire JM, et al.** Esterase electrophoresis compared with biotyping for epidemiological typing of *Acinetobacter baumannii* strains. FEMS Microbiol Lett 1992;75:125–128.

134 **Gerner-Smidt P.** Ribotyping of the *Acinetobacter calcoaceticus-Acinetobacter baumannii* complex. J Clin Microbiol 1992;30:2680–2685.

135 **Kropec A, Hubner J, Daschner FD.** Comparison of three typing methods in hospital outbreaks of *Acinetobacter calcoaceticus* infection. J Hosp Infect 1993;23:133–141.

136 **Hartstein AI, Rashad AL, Liebler JM, et al.** Multiple intensive care unit outbreak of *Acinetobacter calcoaceticus* subspecies *anitratus* respiratory infection and colonization associated with contaminated, reusable ventilator circuits and resuscitation bags. Am J Med 1988;85:624–631.

137 **Crombach WH, Dijkshoorn L, van Noort-**

Klaassen M, et al. Control of an epidemic spread of a multi-resistant strain of *Acinetobacter calcoaceticus* in a hospital. Intensive Care Med 1989;15:166–170.

138 **Rozenberg-Arska M, Dekker AW, Verhoef J.** Ciprofloxacin for selective decontamination of the alimentary tract in patients with acute leukemia during remission induction treatment: the effect on fecal flora. J Infect Dis 1985;152:104–107.

139 **Hugh R, Ryschenkow E.** *Pseudomonas maltophilia*, an Alcaligenes-like species. J Gen Microbiol 1961;26:123–132.

140 **Hugh R.** *Pseudomonas maltophilia* sp. nov., nom. rev. Int J Syst Bacteriol 1981;31:195.

141 **Swings J, DeVos M, Van den Mooter M, DeLey J.** Transfer of *Pseudomonas maltophilia* Hugh 1981 to the genus *Xanthomonas* as *Xanthomonas maltophilia* (Hugh 1981) comb. nov. Int J Syst Bacteriol 1983; 33:409–413.

142 **Palleroni NJ, Bradbury JF.** *Stenotrophomonas*, a new bacterial genus for *Xanthomonas maltophilia*. Int J Syst Bacteriol 1993; 43:606–609.

143 **Burdge DR, Noble MA, Campbell ME, et al.** *Xanthomonas maltophilia* misidentified as *Pseudomonas cepacia* in cultures of sputum from patients with cystic fibrosis: a diagnostic pitfall with major clinical implications. Clin Infect Dis 1995;20:445–448.

144 **Bottone EJ, Reitanot M, Janda JM, Troy K, Cuttner J.** *P. maltophilia* exoenzyme activity as correlate in pathogenesis of ecthyma gangrenosum. J Clin Microbiol 1986;24: 995–997.

145 **Kerr KG, Anson J, Hawkey PM.** Adherence of clinical and environmental strains of *Xanthomonas maltophilia* to plastic material. In: Abstracts of the 94th General Meeting of the American Society for Microbiology. Washington, D.C.: American Society for Microbiology, 1994.

146 **Gilardi GL.** *Pseudomonas maltophilia* infections in man. Am J Clin Pathol 1969;51:58–61.

147 **Khardori N, Elting L, Wong E, et al.** Nosocomial infections due to *Xanthomonas maltophilia* (*Pseudomonas maltophilia*) in patients with cancer. Rev Infect Dis 1990;12: 997–1003.

148 **Oie S, Kamiya A.** Microbial contamination of brushes used for preoperative shaving. J Hosp Infect 1992;21:103–110.

149 **Moffett HL, Allan D, Williams T.** Survival and dissemination of bacteria in nebulizers and incubators. Am J Dis Child 1967;114: 13–20.

150 **Wishart MM, Riley TV.** Infection with *Pseudomonas maltophilia*: hospital outbreak due to contaminated disinfectant. Med J Aust 1976;2:710–712.

151 **Fisher MC, Long SS, Roberts EM, et al.** *Pseudomonas maltophilia* bacteremia in children undergoing open heart surgery. JAMA 1981;246:1571–1574.

152 **Semel JD, Trenholme GM, Harris AA, et al.** *Pseudomonas maltophilia* pseudosepticemia. Am J Med 1978;64:403–406.

153 **Yeh TJ, Anabtawi IN, Cornett VE, et al.** Bacterial endocarditis following open heart surgery. Ann Thorac Surg 1967;3:29–36.

154 **Bassett DCJ, Stokes KJ, Thomas WRG.** Wound infection with *Pseudomonas multivorans*: a water-borne contaminant of disinfectant solutions. Lancet 1970;1:1188–1191.

155 **Chen S, Stroh EM, Wald K, Jalkh A.** *Xanthomonas maltophilia* endophthalmitis after implantation of sustained-release ganciclovir. Am J Ophthalmol 1992;114: 772–773.

156 **Vanholder R, Vanhaecke E, Ringoir S.** *Pseudomonas* septicemia due to deficient disinfectant mixing during reuse. Int J Artif Organs 1992;15:19–24.

157 **Villarino ME, Stevens LE, Schable B, et al.** Risk factors for epidemic *Xanthomonas maltophilia* infection/colonization in intensive care unit patients. Infect Control Hosp Epidemiol 1992;13:201–206.

158 **Nagai T.** Association of *Pseudomonas maltophilia* with malignant lesions. J Clin Microbiol 1984;20:1003–1005.

159 **Jang TN, Wang FD, Wang LS, et al.** *Xanthomonas maltophilia* bacteremia: an analysis of 32 cases. J Formos Med Assoc 1992;91:1170–1176.

160 **Elting LS, Bodey GP.** Septicemia due to *Xanthomonas* species and non-aeruginosa Pseudomonas species: increasing incidence of catheter-related infections. Medicine (Baltimore) 1990;69:296–306.

161 **Morrison AJ, Hoffman KK, Wenzel RP.** Associated mortality and clinical characteristics of nosocomial *Pseudomonas maltophilia* in a university hospital. J Clin Microbiol 1986;24:52–55.

162 **Dismukes WE, Karchmer AW, Buckley MJ, et al.** Prosthetic valve endocarditis: analysis of 38 cases. Circulation 1973;48: 365–377.

163 **Fischer JJ.** *Pseudomonas maltophilia* endocarditis after replacement of the mitral

valve: a case study. J Infect Dis 1973;128: S771–S773.

164 **Berbari N, Johnson DH, Cunha BA.** *Xanthomonas maltophilia* peritonitis in a patient undergoing peritoneal dialysis. Heart Lung 1993;22:282–283.

165 **Muder RR, Yu VL, Dummer JS, et al.** Infections caused by *Pseudomonas maltophilia*: expanding clinical spectrum. Arch Intern Med 1987;147:1672–1674.

166 **Trump DL, Grossman SA, Thompson G, Murray K.** CSF infections complicating the management of neoplastic meningitis: clinical features and results of therapy. Arch Intern Med 1982;142:583–586.

167 **Nguyen MH, Muder RR.** Meningitis due to *Xanthomonas maltophilia*: case report and review. Clin Infect Dis 1994;19:325–326.

168 **Marshall WF, Keating MR, Anhalt JP, Steckerberg JM.** *Xanthomonas maltophilia*: an emerging nosocomial pathogen. Mayo Clin Proc 1989;64:1097–1104.

169 **Elting LS, Khardori N, Bodey GP, Fainstein V.** Nosocomial infection caused by *Xanthomonas maltophilia*: a case-control study of predisposing factors. Infect Control Hosp Epidemiol 1990;11:134–138.

170 **Hulisz DT, File TM.** Predisposing factors and antibiotic use in nosocomial infections caused by *Xanthomonas maltophilia*. Infect Control Hosp Epidemiol 1992;13:489–490.

171 **Laing FPY, Ramotar K, Read RR, et al.** Molecular epidemiology of *Xanthomonas maltophilia* colonization and infection in the hospital environment. J Clin Microbiol 1995;33:513–518.

172 **Vartivarian SE, Papadakis KA, Palacios JA, et al.** Mucocutaneous and soft tissue infections caused by *Xanthomonas maltophilia*. Ann Intern Med 1994;121:969–973.

173 **Zuravleff JJ, Yu VL.** Infections caused by *Pseudomonas maltophilia* with emphasis on bacteremia: case reports and a review of the literature. Rev Infect Dis 1982;4:1236–1246.

174 **Klinger JD, Aronoff SC.** In-vitro activity of ciprofloxacin and other antibacterial agents against *Pseudomonas aeruginosa* and *Pseudomonas cepacia* from cystic fibrosis patients. Antimicrob Agents Chemother 1985;15: 679–684.

175 **Bauernfeind A, Bertele RM, Harms K, et al.** Qualitative and quantitative microbiological analysis of sputa of 102 patients with cystic fibrosis. Infection 1987;15:270–277.

176 **Irifune K, Ishida T, Shimoguchi K, et al.** Pneumonia caused by *Stenotrophomonas maltophilia* with a mucoid phenotype. J Clin Microbiol 1994;32:2856–2857.

177 **Kealey GP, Cram AE.** *Pseuodomonas maltophilia*: an unusual burn wound pathogen. J Burn Care Rehabil 1986;7:409–410.

178 **Agger WA, Cogbill TH, Busch HJ, et al.** Wounds caused by corn-harvesting machines: an unusual source of infection due to gram-negative bacilli. Rev Infect Dis 1986;8:927–931.

179 **Baltimore RS, Jenson HB.** Puncture wound osteochondritis of the foot caused by *Pseudomonas maltophilia*. Pediatr Infect Dis J 1990;9:143–144.

180 **Kato N, Morioka T.** Purpura fulminans secondary to *Xanthomonas maltophilia* sepsis in an adult with aplastic anemia. J Dermatol 1991;18:225–229.

181 **Pham BN, Aractingi S, Dombret H, et al.** *Xanthomonas* (formerly *Pseudomonas*) *maltophilia*-induced cellulitis in a neutropenic patient. Arch Dermatol 1992;128:702–704.

182 **Kerr KG, Corps CM, Hawkey PM.** Infections due to *Pseudomonas maltophilia* in patients with hematologic malignancy. Rev Infect Dis 1991;13:762.

183 **Roilides E, Butler KM, Husson RN, et al.** *Pseudomonas* infections in children with human immunodeficiency virus infection. Pediatr Infect Dis J 1992;11:547–553.

184 **Yu VL, Rumans LW, Wing EJ, et al.** *Pseudomonas maltophilia* causing heroin-associated infective endocarditis. Arch Intern Med 1978;138:1667–1671.

185 **Patrick S, Hindmarch JM, Hague RV, Harris DM.** Meningitis caused by *Pseudomonas maltophilia*. J Clin Pathol 1975;28:741–743.

186 **Denis F, Sow A, David M, et al.** Etude de deux cas de méningites: *Pseudomonas maltophilia* observés au Sénégal. Bull Soc Med Afr Noire Lang Fra 1977;22:135–139.

187 **Sarvamangala Devi JN, Venkatesh A, Shivananda PG.** Neonatal infection due to *Pseudomonas maltophilia*. Indian Pediatr 1984;21:71–74.

188 **Sutter VL.** Identification of *Pseudomonas* species isolated from hospital environment and human sources. Appl Microbiol 1968;16:1532–1538.

189 **Harlowe HD.** Acute mastoiditis following *Pseudomonas maltophilia* infection: case report. Laryngoscope 1972;82:882–883.

190 **Ben-Tovim T, Eylan E, Romano A, Stein R.** Gram-negative bacteria isolated from

external eye infections. Infection 1974;2: 162–165.

191 **Yamazaki E, Ishii J, Sato K, Nakae T.** The barrier function of the outer membrane of *Pseudomonas maltophilia* in the diffusion of saccharides and beta-lactam antibiotics. FEMS Microbiol Lett 1989;51:85–88.

192 **Saino Y, Kobayashi F, Inoue M, Mitsuhashi S.** Purification and properties of inducible penicillin beta-lactamase isolated from *Pseudomonas maltophilia*. Antimicrob Agents Chemother 1982;22:564–570.

193 **Saino Y, Inoue M, Mitsuhashi S.** Purification and properties of an inducible cephalosporinase from *Pseudomonas maltophilia* GN12873. Antimicrob Agents Chemother 1984;25:362–365.

194 **Mett H, Rosta S, Schacher B, Frei R.** Outer membrane permeability and beta-lactamase content in *Pseudomonas maltophilia* clinical isolates and laboratory mutants. Rev Infect Dis 1988;10:765–769.

195 **Cullmann W, Dick W.** Heterogenity of beta-lactamase production in *Pseudomonas maltophilia,* a nosocomial pathogen. Chemotherapy 1990;36:117–126.

196 **Akova M, Bonfiglio G, Livermore DM.** Susceptibility to beta-lactam antibiotics of mutant strains of *Xanthomonas maltophilia* with high- and low-level constitutive expression of L1 and L2 beta-lactamases. J Med Microbiol 1991;35:208–213.

197 **Dufresne J, Vezina G, Levesque RC.** Cloning and expression of the imipenem-hydrolyzing beta-lactamase operon from *Pseudomonas maltophilia* in *Escherichia coli*. Antimicrob Agents Chemother 1988;32: 819–826.

198 **Paton R, Miles RS, Amyes SGB.** Biochemical properties of inducible β-lactamases produced from *Xanthomonas maltophilia*. Antimicrob Agents Chemother 1994;38: 2143–2149.

199 **Neu HC, Saha G, Chin NX.** Resistance of *Xanthomonas maltophilia* to antibiotics and the effect of beta-lactamase inhibitors. Diagn Microbiol Infect Dis 1989;12:283–285.

200 **Hupková M, Blahová J, Králiková J, Krcméry V.** Transferable resistance to β-lactams in a nosocomial strain of *Xanthomonas maltophilia*. Antimicrob Agents Chemother 1995;39:1011–1012.

201 **Krcméry V, Antal M, Langsadl L, Knothe H.** Transferable amikacin resistance in *Pseudomonas maltophilia* and *Acinetobacter calcoaceticus*. Infection 1985;13:89–90.

202 **Khardori N, Reuben A, Rosenbaum B, et al.** In vitro susceptibility of *Xanthomonas (Pseudomonas) maltophilia* to newer antimicrobial agents. Antimicrob Agents Chemother 1990;34:1609–1610.

203 **Garcia-Rodriguez JA, Garcia-Sanchez JE, Garcia-Garcia MI, et al.** Antibiotic susceptibility profile of *Xanthomonas maltophilia*: in-vitro activity of beta-lactam/beta-lactamase inhibitor combinations. Diagn Microbiol Infect Dis 1991;14:239–243.

204 **Vartivarian S, Anaissie E, Bodey G, et al.** A changing pattern of susceptiblity of *Xanthomonas maltophilia* to antimicrobial agents: implications for therapy. Antimicrob Agents Chemother 1994;38:624–7.

205 **Traub WH, Spohr M.** Comparative disk and broth dilution susceptibility test results with ticarcillin and timentin against *Pseudomonas aeruginosa* and *Pseudomonas maltophilia*. Chemotherapy 1987;33:340–346.

206 **Hohl P, Frei R, Aubry P.** In vitro susceptibility of 33 clinical isolates of *Xanthomonas maltophilia*: inconsistent correlation of agar dilution and of disk diffusion test results. Diagn Microbiol Infect Dis 1991;14:447–450.

207 **Papadakis KA, Vartivarian SE, Anaissie EJ, Samonis G.** *Xanthomonas maltophilia* bacteremia in cancer patients: an analysis of 44 episodes. Clin Infect Dis 1994;19:588. Abstract.

208 **Cullmann W.** Antibiotic susceptibility and outer membrane proteins of clinical *Xanthomonas maltophilia* isolates. Chemotherapy 1991; 37:246–250.

209 **Matsuyama JR, Beail B, Wallis C, et al.** Susceptibility of *Xanthomonas maltophilia* and amikacin-resistant gram-negative bacteria to newer antimicrobials. Clin Pharm 1991;10:544–548.

210 **Lecso-Bornet M, Pierre J, Sarkis-Karam D, et al.** Susceptibility of *Xanthomonas maltophilia* to six quinolones and study of outer membrane proteins in resistant mutants selected in vitro. Antimicrob Agents Chemother 1992;36:669–671.

211 **Bauer AW, Kirby WMM, Sherris JC, et al.** Antibiotic susceptibility testing by a standardized single disk method. Am J Clin Pathol 1966;45:493–496.

212 **Rolston KV, Messer M, Ho DH.** Comparative in vitro activities of newer quinolones against *Pseudomonas* species and *Xanthomonas maltophilia* isolated from patients with cancer. Antimicrob Agents Chemother 1990;34:1812–1813.

213 **Pankuch GA, Jacobs MR, Appelbaum PC.** Susceptibilities of 123 *Xanthomonas maltophilia* strains to clinafloxacin, PD 131628, PD 138312, PD 140248, ciprofloxacin, and ofloxacin. Antimicrob Agents Chemother 1994;38:369–370.

214 **Louie A, Baltch AL, Ritz WJ, Smith RP.** Comparative in-vitro susceptibilities of *Pseudomonas aeruginosa*, *Xanthomonas maltophilia*, and *Pseudomonas* spp. to sparfloxacin (CI-978, AT-4140, PD131501) and reference antimicrobial agents. J Antimicrob Chemother 1991;27:793–799.

215 **Ford AS, Baltch AL, Smith RP, Ritz W.** In-vitro susceptibilities of *Pseudomonas aeruginosa* and *Pseudomonas* spp. to the new fluoroquinolones clinafloxacin and PD 131628 and nine other antimicrobial agents. J Antimicrob Chemother 1993;31:523–532.

216 **Schoch PE, Cunha BA.** *Pseudomonas maltophilia*. Infect Control 1987;8:169–172.

217 **Schable B, Rhoden DL, Jarvis WR, Miller JM.** Prevalence of serotypes of *Xanthomonas maltophilia* from world-wide sources. Epidemiol Infect 1992;108:337–341.

218 **Schable B, Villarino ME, Favero MS, Miller JM.** Application of multilocus enzyme electrophoresis to epidemiologic investigations of *Xanthomonas maltophilia*. Infect Control Hosp Epidemiol 1991;12: 163–167.

219 **Bingen EH, Denamur E, Lambert-Zechovsky NY, et al.** DNA restriction fragment length polymorphism differentiates crossed from independent infections in nosocomial *Xanthomonas maltophilia* bacteremia. J Clin Microbiol 1991;29:1348–1350.

220 **VanCouwenberghe C, Cohen S.** Analysis of epidemic and endemic isolates of *Xanthomonas maltophilia* by contour-clamped homogeneous electric field gel electrophoresis. Infect Control Hosp Epidemiol 1994;15:691–696.

221 **Chatelut M, Dournes JL, Chabanon G, Marty N.** Epidemiological typing of *Stenotrophomonas (Xanthomonas) maltophilia* by PCR. J Clin Microbiol 1995;33:912–914.

222 **Orr K, Gould FK, Sisson PR, et al.** Rapid inter-strain comparison by pyrolysis mass spectrometry in nosocomial infection with *Xanthomonas maltophilia*. J Hosp Infect 1991;17:187–195.

223 **Burkholder WH.** Sour skin, a bacterial rot of onion bulbs. Phytopathology 1950;40: 115–117.

224 **DeVos P, Goor M, Gillis M, et al.** Ribosomal ribonucleic-acid cistron similarities of phytopathogenic *Pseudomonas* species. Int J Syst Bacteriol 1985;35:169–184.

225 **Yabuuchi E, Kosako Y, Oyaizu H, et al.** Proposal of *Burkholderia* gen. nov. and transfer of seven species of the genus *Pseudomonas* homology group II to the new genus, with the type species *Burkholderia cepacia* (Palleroni and Holmes 1981) comb. nov. Microbiol Immunol 1992;36:1251–1275.

226 **Richards RM, Richards JM.** *Pseudomonas cepacia* resistance to antibacterials. J Pharm Sci 1979;68:1436–1438.

227 **Simpson IN, Finaly J, Winstanley DJ, et al.** Multi-resistant isolates possessing characteristics of both *Burkholderia (Pseudomonas) cepacia* and *Burkholderia gladioli* from patients with cystic fibrosis. J Antimicrob Chemother 1994;34:353–361.

228 **Welch DF, Muszynski MJ, Pai CH, et al.** Selective and differential medium for recovery of *Pseudomonas cepacia* from the respiratory tracts of patients with cystic fibrosis. J Clin Microbiol 1987;25:1730–1734.

229 **LiPuma JJ, Marks-Austin KA, Holsclaw DS Jr, et al.** Inapparent transmission of *Pseudomonas (Burkholderia) cepacia* among patients with cystic fibrosis. Pediatr Infect Dis J 1994;13:716–719.

230 **O'Callaghan EM, Tanner MS, Boulnois GJ.** Development of a PCR probe test for identifying *Pseudomonas aeruginosa* and *Pseudomonas (Burkholderia) cepacia*. J Clin Pathol 1994;47:222–226.

231 **Nelson JW, Butler SL, Krieg D, Govan JR.** Virulence factors of *Burkholderia cepacia*. FEMS Immunol Med Microbiol 1994;8:89–97.

232 **Jonsson V.** Proposal of a new species *Pseudomonas kingii*. Int J Syst Bacteriol 1970;20:255–257.

233 **Mckevitt AI, Woods DE.** Characterization of *Pseudomonas cepacia* isolates from patients with cystic fibrosis. J Clin Microbiol 1984;19:291–293.

234 **Vasil ML, Krieg DP, Kuhns JS, et al.** Molecular analysis of hemolytic and phospholipase C activities of *Pseudomonas cepacia*. Infect Immun 1990;58:4020–4029.

235 **Pennington JE, Miller JJ.** Evaluation of a new polyvalent *Pseudomonas* vaccine in respiratory infections. Infect Immun 1979;25:1029–1034.

236 **Stover GB, Drake DR, Montie TC.** Virulence of different *Pseudomonas* species in a burned mouse model: tissue colonization

by *Pseudomonas cepacia*. Infect Immun 1983; 41:1099–1104.

237 **Goldmann DA, Klinger JD.** *Pseudomonas cepacia*: biology, mechanisms of virulence, epidemiology. J Pediatr 1986;108: 806–812.

238 **McKevitt AI, Bajaksouzian S, Klinger JD, Woods DE.** Purification and characterization of an extracellular protease from *Pseudomonas cepacia*. Infect Immun 1989;57: 771–778.

239 **Speert DP, Bond M, Woodman RC, Curnutte JT.** Infection with *Pseudomonas cepacia* in chronic granulomatous disease. Role of nonoxidative killing by neutrophils in host defense. J Infect Dis 1994;170:1524–1531.

240 **Sajjan US, Corey M, Karmali MA, et al.** Binding of *Pseudomonas cepacia* to normal human intestinal mucin and respiratory mucin from patients with cystic fibrosis. J Clin Invest 1992;84:648–656.

241 **Gilardi GL.** *Pseudomonas cepacia*: culture and laboratory identification. Lab Management 1983;21:29–32.

242 **Butler SL, Doherty CJ, Hughes JE, et al.** *Burkholderia cepacia* and cystic fibrosis: do natural environments present a potential hazard? J Clin Microbiol 1995;33:1001–1004.

243 **Walsh DM, Eberiel DT.** *Pseudomonas cepacia* isolated from crystal violet solution in a hospital laboratory. J Clin Microbiol 1986;23:962.

244 **Geftic SG, Heymann H, Adair FW.** Fourteen-year survival of *Pseudomonas cepacia* in a salts solution preserved with benzalkonium chloride. Appl Environ Microbiol 1979;37:507–510.

245 **Carson LA, Favero MS, Bond WW, et al.** Morphological, biochemical, and growth characteristics of *Pseudomonas cepacia* from distilled water. Appl Microbiol 1973;25: 476–483.

246 **Beckman W, Lessie TG.** Response of *Pseudomonas cepacia* to β-lactam antibiotics: utilization of penicillin G as the carbon source. J Bacteriol 1979;140:1136–1138.

247 **Phillips I, Eykyn S, Curtis MA, et al.** *Pseudomonas cepacia* (*multivorans*) septicaemia in an intensive care unit. Lancet 1971;1:375–377.

248 **Schaffner W, Reisig G, Verrall RA.** Outbreak of *Pseudomonas cepacia* infection due to contaminated anaesthetics. Lancet 1973; 1:1050–1051.

249 **Gelbart SM, Reinhardt GF, Greenlee HB.** *Pseudomonas cepacia* strains isolated from water reservoirs of unheated nebulizers. J Clin Microbiol 1976;3:62–66.

250 **Rapkin RH.** *Pseudomonas cepacia* in an intensive care nursery. Pediatrics 1976;57: 239–243.

251 **Siboni K, Olsen H, Ravn E, et al.** *Pseudomonas cepacia* in 16 nonfatal cases of postoperative bacteremia derived from intrinsic contamination of the anesthetic fentanyl: clinical and epidemiologic observations in Denmark and Holland. Scand J Infect Dis 1979;11:39–45.

252 **Conly JM, Klass L, Larson L, et al.** *Pseudomonas cepacia* colonization and infection in intensive care units. J Can Med Assoc 1986;134:363–366.

253 **Henderson DK, Baptiste R, Parrillo J, Gill VJ.** Indolent epidemic of *Pseudomonas cepacia* bacteremia and pseudobacteremia in an intensive care unit traced to a contaminated blood gas analyzer. Am J Med 1988;84:75–81.

254 **George SE, Kohan MJ, Whitehouse DA, et al.** Prolonged survival of *Pseudomonas cepacia* in commercially manufactured povidone-iodine. Appl Environ Microbiol 1990;56:3598–3600.

255 **Weems JJ.** Nosocomial outbreak of *Pseudomonas cepacia* associated with contamination of reusable electronic ventilator temperature probes. Infect Control Hosp Epidemiol 1993;14:583–586.

256 **Wilson JA, Viggars S, Parsons A.** *Pseudomonas cepacia* pseudobacteremia associated with a contaminated blood gas analyzer. J Hosp Infect 1987;10:314–315.

257 **Panlilio AL, Beck-Sague CM, Siegel JD, et al.** Infections and pseudoinfections due to povidone-iodine solution contaminated with *Pseudomonas cepacia*. Clin Infect Dis 1992;14:1078–1083.

258 **Yamagishi Y, Fujita J, Takigawa K, et al.** Clinical features of *Pseudomonas cepacia* pneumonia in an epidemic among immunocompromised patients. Chest 1993;103: 1706–1709.

259 **Brauner A, Hfiby N, Kjartansson J, et al.** *Pseudomonas cepacia* septicemia in patients with burns: report of two cases. Scand J Infect Dis 1985;17:63–66.

260 **Bottone EJ, Douglas SD, Rausen AR, et al.** Association of *Pseudomonas cepacia* with chronic granulomatous disease. J Clin Microbiol 1975;1:425–428.

261 **Denney D, Bigley RH, Rashad AL.** Recurrent pneumonitis due to *Pseudomonas*

cepacia: an unexpected phagocyte dysfunction. West J Med 1975;122:160–164.

262 **Sieber OF, Fulginiti VA.** *Pseudomonas cepacia* pneumonia in a child with chronic granulomatous disease and selective IgA deficiency. Acta Paediatr Scand 1976;65: 519–520.

263 **Noriega ER, Rubinstein E, Simberkoff MS, et al.** Subacute and acute endocarditis due to *Pseudomonas cepacia* in heroin addicts. Am J Med 1975;59:29–36.

264 **Berry MD, Asmar BI.** *Pseudomonas cepacia* bacteremia in children with sickle cell hemoglobinopathies. Pediatr Infect Dis J 1991;10:696–699.

265 **Govan JR, Brown PH, Maddison J, et al.** Evidence for transmission of *Pseudomonas cepacia* by social contact in cystic fibrosis. Lancet 1993;342:15–19.

266 **Corey M, Alison L, Prober C, et al.** Sputum bacteriology in patients with cystic fibrosis in a Toronto hospital during 1970–81. J Infect Dis 1984;149:283.

267 **Isles A, Maclusky I, Corey M, et al.** *Pseudomonas cepacia* infection in cystic fibrosis: an emerging problem. J Pediatr 1984;104:206–210.

268 **Thomassen MJ, Demko CA, Klinger JD, Stern RC.** *Pseudomonas cepacia* colonization among patients with cystic fibrosis: a new opportunist. Am Rev Respir Dis 1985;131: 791–796.

269 **Tablan OC, Martone WJ, Doershuk CF, et al.** Colonization of the respiratory tract with *Pseudomonas cepacia* in cystic fibrosis: risk factors and outcomes. Chest 1987;91: 527–532.

270 **Thomassen MJ, Demko CA, Doershuk CF, et al.** *Pseudomonas cepacia*: decrease in colonization in patients with cystic fibrosis. Am Rev Respir Dis 1986;134:669–671.

271 **Gilligan PH.** Microbiology of airway disease in patients with cystic fibrosis. Clin Microbiol Rev 1991;4:35–51.

272 **Ramirez JC, Patterson GA, Winton TL, et al.** Bilateral lung transplantation for cystic fibrosis. J Thorac Cardiovasc Surg 1992;103: 287–294.

273 **Knight SR, Dresler C.** Results of lung transplantation. Semin Thorac Cardiovasc Surg 1992;4:107–112.

274 **Noyes BE, Kurland G, Orenstein DM, et al.** Experience with pediatric lung transplantation. J Pediatr 1994;124:261–268.

275 **LiPuma JJ, Dasen SE, Nielson DW, et al.** Person-to-person transmission of *Pseudomonas cepacia* between patients with cystic fibrosis. Lancet 1990;336:1094–1096.

276 **Centers for Disease Control and Prevention.** *Pseudomonas cepacia* at summer camps for persons with cystic fibrosis. MMWR 1993;42:456–459.

277 **Pegues DA, Carson LA, Tablan OC, et al.** Acquisition of *Pseudomonas cepacia* at summer camps for patients with cystic fibrosis. J Pediatr 1994;124:694–702.

278 **LiPuma JJ, Mortensen JE, Dasen SE, et al.** Ribotype analysis of *Pseudomonas cepacia* from cystic fibrosis treatment centers. J Pediatr 1988;113:859–862.

279 **Lipuma JJ, Stull TL.** *Burkholderia cepacia* in cystic fibrosis. N Engl J Med 1995;332:820.

280 **Smith DL, Gumery LB, Smith EG, et al.** Epidemic of *Pseudmonas cepacia* in an adult cystic fibrosis unit: evidence of person-to-person transmission. J Clin Microbiol 1993;31:3017–3022.

281 **Burdge DR, Nakielna EM, Noble MA.** Case-control and vector studies of nosocomial acquisition of *Pseudomonas cepacia* in adult patients with cystic fibrosis. Infect Control Hosp Epidemiol 1993;14:127–130.

282 **Steinbach S, Sun L, Jiang RZ, et al.** Transmissibility of *Pseudomonas cepacia* infection in clinic patients and lung-transplant recipients with cystic fibrosis. N Engl J Med 1994;331:981–987.

283 **Govan JRW.** *Burkholderia cepacia* in cystic fibrosis. N Engl J Med 1995;332:819–820.

284 **Steinbach SF, Goldstein R.** *Burkholderia cepacia* in cystic fibrosis. N Engl J Med 1995;332:820–821.

285 **Jarvis WR, Olson D, Tablan O, Martone WJ.** The epidemiology of nosocomial *Pseudomonas cepacia* infections: endemic infections. Eur J Epidemiol 1987;3:233–236.

286 **Weinstein AJ, Moellering RC, Hopkins CC, et al.** *Pseudomonas cepacia* pneumonia. Am J Med Sci 1973;265:491–504.

287 **Poe RH, Marcus HR, Emerson GL.** Lung abscess due to *Pseudomonas cepacia*. Am Rev Respir Dis 1977;115:861–865.

288 **Gold R, Overmeyer A, Knie B, et al.** Controlled trial of ceftazidime vs. ticarcillin and tobramycin in the treatment of acute respiratory exacerbations in patients with cystic fibrosis. Pediatr Infect Dis J 1985;4:172–177.

289 **Tablan OC, Chorba TL, Schidlow DV, et al.** *Pseudomonas cepacia* colonization in patients with cystic fibrosis: risk factors and clinical outcome. J Pediatr 1985;107:382–387.

290 **Boxerbaum B, Klinger JD.** *Pseudomonas cepacia* bacteremia in cystic fibrosis. Pediatr Res 1984;18:269A.

291 **Dailey RH, Benner EJ.** Necrotizing pneumonitis due to the pseudomonad "Eugonic Oxidizer-Group I". N Engl J Med 1968;279: 361–362.

292 **Styrt B, Klempner MS.** Late-presenting variant of chronic granulomatous disease. Pediatr Infect Dis 1984;3:556–559.

293 **Clegg HW, Ephros M, Newburger PE.** *Pseudomonas cepacia* pneumonia in chronic granulomatous disease. Pediatr Infect Dis 1986;5:111.

294 **O'Neill KM, Herman JH, Modlin JF, et al.** *Pseudomonas cepacia*: an emerging problem in chronic granulomatous disease. J Pediatr 1986;108:940–942.

295 **Schapiro BL, Newburger PE, Klempner MS.** Chronic granulomatous disease presenting in a 69 year-old man. N Engl J Med 1991;325:1786–1790.

296 **Gladman G, Connor PJ, Williams RF, David TJ.** Controlled study of *Pseudomonas cepacia* and *Pseudomonas maltophilia* in cystic fibrosis. Arch Dis Child 1992;67:192–195.

297 **Snell GI, deHoyos A, Krajden M, et al.** *Pseudomonas cepacia* in lung transplant recipients with cystic fibrosis. Chest 1993; 103:466–471.

298 **Flume PA, Egan TM, Paradowski LJ, et al.** Infectious complications of lung transplantation: impact of cystic fibrosis. Am J Respir Crit Care Med 1994;149:1601–1607.

299 **Egan TM, Detterbeck FC, Mill MR, et al.** Improved results of lung transplantation for patients with cystic fibrosis. J Thorac Cardiovasc Surg 1995;109:224–235.

300 **Sobel JD, Hashman N, Reinherz G, et al.** Nosocomial *Pseudomonas cepacia* infection associated with chlorhexidine contamination. Am J Med 1982;73:183–186.

301 **Pallent LJ, Hugo WB, Grant DJW, et al.** *Pseudomonas cepacia* as a contaminant and infective agent. J Hosp Infect 1983;4:9–13.

302 **Mandell IN, Feiner HD, Price NM, Simberkoff M.** *Pseudomonas cepacia* endocarditis and ecthyma gangrenosum. Arch Dermatol 1977;113:199–202.

303 **Taplin D, Bassett DCJ, Mertz PM.** Foot lesions associated with *Pseudomonas cepacia*. Lancet 1971;2:568–571.

304 **Meyer GW.** *Pseudomonas cepacia* septicemia associated with intravenous therapy. Calif Med 1973;119:15–18.

305 **Pegues DA, Carson LA, Anderson RL, et al.** Outbreak of *Pseudomonas cepacia* bacteremia in oncology patients. Clin Infect Dis 1993;16:407–411.

306 **Borghans JG, Hosli MT, Olsen H, el al.** *Pseudomonas cepacia* bacteraemia due to intrinsic contamination of an anaesthetic: bacteriological and serological observations. Acta Path Microbiol Scand 1979; 87(suppl B):15–20.

307 **Wanaying B.** An epidemic of *Pseudomonas cepacia* bacteraemia in Ramathibodi Hospital. J Med Assoc Thai 1989;72(suppl 2):20–22.

308 **Steere AC, Tenney JH, Mackel DC, et al.** *Pseudomonas* species bacteremia caused by contaminated normal human serum albumin. J Infect Dis 1977:135:729–735.

309 **Ishidate T, Iitaka K, Yoshida S, Sakai T.** *Pseudomonas cepacia* infection in children. Int J Pediatr Nephrol 1982;3:99–102.

310 **Weinstein RA, Jones EL, Schwarzmann SW, et al.** Sternal osteomyelitis and mediastinitis after open-heart operation: pathogenesis and prevention. Ann Thorac Surg 1976;21:442–444.

311 **Rutala WA, Weber DJ, Thomann CA, et al.** An outbreak of *Pseudomonas cepacia* bacteremia associated with a contaminated intra-aortic balloon pump. J Thorac Cardiovasc Surg 1988;96:157–161.

312 **Sorrell WB, White LV.** Acute bacterial endocarditis by a variant of the genus *Herellea*. Am J Clin Pathol 1953;23:134–138.

313 **Hamilton J, Burch W, Grimmett G, et al.** Successful treatment of *Pseudomonas cepacia* endocarditis with trimethoprim-sulfamethoxazole. Antimicrob Agents Chemother 1973;4:551–554.

314 **Speller DC.** *Pseudomonas cepacia* endocarditis treated with cotrimoxazole and kanamycin. Br Heart J 1973;35:47–48.

315 **Speller DC, Stephens ME, Viant AC.** Hospital infection by *Pseudomonas cepacia*. Lancet 1971;1:798–799.

316 **Kaslow RA, Mackel DC, Mallison GF.** Nosocomial pseudobacteremia: positive blood cultures due to contaminated benzalkonium antiseptic. JAMA 1976;236:2407–2409.

317 **Berkelman RL, Lewin S, Allen JR, et al.** Pseudobacteremia attributed to contamination of povidone-iodine with *Pseudomonas cepacia*. Ann Intern Med 1981;95:32–36.

318 **Craven DE, Moody B, Connolly MG, et al.** Pseudobacteremia caused by povidone-iodine solution contaminated with *Pseudomonas cepacia*. N Engl J Med 1981;305:621–623.

319 **Anderson RL, Vess RW, Carr JH, et al.** Investigations of intrinsic *Pseudomonas cepacia* contamination in commercially manufactured povidone-iodine. Infect Control Hosp Epidemiol 1991;12:297–302.

320 **Darby CP.** Treating *Pseudomonas cepacia*

meningitis with trimethoprim-sulfamethoxazole. Am J Dis Child 1976;130:1365–1366.

321 **Krcméry V, Havlik J, Vicianova L.** Nosocomial meningitis caused by multiply resistant *Pseudomonas cepacia*. Pediatr Infect Dis J 1987;6:769.

322 **Bassett DCJ, Pickson JAS, Hunt GH.** Infection of Holter valve by *Pseudomonas*-contaminated chlorhexidine. Lancet 1973;1: 1263–1264.

323 **Berkelman RL, Godley J, Weber JA, et al.** *Pseudomonas cepacia* peritonitis associated with contamination of automatic peritoneal dialysis machines. Ann Intern Med 1982;96:456–458.

324 **Matteson EL, McCune WJ.** Septic arthritis caused by treatment resistant *Pseudomonas cepacia*. Ann Rheum Dis 1990;49:258–259.

325 **Kothari T, Reyes MP, Brooks N, et al.** *Pseudomonas cepacia* septic arthritis due to intra-articular injections of methylprednisolone. Can Med Assoc J 1977;116:1230–1232.

326 **Mitchell RG, Hayward AC.** Postoperative urinary-tract infections caused by contaminated irrigating fluid. Lancet 1966;1:793–795.

327 **Hardy PC, Ederer GM, Matsen JM.** Contamination of commercially packaged urinary catheter kits with the pseudomonad EO-1. N Engl J Med 1970;282:33–35.

328 **Keizur JJ, Lavin B, Leidich RB.** Iatrogenic urinary tract infection with *Pseudomonas cepacia* after transrectal ultrasound guided needle biopsy of the prostate. J Urol 1993; 149:523–526.

329 **Gregory WJ, McNabb PC.** *Pseudomonas cepacia*. Infect Control 1986;7:281–284.

330 **Moore RA, Hancock RE.** Involvement of outer membrane of *Pseudomonas cepacia* in aminoglycoside and polymyxin resistance. Antimicrob Agents Chemother 1986;30: 923–926.

331 **Manniello JM, Heymann H, Adair FW.** Resistance of spheroplasts and whole cells of *Pseudomonas cepacia* to polymyxin B. Antimicrob Agents Chemother 1978;14: 500–504.

332 **Aronoff SC.** Derepressed beta-lactamase production as a mediator of high-level beta-lactam resistance in *Pseudomonas cepacia*. Pediatr Pulmonol 1988;4:72–77.

333 **Parr TRJ, Moore RA, Moore LV, Hancock RE.** Role of porins in intrinsic antibiotic resistance of *Pseudomonas cepacia*. Antimicrob Agents Chemother 1987;31:121–123.

334 **Burns JL, Wadsworth C, Barry J.** A multiple antibiotic resistance gene from *Pseudomonas cepacia* is homologous with an outer membrane protein from *Pseudomonas aeruginosa*. In: Abstracts of the 94th General Meeting of the American Society for Microbiology. Washington, D.C.: American Society for Microbiology, 1994.

335 **Santos Ferreira MO, Canica MM, Bacelar MJ.** *Pseudomonas cepacia*: the sensitivity of nosocomial strains to new antibiotics. J Int Med Res 1985;13:270–275.

336 **Burns JL, Lien DM, Hedin LA.** Isolation and characterization of dihydrofolate reductase from trimethoprim-susceptible and trimethoprim-resistant *Pseudomonas cepacia*. Antimicrob Agents Chemother 1989;33:1247–1251.

337 **Kumar A, Wofford-McQueen R, Gordon RC.** In vitro activity of multiple antimicrobial combinations against *Pseudomonas cepacia* isolates. Chemotherapy 1989:35: 246–253.

338 **Bhakta DR, Leader I, Jacobson R, et al.** Antibacterial properties of investigational, new, and commonly used antibiotics against isolates of *Pseudomonas cepacia* isolates in Michigan. Chemotherapy 1992;38: 319–323.

339 **Jacoby GA, Sutton L.** *Pseudomonas cepacia* susceptibility to sulbactam. Antimicrob Agents Chemother 1989;33:583–584.

340 **Gold R, Jim E, Levison H, et al.** Ceftazidime alone and in combination in patients with cystic fibrosis: lack of efficacy in treatment of severe respiratory infections caused by *Pseudomonas cepacia*. J Antimicrob Chemother 1983;12(suppl A): 331–336.

341 **Iaconis J, Tabinowski A, Nadler H, Sheikh W.** Lack of cross-resistance between imipenem-resistant (IPM^r) *Pseudomonas cepacia* isolates and meropenem. In: Abstracts of the 33rd Interscience Conference on Antimicrobial Agents and Chemotherapy. Washington, D.C.: American Society for Microbiology, 1993.

342 **Aronoff SC, Klinger JD.** In vitro activities of aztreonam, piperacillin, and ticarcillin combined with amikacin against amikacin-resistant *Pseudomonas aeruginosa* and *P. cepacia* isolates from children with cystic fibrosis. Antimicrob Agents Chemother 1984;25:279–280.

343 **Bosso JA, Saxon BA, Matsen JM.** In vitro activity of aztreonam combined with tobramycin and gentamicin against clinical isolates of *Pseudomonas aeruginosa* and

Pseudomonas cepacia from patients with cystic fibrosis. Antimicrob Agents Chemother 1987;31:1403.

344 **Kumar A, Wofford-McQueen R, Gordon RC.** Ciprofloxacin, imipenem, and rifampicin: in-vitro synergy of two and three drug combinations against *Pseudomonas cepacia*. J Antimicrob Chemother 1989;23: 831–835.

345 **Martone WJ, Osterman CA, Fisher KA, et al.** *Pseudomonas cepacia*: implications and control of epidemic nosocomial colonization. Rev Infect Dis 1981;3:708–715.

346 **Martone WJ, Tablan OC, Jarvis WR.** The epidemiology of nosocomial epidemic *Pseudomonas cepacia* infections. Eur J Epidemiol 1987;3:222–232.

347 **Pierce AK, Sanford JP.** Bacterial contamination of aerosols. Arch Intern Med 1973;131:156–159.

348 **Berthelot P, Grattard F, Mahul P, et al.** Ventilator temperature sensors: an unusual source of *Pseudomonas cepacia* in nosocomial infection. J Hosp Infect 1993;25:33–43.

349 **Walters S, Smith EG.** *Pseudomonas cepacia* in cystic fibrosis: transmissibility and its implications. Lancet 1993;342:3–4.

350 **Mahenthiralingam E, Campbell M, Speert DP.** *Burkholderia cepacia* in cystic fibrosis. N Engl J Med 1995;332:819.

351 **Heidt A, Monteil H, Richard C.** O and H serotyping of *Pseudomonas cepacia*. J Clin Microbiol 1983;18:738–740.

352 **Nakamura Y, Shigeta S, Yabuuchi E.** Serological classification of *Pseudomonas cepacia*. Kansenshogaku Zasshi 1984;58:491–494.

353 **Richard G, Monteil H, Megraud F, et al.** Caracteres phenotypiques de 100 souches de *Pseudomonas cepacia*: proposition d'un schema de biovars. Ann Biol Clin 1981; 39:9–15.

354 **Carson LA, Anderson RL, Panlilio AL, et al.** Isoenzyme analysis of *Pseudomonas cepacia* as an epidemiologic tool. Am J Med 1991;91(suppl 3B):S252–S255.

355 **Johnson WM, Tyler SD, Rozee KR.** Linkage analysis of geographic and clinical clusters in *Pseudomonas cepacia* infections by multilocus enzyme electrophoresis and ribotyping. J Clin Microbiol 1994;32:924–930.

356 **Govan JRW, Harris G.** Typing of *Pseudomonas cepacia* by bacteriocin susceptibility and production. J Clin Microbiol 1985;22:490–494.

357 **Rabkin CS, Jarvis WR, Martone WJ.** Current status of *Pseudomonas cepacia* typing systems. Eur J Epidemiol 1987;3:343–346.

358 **Anderson DJ, Kuhns JS, Vasil ML, et al.** DNA fingerprinting by pulsed field gel electrophoresis and ribotyping to distinguish *Pseudomonas cepacia* isolates from a nosocomial outbreak. J Clin Microbiol 1991;29:648–649.

359 **Bingen EH, Weber M, Derelle J, et al.** Arbitrarily primed polymerase chain reaction as a rapid method to differentiate crossed from independent *Pseudomonas cepacia* infections in cystic fibrosis patients. J Clin Microbiol 1993;31:2589–2593.

360 **Fisher MC, LiPuma JJ, Dasen SE, et al.** Source of *Pseudomonas cepacia*: ribotyping of isolates from patients and from the environment. J Pediatr 1993;123:745–747.

361 **Kostman JR, Edlind TB, LiPuma JJ, Stull TL.** Molecular epidemiology of *Pseudomonas cepacia* determined by polymerase chain reaction ribotyping. J Clin Microbiol 1992;30:2084–2087.

362 **Bingen EH, Denamur E, Elion J.** Use of ribotyping in epidemiological surveillance of nosocomial outbreaks. Clin Microbiol Rev 1994;7:311–327.

363 **Maslow JN, Mulligan ME, Arbeit RD.** Molecular epidemiology: application of contemporary techniques to the typing of microorganisms. Clin Infect Dis 1993;17: 153–164.

Human Immunodeficiency Virus Type 2: Human Biology of the Other AIDS Virus

RICHARD T. D'AQUILA

Human immunodeficiency virus type 2 (HIV-2) remains the only virus other than human immunodeficiency virus type 1 (HIV-1) that has been documented to cause the acquired immunodeficiency syndrome (AIDS). The existence of a second human lentivirus was initially suspected because healthy Senegalese persons had some serologic cross-reactivity to HIV-1, with stronger antibody reactivity to simian immunodeficiency virus (SIV) antigens than to HIV-1 antigens (1,2). Subsequently, HIV-2 was isolated from patients with severe immunodeficiency clinically indistinguishable from that caused by HIV-1 (3–7) as well as from healthy persons in west Africa (8). The HIV-2 genome was shown to be more closely related to SIVs than to HIV-1 (5,9–11).

HIV-1 and HIV-2 can now be classified with some phylogenetic accuracy within a large family of primate lentiviruses that differ from most other exogenous retroviruses in having a more complex genome and an enormous potential for genetic diversification. Study of the genetic diversity of the primate lentiviruses has led to consensus on the origins of these viruses in nonhuman primates and a suggestion that adaptation to a new host species is associated with ability to cause disease. But biologic differences between these related viruses delineated in just the past few years are of even greater interest than their similarities. Although HIV-2 is endemic in west Africa and transmitted by the same routes as HIV-1, a second pandemic of HIV-2 disease in humans on the scale caused by HIV-1 has not yet materialized. HIV-2 is less efficiently transmitted than HIV-1 and causes immunodeficiency at a decreased rate compared with HIV-1 (12,13). The differences in HIV-2 phylogeny, epidemiology, transmissibility, pathogenesis, and molecular virology from HIV-1 suggest that viral factors can attenuate lentiviral replication in humans. Future identification of such viral factors is likely to suggest public health and medical strategies to limit the epidemic spread and pathogenicity of HIV-1. In contrast to the guarded optimism engendered by this prospect and the increasing evidence that HIV-2 may not spread globally, the apparent evolutionary interrelationships among the primate lentiviruses suggest the possibility of future spread of zoonotic human disease due to as yet unrecognized lentiviruses.

PHYLOGENY OF HIV-2 AND OTHER PRIMATE RETROVIRUSES

Simpler retroviruses have coevolved with their host animal, such as mouse or chicken, for millions of years and only rarely cause disease. But viruses of two of the five currently identified primate lentivirus lineages (Figure 4.1) have apparently been more recently introduced into humans and Asian primates (macaques) and are clearly pathogens (Table 4.1) (11). These lineages also encompass viruses that have been widely prevalent and nonpathogenic among a number of African primate species for some time ("natural infections," see Table 4.1). The molecular anatomy of numerous viruses from feral nonhuman primates, as well as some unusual human isolates, has led to this phylogenetic tree and the following generalizations, which are further detailed by Sharp et al (11).

HIV-2 Is Not in the Same Evolutionary Lineage as HIV-1

This fact is obscured by current biologically uninformative nomenclature, but each human virus is more closely related to viruses found in nonhuman primates than to each other. Viruses labeled as "HIVs" and "SIVs" exist together in two of the major lineages. The human pathogen HIV-1 clusters in the same lineage as nonpathogenic SIV_{CPZ} isolated from healthy chimpanzees (14,15).

Table 4.1. Primate Lentiviruses Characterized at the Sequence Level

Virus	*Host*	*Natural Infection*	*Pathogenic Infection*	*Lineage*
HIV-1	Human	No	Yes	1
SIV_{CPZ}	Chimpanzee	?	No	1
HIV-2	Human	No	Yes	2
SIV_{SM}	Sooty mangabey	Yes	No	2
SIV_{MAC}	Rhesus macaque	No	Yes	2
SIV_{MNE}	Pig-tailed macaque	No	Yes	2
SIV_{STM}	Stump-tailed macaque	No	Yes	2
SIV_{AGM}ver	Vervet monkey	Yes	No	3
SIV_{AGM}gri	Grivet monkey	Yes	No	3
SIV_{AGM}sab	Sabaeus monkey	Yes	No	3
SIV_{AGM}tan	Tantalus monkey	Yes	No	3
SIV_{MND}	Mandrill	Yes?	No	4
SIV_{SYK}	Sykes' monkey	Yes	No	5

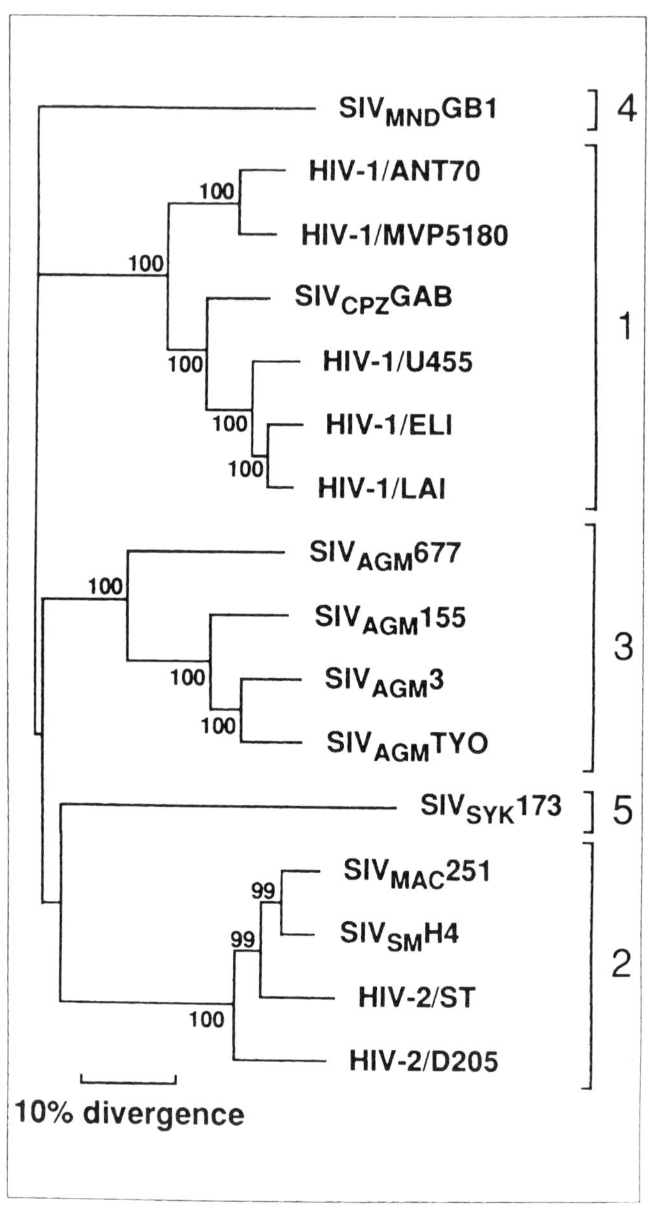

$SIV_{MND}GB1$
4
HIV-1/ANT70
HIV-1/MVP5180
$SIV_{CPZ}GAB$
HIV-1/U455
HIV-1/ELI
HIV-1/LAI
1
$SIV_{AGM}677$
$SIV_{AGM}155$
$SIV_{AGM}3$
$SIV_{AGM}TYO$
3
$SIV_{SYK}173$
5
$SIV_{MAC}251$
$SIV_{SM}H4$
HIV-2/ST
HIV-2/D205
2
100
100
100
100
100
100
100
100
99
99
100
10% divergence

HIV-2 is in a distinct and different grouping and is most closely related to SIV_{SM} viruses from sooty mangabeys (10,16–18). Although the primate relative of HIV-2, SIV_{SM}, does not cause disease in sooty mangabeys (18,19), it is also the closest genetic relative of another virus that does cause disease in nonhuman primates, SIV_{MAC}. SIV_{MAC} has caused epidemic immunodeficiency disease in a number of colonies of captive Asian macaques and allowed development of one of the best available animal models of HIV-1 (20,21). HIV-2 is more closely related to SIV_{SM} and/or SIV_{MAC} than it is to HIV-1. The other primate lentivirus groups (SIV_{AGM} from African green monkeys, SIV_{MND} from mandrills, and SIV_{SYK} from Sykes monkeys) do not cause disease in their natural hosts and each represent distinct groupings genetically quite different from either of the human immunodeficiency lentiviruses (11).

Figure 4.1. A phylogenetic tree of primate lentiviruses derived from polymerase protein sequences (11) illustrates a statistical estimate of the evolutionary relationships among these viruses. Amino acids at 871 positions in different polymerase proteins were compared. There are two important aspects of this tree: horizontal branch lengths and the relative vertical order of the branch points separating the five main lineages (indicated by the numbered brackets on the right). (**A**) The length between branching points ("nodes") indicates the extent of sequence change and, assuming a roughly constant "molecular clock," the approximate evolutionary time between branching points. The horizontal branch lengths are drawn to scale and the scale bar indicates the length that represents a 10% divergence between sequences. There are two lines of evidence that support the clustering within each of the lineages containing multiple viruses (lineages 1, 2, and 3): the presence of a long branch before the divergence within each lineage and a statistical assessment of how often particular clusters of sequences are found when the sequence data are randomly resampled, called "the bootstrap" (82). Numbers at the nodes in the tree are the percentage of the 1000 bootstrap samples examined in which the cluster to the right was found; only values greater than 90% are shown. (**B**) The relative order of the branching points separating the five major lineages has not yet been resolved because there are only short statistically uncertain branches between successive divergence points at the root of the tree (at the extreme left). Indeed, vertical branches are drawn only for clarity and may not accurately reflect real relationships. Construction of this tree was described by Sharp et al. (11) in a methodologic appendix. Sequences were aligned using CLUSTAL (83) with minor manual adjustment; pairwise distances among protein sequences were estimated by an empirical method (84). Each tree was constructed by the neighbor-joining method (85) applied to the matrix of pairwise distances and 1000 bootstrap samples were examined (86). Reprinted with permission from Sharp PM, Robertson DL, Gao F, et al. Origins and diversity of human immunodeficiency viruses. AIDS 1994;8(suppl 1):S27–S42.

Both HIVs Probably Originated as Zoonotic Infections of Humans from Monkeys

The primate lentiviral tree must reflect a number of cross-species transmission events because primate lentivirus phylogeny does not follow primate species lines (see Figure 4.1). Times of divergence between different viruses do not correspond to when their hosts diverged. Human viruses seem most closely related to those of evolutionarily distant nonhuman primates, and nonhuman primate species that are closely related to each other do not harbor closely related viruses. African green monkeys and Sykes monkeys are both classified in the genus Cercopithecus. However, their viruses are no more similar to each other than they are to viruses from primates of different genera, such as mandrills from the genus Papio and sooty mangabeys from the genus Cercocebus. This leads to the inescapable conclusion that different viruses entered the same or closely related host species at different times and that a single virus was not evolving along with one particular species. Nonhuman primates have been hunted for food by humans and sometimes kept as pets. The most likely route for a zoonotic infection of humans involves exposure to infectious nonhuman primate blood and/or tissues during hunting or food preparation.

Although the speculation that a monkey virus was transmitted to humans by hunting remains unproven, the risk of transmission of an SIV into humans is no longer theoretical. Two seroconversions of different workers in SIV research laboratories have been documented in which clear reactivity to SIV, but not HIV-1 or -2, antigens developed after SIV exposure (22,23). One case is particularly instructive, in considering the potential for transmission to humans in a more "natural" setting. The worker's only reported exposure risk involved performing serologic assays on samples of experimentally infected macaque blood without wearing gloves while having a severe hand dermatitis (23). In that case, a virus (SIV_{HU}) isolated from the persistently infected human was shown to be genetically nearly identical to the SIV_{SM} strain being used in the researcher's experiments after isolation from a sooty mangabey (23). There were a large number of distinct differences between these SIV_{HU} sequences and those of HIV-2 strains (23). Cross-species transmission of a lentivirus between different monkeys in the wild has also been directly documented (24), as well as inferred from many different SIV_{MAC} sequences. In addition, it is hypothesized that SIV_{MAC} was generated by transfer of SIV_{SM} from infected sooty mangabeys to macaques in primate centers, because SIV_{MAC} is not found in Asian macaques in the wild.

Strong indirect evidence that HIV-2 entered humans as an ancestor virus acquired from sooty mangabeys is the phylogenetic relatedness of the two currently circulating viruses, which are much more similar to each other than HIV-2 is to HIV-1 (10,16–18). This is supported by the geographic distribution of sooty mangabeys, which overlaps with the west African pattern of HIV-2 endemicity in humans. Furthermore, it has been estimated that 30% of feral sooty mangabeys are infected with SIV_{SM} (Marx, P cited in reference 1). Indeed, one recent genetic analysis of the five so far identified subtypes of HIV-2 suggests that these divergent subtypes may have arisen from independent introductions of different sooty mangabey viruses into humans (25). It is less clear what primate species was the natural host for the virus from which HIV-1 descended; it is not yet known if chimpanzees have ever been a natural reservoir of an SIV. It is possible that a third as yet unidentified primate species served as the source for the ancestral virus that infected both chimpanzees and humans. Chimpanzees do hunt small monkeys for food in the wild.

HIV-1 and HIV-2 May Differ from Each Other Because of Long Periods of Evolution of Their Respective Ancestors in Monkeys

A number of estimates based on quite different data and methodologies suggest HIV-1 and HIV-2 emerged relatively recently (10,11). It has been roughly estimated that HIV-2 and SIV_{MAC}, respectively, may have each diverged from SIV_{SM} as recently as the 1960s, although this is controversial (10). Estimates of the time when HIV-1 diverged from SIV_{CPZ} are based on less good data but also suggest HIV-1 may have evolved as recently as 30 to 50 years ago (10). Although these estimates may be pushed back to earlier dates as more diverse viruses are characterized, the genetic differences between HIV-1 and HIV-2 seem unlikely to have all evolved in the relatively short time period since each virus separately crossed a species barrier to human hosts.

There are two different ways to estimate when the initial virus ancestral to all the lineages depicted in Figure 4.1 first evolved, and they yield very different estimates. If the rate of sequence change over time is used, the ancestor can be dated to have existed only 150 years ago (11,26). This is based on use of a uniform rate of sequence change (on the order of 10^{-3} to 10^{-2} nucleotide substitutions per site per year) determined from the current rate of evolution of HIV-1 subtypes (11,27). However, there is some evidence that rates of primate lentivirus evolution are nonlinear (10); that is, some branches within the tree may have evolved much more slowly than HIV-1s are currently changing.

The alternative way to estimate when the progenitor of all primate lentiviruses existed is based on speculation in the literature that the currently known genetically diverse lineages of primate lentiviruses may have each had their origins in Cercopithecus monkeys (11). In other words, all the presently known lineages may have evolved and diverged from each other within Cercopithecus monkeys coincident with speciation events in that genus. This is based on the following points. [1] Two of the five known major lineages are from the Cercopithecus genus, including the Sykes' monkey (*C. mitis*) (28) and the African green monkeys (the *C. aethiops* "superspecies") (29–32). [2] The diversity of SIVs is greatest among those isolated from African green monkeys, relative to that seen in other major lineages (29–32). Indeed, the subtyping of

SIV_{AGM}s isolated from the four major African green monkey species (vervet, grivet, sabaeus, and tantalus monkeys) revealed that each of these African green monkey species harbors its own distinct, but related, SIV_{AGM} subtype (32). [3] The four major species of African green monkey are estimated to have diverged from each other from 10,000 to millions of years ago and are thought to have entered separate geographic niches when they diverged (10). The vervets and grivets reside in east and southeast Africa, the sabaeus species in west Africa, and the tantalus species in central Africa overlapping the mangabey range. It is difficult to explain how the geographically separated species could have each been infected by a common viral source after they had dispersed to their separate niches (10). [4] These SIVs are now quite prevalent in these monkeys in the wild and do not cause any disease (29–31). All of these points suggest that the relationship between SIV_{AGM}s and their hosts is the most ancient of the currently known virus-host relationships, dating back perhaps millions of years.

HIV-1 and HIV-2 May Not Be the Only Zoonotic Infections of Humans from Monkeys

Interaction between humans and nonhuman primates in Africa does clearly date quite far into the distant past. One might suspect that primate lentivirus pathogenicity is a recent acquisition or an aberration. But it does seem plausible that other cross-species virus transmissions are likely to have occurred (or may occur in the future), especially in light of recent speculation that multiple monkey-to-human transmission events explain the sequence differences in HIV-2 subtypes (25). One must then assume that virus descendants of other cross-species transmission events either no longer exist in humans or they have not yet been detected. It must be emphasized that this is a hypothesis that merits investigation, but there is no direct evidence to support it as yet. This does suggest the prudence of careful surveillance for newly emerging infections.

EPIDEMIOLOGY OF HIV-2

HIV-2 Seroprevalence Studies Show Only Limited Spread Beyond West Africa

Urban centers in certain west African countries (Figure 4.2) have the highest seroprevalence of HIV-2 infection, with the predominance of evidence suggesting that most infections are acquired through heterosexual intercourse (33,34). Some countries elsewhere in Africa (see Figure 4.2), in Europe, and in South America have also had appreciable prevalence of HIV-2 infection. Links between some of these other nations and Guinea-Bissau or Cape Verde have been based on mutual former Portuguese colonial status. Cases of HIV-2 in-

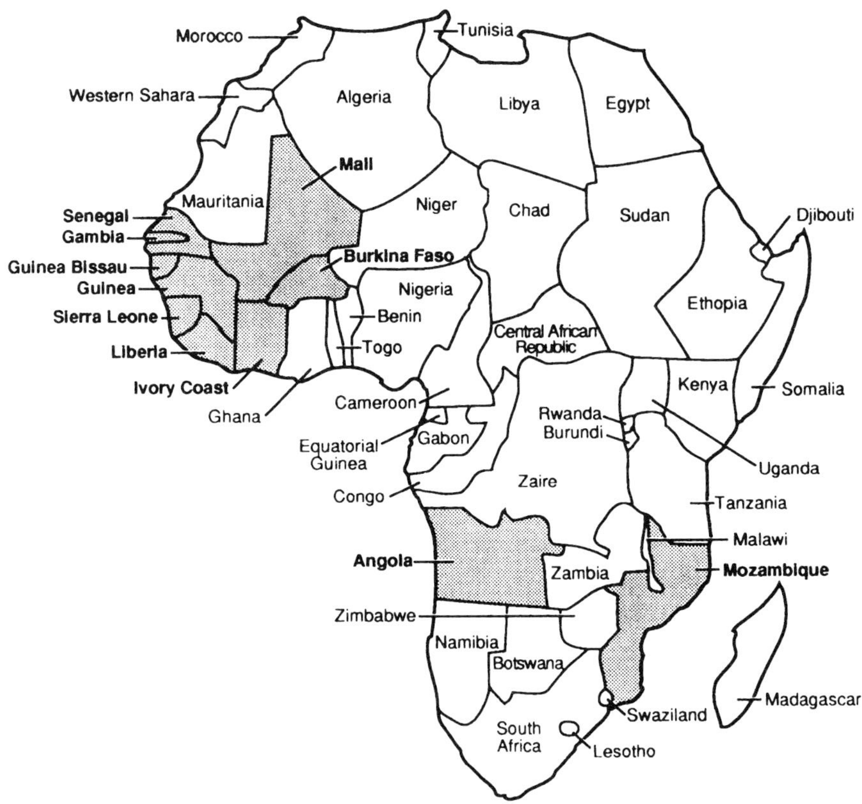

Figure 4.2. Distribution of HIV-2 in Africa. Shaded areas represent regions where significant rates of HIV-2 infection have been reported. Reprinted with permission from Markovitz DM. Infection with the human immunodeficiency virus type 2. Ann Intern Med 1993;118:211–218.

fection have also been diagnosed in the United States, initially in persons presenting with AIDS (35,36) and later because of routine screening of all blood donors (37,38). In all of these areas other than west Africa, infected persons have generally either lived in one of the west African nations where HIV-2 is established or had sexual contact with a person from such a country. Spread by blood transfusion has not yet been documented within the United States.

Until recently there was little evidence that HIV-2 was becoming established as a locally growing epidemic anywhere beyond west Africa. Putative direct spread from west Africa in virtually every case differentiated HIV-2 from the rapid worldwide dissemination seen with HIV-1. However, HIV-2 spread has now been documented within India, primarily via heterosexual intercourse without apparent direct contact with west Africans (39). A genetic analysis has shown relatively close relatedness of a small number of these Indian HIV-2 sequences, consistent with recent introduction from a single point of entry as suggested by the seroepidemiology (40). Thus, although the global spread of HIV-2 is markedly slower than the blinding pace of the intercontinental HIV-1 pandemic, it has spread beyond the confines of the original African source of the epidemic, at least to India.

Infectivity Potential of HIV-2 Is Lower than that of HIV-1

Horizontal Transmission of HIV-2 Evidence for a slow pace of HIV-2 spread also comes from long-term studies monitoring population prevalence and incidence in west Africa. Between 1988 and 1992, 19,701 women of reproductive age were tested in Abidjan, Ivory Coast (34). Although prevalence of HIV-1 increased from 5% to 9%, frequency of HIV-2 infection trended down from 2.6% to 1.5% (34). An increase in risk of seropositivity with age and increased years of sexual activity was noted among a higher risk population, female sex workers in Dakar, Senegal (41). This is consistent with the presence of the virus for several decades in that locale despite stable prevalence rates. However, these types of studies are prone to possible biases and only indirectly evaluate the variable of interest, incidence of HIV-2 infection.

A prospective study of HIV-1 and HIV-2 incidence among 1452 registered female sex workers in Dakar followed from 1985 to 1993 provides the most convincing evidence that HIV-2 has a lower infectivity potential than HIV-1 (13). The overall incidence of both viruses was low over the entire study period. However, the annual incidence of HIV-1 increased 1.4-fold per year or 12-fold over the 8-year study period of 1985 to 1993. In contrast, the annual incidence of HIV-2 remained stable over these years, as did the HIV-2 seroprevalence. This occurred in the setting of a higher overall HIV-2 seroprevalence over the entire study period (11.3% for HIV-2 vs. 6.2% for HIV-1). The annual incidence rate for heterosexually acquired HIV-1 infection in this study in Senegal is similar to that seen in cohorts of homosexual men in the United States (42), although much lower than that reported from a study of female sex workers in Nairobi, Kenya (43). In the high-risk Senegal cohort, HIV-2 prevalence seems to have plateaued at a much lower level (11%) than the plateau level observed and calculated for HIV-1 in other high risk populations (65% to 97%) (44). Mathematical modeling of seroincidence data suggest a five- to ninefold decreased infectivity of HIV-2 per sexual act, compared with HIV-1 (45).

Vertical Transmission of HIV-2 Spread of HIV-2 from an infected mother to infant has been documented, but it occurs 15- to 20-fold less frequently for HIV-2 than for HIV-1 (46–50). In a prospective cohort including 86 infants born to 68 HIV-2–infected mothers and 1758 infants born to 1589 HIV-1–infected mothers, transmission was assessed by the infant's serologic status at 18 months. No HIV-2 transmissions were seen (95% confidence interval 0 to 11%) (50). In contrast, the HIV-1 transmission rate in this cohort was 21% (95% confidence interval 16% to 26%) (50), similar to the HIV-1 vertical transmission rate seen in many other studies.

These studies of both horizontal and vertical transmission are consistent with the conclusion that the biologic efficiency of HIV-2 transmission is lower than that of HIV-1. Attenuated HIV-2 replication in vivo appears to explain these findings and is detailed after discussion of HIV-2 pathogenesis in the next section. However, human biology and sociology are inextricably linked to the ongoing epidemics of HIV-1 and HIV-2 infection, in addition to lentivirus biology. HIV-2 spread is driven by the same social, cultural, and economic factors that propelled HIV-1 so much more rapidly. These factors, and their public health implications for attempts to limit the HIV epidemics, have been eloquently summarized by Quinn: ". . . the migration of poor, rural, and young sexually active individuals to urban centers coupled with large international movements of HIV-infected individuals played a prominent role in the dissemination of HIV globally. The economic recession has aggravated the transmission of HIV by directly increasing the population at risk through increased urban migration, disruption of rural families and cultural values, poverty, and prostitution and indirectly through a decrease in health care provision. Consequently, social and economic reform as well as sexual behavior education needs to be intensified if HIV transmission is to be controlled (51)."

PATHOGENESIS OF HIV-2

The proximate pathogenetic mechanism of CD4+ T-lymphocyte depletion appears identical for both HIV-1 and HIV-2, although the complex biology underlying that mechanism is still being defined for both viruses. Disease manifestations include virtually the same opportunistic infections for both viruses, as well as Kaposi's sarcoma. However, there are some key differences of HIV-2 from HIV-1 pathogenesis.

Risk of Disease Development After HIV-2 Infection is Reduced Compared with HIV-1 Infection

Early anecdotal case reports first suggested that there may be a longer time from infection to development of AIDS for HIV-2 than for HIV-1 (36,52,53). There have been fewer AIDS cases reported in west Africa, where HIV-2 is more prevalent than HIV-1, than in central or east Africa, where HIV-1 predominates (54). The well-studied cohort of HIV-2–infected female sex workers in Dakar, Senegal, was reported to be relatively free of disease compared with female sex workers in HIV-1–predominant areas of Africa (55).

A cross-sectional comparison of HIV-1 and HIV-2 disease in the same population also found that HIV-2–infected persons were healthier than HIV-1–infected persons (56). These studies raised the hypothesis that HIV-2 had reduced disease-causing potential but could not prove it conclusively.

A case series also suggested that progression to death after development of full-blown AIDS was slower for HIV-2 than HIV-1 (6). A more recent study involved identifying patients hospitalized in The Gambia with either HIV-1 or HIV-2 infection and following them prospectively. The mortality rate of the HIV-2 patients was two thirds that of the HIV-1 patients, even after adjusting for differences in mortality risk attributable to age, sex, World Health Organization clinical classification, and CD4+ T-lymphocyte count (57). However, such hospital-based identification of already ill infected persons may be prone to selection bias and either under- or overestimate the apparent relative pathologic effects of HIV-2.

A prospective study of disease outcomes among Dakar female sex workers from 1985 to 1993 has recently provided the best, and least-biased, comparison yet of the natural history of HIV-2 and HIV-1 infection in a cohort of initially asymptomatic individuals (12). Rates of AIDS development were lower for HIV-2 than HIV-1 among subjects who were seroprevalent and those who were seroincident (i.e., seronegative at enrollment and seroconverted during observation in the study). No seroincident HIV-2 women developed AIDS over 112 person-years of observation. This 100% probability (with inestimable SD) of greater than 5 years AIDS-free survival with HIV-2 compared with an estimate of 67% (SD, 14%) 5 years AIDS-free survival with HIV-1 (12). The latter is similar to the 5 years AIDS-free survival rate noted in other HIV-1 incidence studies (58). Less-severe disease outcomes did occur in the HIV-2 subgroup and allowed better comparisons to HIV-1 infection outcomes. Centers for Disease Control and Prevention stage IV disease includes non-AIDS-defining as well as AIDS-defining conditions (59) and was seen in two HIV-2–seroincident women, compared with eight HIV-1–seroincident women (12). Development of a CD4+ T-lymphocyte count less than 400/mm^3 was seen in one HIV-2– and seven HIV-1–seroincident women (12). Among those who were purified protein derivative skin test positive at enrollment, 2 of 20 HIV-2– and 6 of 17 HIV-1–seroincident women became anergic (12). Each difference in disease outcome after HIV-2 versus HIV-1 infection was statistically significant (12). This report provides definitive evidence that HIV-2 infection has a reduced rate of disease development, compared with HIV-1. However, the small number of events led to rather wide confidence intervals around the estimates of relative hazard of HIV-2–related disease development, which limited ability to estimate how much more slowly disease develops after HIV-2 infection compared with HIV-1. In addition, it remains difficult to judge from these data whether there are differences in natural history among HIV-2–infected persons. It is possible either that some HIV-2 infections are markedly less virulent than other HIV-2 infections (and perhaps even avirulent) or that most HIV-2 infections have similar virulence, which is lower than the virulence of HIV-1 infection.

HIV-2 Replication Appears Attenuated In Vivo Compared with HIV-1

Decreased pathogenicity and infectivity of HIV-2, relative to HIV-1, may be explainable by attenuated viral replication in vivo if an intriguing, somewhat speculative, cross-study comparison is confirmed. This study suggested that circulating virus isolation rate is lower in HIV-2–infected individuals than in HIV-1–infected persons at early stages of the disease process (60). At more advanced stages of immunodeficiency, virus load appeared equivalent in HIV-2 and HIV-1 infection. A standardized assay of circulating peripheral blood mononuclear cells (PBMC) that indicates whether a virus culture is positive and quantitates the number of infectious units of virus per 10^6 cells cultured, Tissue Culture Infectious Doses (TCID/10^6 cells), was used, as well as a qualitative plasma culture assay. These assays were used in this study of selected French HIV-2–infected patients (60) and had previously been used in a study of a different group of French HIV-1–infected patients (61). Although one cannot ignore possible influence of selection bias in such a cross-study comparison, the frequency of isolation of any amount of virus from either circulating cells or plasma was lower among the HIV-2–infected patients compared with the HIV-1–infected patients at CD4+ T lymphocyte counts from 200 to 500/μL and similar among patients with more advanced immunodeficiency, less than 200 cells/μL (60) (Table 4.2). There was no significant difference in mean cell infectivity titer (TCID/10^6 cells) between HIV-2– and HIV-1–infected patients with less than 200 CD4 cells/μL, but there was about a 10-fold lower cellular virus load for the HIV-2–infected patients with 200 to 500 CD4 cells/μL (60). In another study, a sensitive and quantitative nested RNA polymerase chain reaction method was used and a correlation between CD4 count and amount of

Table 4.2. HIV-1[a] and HIV-2 Cell and Plasma Viremia According to the French National Agency for AIDS Research Action Coordonée No. 11 (AC 11) Protocol in Relation to the CD4+ Cell Count (as Determined by Flow Cytometry) in 54 HIV-1–Infected and 40 HIV-2–Infected Patients

	CD4 count × 10^6/liter					
	<200		*200–500*		*>500*	
	HIV-1 (n = 23)	*HIV-2 (n = 10)*	*HIV-1 (n = 18)*	*HIV-2 (n = 8)*	*HIV-1 (n = 13)*	*HIV-2 (n = 22)*
Cell viraemia (%)	23(100)	10(100)	17(94)	5(62)	12(92)	4(18)
P[b]			<0.07>		<0.01	
Plasma viraemia (%)	19(83)	4(40)	11(61)	0	0	0
P[b]	0.03		<<0.01>			

[a] Data for HIV-1 from the AC 11 protocol were reported previously (61).
[b] Fisher's exact test.

HIV-2 plasma RNA was noted (62). The absolute levels of RNA appeared relatively low, but they were not directly compared with levels in HIV-1 infection (62).

If it is indeed the case that virus replication is reduced in vivo for all HIV-2 strains only until a certain degree of immunodeficiency is reached, it suggests that HIV-2 will eventually spread globally as did HIV-1, albeit with some delay. However, other data suggest the possibility that only some genetic subtypes of HIV-2 replicate in laboratory cultures (25). Some of the viruses that do not replicate in vitro were isolated from healthy individuals with normal immunity who live in rural communities of west Africa where HIV-2 AIDS has not yet been recognized (16,25). It has recently been documented that some HIV-1–infected persons who are long-term survivors have a clearly biologically different virus-host interaction than most HIV-1–infected persons (63). Thus, there may be a precedent for the intriguing hypothesis that there are biologic differences between HIV-2 genetic subtypes such that only some subtypes replicate in vitro and are pathogenic in vivo. The implications of this alternative scenario are that the HIV-2 epidemic may not spread and some HIV-2–infected persons will never develop disease. However, there are no data as yet correlating variation in any viral function with genetic subtypes of HIV-2. In either scenario, characterization of the mechanisms that cause comparatively attenuated HIV-2 replication in vivo will yield crucial insight into pathogenesis for both HIV-1 and HIV-2.

Molecular Virologic Factors May Relatively Attenuate HIV-2 Replication

Although a number of differences in the HIV-2 genome, protein structure, and possibly host immune response have been noted, more systematic study is needed to identify the factors that operate in vivo to either directly attenuate viral replication or indirectly allow better host immune control of the infection. The situation in vivo is likely to be quite complex.

Differences in HIV-2 Genome Structure and Diversity from HIV-1 HIV-2 has an additional gene, *vpx*, than HIV-1 that may have been acquired by duplication of the *vpr* gene present in an ancestral primate lentivirus (64). The *vpx* gene product may play a role early in the viral life cycle. This function is dispensable for HIV-2 replication in vitro, however, in T-cell lines and primary monocyte/macrophages, although it may slightly augment replication in PBMC (65,66). The degree of viral genetic diversity has been suggested to correlate with pathogenicity, but similar genetic variation has been noted in envelope genes of both pathogenic and nonpathogenic strains of SIV_{MAC} (67). Some of the genetically complex quasi-species present in primate lentivirus-infected hosts are defective for virus production. It is intriguing that many genetically defective molecular clones were noted during sequencing of some nonpathogenic HIV-2s (16).

Differences in Function of Regulatory Proteins or Enzymes A number of differences in some regulatory genes (*tat* and *rev*) and their viral genomic targets (TAR and RRE) have been noted between HIV-2 and HIV-1 (68,69). There are also differences in regulation of viral transcription based on the structure and function of the viral promoter/enhancer in the long terminal repeat (LTR) (succinctly reviewed in reference 70). Different cellular factors bind to different enhancer sequences in the HIV-2 LTR, compared with the HIV-1 LTR (71–73). Some physiologic T-cell activation signals (antigen presentation) strongly induce the HIV-2 transcription, whereas other signals that strongly induce HIV-1 enhancer (tumor necrosis factor-α (TNF-α) and NFκ B) do not induce HIV-2 transcription (73). Differences in HIV-2 replicative enzymes have also been noted, although it remains unclear how they might explain HIV-2's attenuated replication. HIV-2 is not susceptible to nonnucleoside reverse transcriptase inhibitors and less susceptible to some protease inhibitors, although there is less data comparing levels of functional activity of these enzymes in the absence of inhibitors. There is evidence that HIV-2 integrase cleaves the two ends of linear reverse transcribed DNA asymmetrically (74), whereas the HIV-1 integrase cleaves symmetrically.

Differences in CD4 Cell Receptor and Envelope Protein Interaction In vitro, genetic determinants in the envelope gene contribute to the differential cytopathogenicity in T-cell lines of HIV-2 strains, including the tendency for noncytopathic variants to have truncated transmembrane envelope proteins and lower CD4 affinity (75–77).

Differences in Immune Recognition and Control It has been speculated that a more effective immune response to HIV-2 limits its replication in the infected human. This must be due to differences in virus biology that lead to better immune control rather than to host-related differences in immunity. Lower levels of plasma TNF-α were found in HIV-2–infected than in HIV-1–infected African patients who were prospectively followed over 3 years (78). The lower TNF-α levels correlated with lower virus loads and higher CD4 counts and are consistent with a more appropriate immune response to HIV-2 infection (78). An intriguing recent study showed HIV-1/HIV-2 cross-reactive, specific cytotoxic T lymphocytes (CTL) in repeatedly HIV-exposed but uninfected seronegative Gambian female sex workers (79). The controversial unproven presumption is that this CTL response has protected these women from infection. The authors speculate that exposure to low doses of virus primes primarily cellular T-helper type 1 (TH-1) immune responses at the expense of humoral T-helper type 2 (TH-2) immune responses and that these women were likely to have been first exposed to HIV-2, which has a lower in vivo virus load than HIV-1. HIV-1 was introduced into The Gambia more recently, and they postulate that those who had made a cross-reactive CTL response to low-dose HIV-2 exposure were subsequently protected from infection with either virus. If an effective CTL response could clear an infection with a second HIV, this may explain why both HIV-1 and HIV-2 cannot be isolated from some patients with dual seroreactivity to HIV-1 and HIV-2 (80).

CONCLUSIONS

Continuing comparison of HIV-2 and HIV-1 biology may elucidate pathogenic mechanisms needed to improve treatment and limit spread of the current HIV-1 pandemic, as well a potential future epidemic that may be caused by HIV-L or by another lentivirus zoonotically infecting humans. In practical terms, the need for U.S. physicians to treat HIV-2 AIDS is currently unlikely, although it is reasonable to treat it identically to HIV-1 AIDS. Clinicians are more likely to be confronted with asymptomatic HIV-2–seropositive blood donors, because all donated blood is now screened using a combination HIV-1/HIV-2 enzyme-linked immunosorbent assay and persons from sub-Saharan Africa are no longer excluded from donating blood (81). At present, all such HIV-2–infected persons must be considered potentially infectious and counseled to prevent transmission the same way an HIV-1–infected person would be counseled. It is reasonable to inform HIV-2–infected women of childbearing age that there is a lower risk of transmitting the virus to an infant than for HIV-1 but that there is still a risk. All HIV-2–infected persons must also currently be considered likely to eventually progress to AIDS, although at least some will probably do so at a relatively slow pace. There are no available guidelines for use of antiretrovirals in such patients. When faced with advancing immunodeficiency, it appears reasonable to follow accepted practice for HIV-1. All of these recommendations may change, however, if future work supports the optimistic, as yet unsupported, speculation that some HIV-2–infected persons can be identified who are not infectious and/or will not progress to AIDS.

REFERENCES

1 **Barin FM, 'Boup S, Denis F, et al.** Serological evidence for virus related to simian T-lymphotropic retrovirus III in residents of west Africa. Lancet 1985;2:1387–1389.

2 **Kanki PJ, McLane MF, King NW Jr, et al.** Serologic identification and characterization of a macaque T-lymphotropic retrovirus closely related to HTLV-III. Science 1985; 228:1199–1201.

3 **Clavel F, Mansinho K, Chamaret S, et al.** Human immunodeficiency virus type 2 infection associated with AIDS in West Africa. N Engl J Med 1987;316:1180–1185.

4 **Clavel F, Guetard D, Brun-Vezinet F, et al.** Isolation of a new human retrovirus from West African patients with AIDS. Science 1986;233:343–346.

5 **Clavel F, Guyader M, Guetard D, et al.** Molecular cloning and polymorphism of the human immune deficiency virus type 2. Nature 1986;324:691–695.

6 **Brun-Vezinet F, Rey MA, Katlama C, et al.** Lymphadenopathy-associated virus type 2 in AIDS and AIDS-related complex. Clinical and virological features in four patients. Lancet 1987;1:128–132.

7 **Denis F, Barin F, Gershy-Damet G, et al.** Prevalence of human T-lymphotropic retroviruses type III (HIV) and type IV in Ivory Coast. Lancet 1987;1:408–411.

8 **Kanki PJ, Barin FM, 'Boup S, et al.** New human T-lymphotropic retrovirus related to simian T-lymphotropic virus type III (STLV-IIIAGM). Science 1986;232:238–243.

9 **Guyader M, Emerman M, Sonigo P, et al.** Genome organization and transactivation of the human immunodeficiency virus type 2. Nature 1987;326:662–669.

10 **Myers G, MacInnes K, Korber B.** The emergence of simian/human immunodeficiency viruses. AIDS Res Hum Retroviruses 1992;8: 373–386.

11 **Sharp PM, Robertson DL, Gao F, Hahn BH.** Origins and diversity of human immunodeficiency viruses. AIDS 1994;8(suppl 1):S27–S42.

12 **Marlink R, Kanki P, Thior I, et al.** Reduced rate of disease development after HIV-2 infection as compared to HIV-1. Science 1994; 265:1587–1590.

13 **Kanki PJ, Travers KUM, Boup S, et al.** Slower heterosexual spread of HIV-2 than HIV-1. Lancet 1994;343:943–946.

14 **Peeters M, Fransen K, Delaporte E, et al.** Isolation and characterization of a new chimpanzee lentivirus (simian immunodeficiency virus isolate cpz-ant) from a wild-captured chimpanzee. AIDS 1992;6:477–451.

15 **Huet T, Cheynier R, Meyerhans A, et al.** Genetic organization of a chimpanzee lentivirus related to HIV-1. Nature 1990;345: 356–359.

16 **Gao F, Yue L, White AT, et al.** Human infection by genetically diverse SIV_{SM}-related HIV-2 in west Africa. Nature 1992;358:495–499.

17 **Hirsch VJ, Olmstead RA, Murphey-Corb M, et al.** An African primate lentivirus (SIV_{SM}) closely related to HIV-2. Nature 1989;339:389–392.

18 **Marx PA, Li Y, Lerche NW, et al.** Isolation of a simian immunodeficiency virus related to human immunodeficiency virus type 2 from a west African pet sooty mangabey. J Virol 1991;65:4480–4485.

19 **Fultz PN, McClure HM, Anderson DC, et al.** Isolation of a T-lymphotropic retrovirus from naturally infected sooty mangabey monkeys (*Cercocebus atys*). Proc Natl Acad Sci USA 1986;83:5286–5290.

20 **Letvin NL, Daniel MD, Sehgal PK, et al.** Induction of AIDS-like disease in macaque monkeys with T-cell tropic retrovirus STLV-III. Science 1985;230:71–73.

21 **Daniel MD, Letvin NL, King NW, et al.** Isolation of T-cell tropic HTLV-III-like retrovirus from macaques. Science 1985; 228:1201–1204.

22 **Khabbaz RF, Rowe T, Murphey-Corb M, et al.** Simian immunodeficiency virus needle-stick accident in a laboratory worker. Lancet 1992;340:271–273.

23 **Khabbaz RF, Heneine W, George JR, et al.** Brief report: infection of a laboratory worker with simian immunodeficiency virus. N Engl J Med 1994;330:172–177.

24 **Jin MJ, Rogers J, Phillips-Conroy JE, et al.** Infection of a yellow baboon with simian immunodeficiency virus from African green monkeys: evidence for cross-species transmission in the wild. J Virol 1994;68:8454–8460.

25 **Gao F, Yue L, Robertson DL, et al.** Genetic diversity of human immunodeficiency virus type 2: evidence for distinct sequence subtypes with differences in virus biology. J Virol 1994;68:7433–7447.

26 **Sharp PM, Li W-H.** Understanding the origins of AIDS viruses. Nature 1988;336:315.

27 **Li W-H, Tanimura M, Sharp PM.** Rates and dates of divergence between AIDS virus nucleotide sequences. Mol Biol Evol 1988;5: 313–330.

28 **Hirsch VM, Dapolito GA, Goldstein S, et al.** A distinct African lentivirus from Sykes' monkeys. J Virol 1993;67:1517–1528.

29 **Hirsch VM, McGann C, Dapolito G, et al.** Identification of a new subgroup of SIVagm in tantalus monkeys. Virology 1993;197:426–430.

30 **Muller MC, Saksena NK, Nerrienet E, et al.** Simian immunodeficiency viruses from central and western Africa: evidence for a new species-specific lentivirus in tantalus monkeys. J Virol 1993;67:1227–1235.

31 **Allan JS, Short M, Taylor ME, et al.** Species-specific diversity among simian immunodeficiency viruses from African green monkeys. J Virol 1991;65:2816–2828.

32 **Jin MJ, Hui H, Robertson DL, et al.** Mosaic genome structure of simian immunodeficiency virus from west African green monkeys. EMBO J 1994;13:2935–2947.

33 **De Cock KM, Brun-Vezinet F.** Epidemiology of HIV-2 infection. AIDS 1989;3(suppl 1):S89–S95.

34 **De Cock KM, Adjorlolo G, Ekpini E, et al.** Epidemiology and transmission of HIV-2. Why there is no HIV-2 pandemic [published erratum appears in JAMA 1994;271:196]. JAMA 1993;270:2083–2086.

35 **Ayanian JZ, Maguire JH, Marlink RG, et al.** HIV-2 infection in the United States. N Engl J Med 1989;320:1422–1423.

36 **Ruef C, Dickey P, Schable CA, et al.** A second case of the acquired immunodeficiency

syndrome due to human immunodeficiency virus type 2 in the United States: the clinical implications. Am J Med 1989;86:709–712.

37 **Centers for Disease Control and Prevention.** Surveillance for HIV-2 infection in blood donors—United States, 1987–1989. MMWR 1990;39:829–831.

38 **Busch MP, Tobler L, Schable C, Petersen L.** Continued monitoring for human immunodeficiency virus type 2 infections in California. Transfusion 1992;32:873. Letter.

39 **Rubsamen-Waigmann H, Briesen HV, Maniar JK, et al.** Spread of HIV-2 in India. Lancet 1991;337:550–551. Letter.

40 **Grez M, Dietrich U, Balfe P, et al.** Genetic analysis of human immunodeficiency virus type 1 and 2 (HIV-1 and HIV-2) mixed infections in India reveals a recent spread of HIV-1 and HIV-2 from a single ancestor for each of these viruses. J Virol 1994;68:2161–2168.

41 **Kanki PM, 'Boup S, Marlink R, et al.** Prevalence and risk determinants of human immunodeficiency virus type 2 (HIV-2) and human immunodeficiency virus type 1 (HIV-1) in west African female prostitutes. Am J Epidemiol 1992;136:895–907.

42 **Winkelstein W Jr, Samuel M, Padian NS, et al.** The San Francisco Men's Health Study. III. Reduction in human immunodeficiency virus transmission among homosexual/bisexual men, 1982–86. Am J Public Health 1987;77:685–689.

43 **Plummer FA, Simonsen JN, Cameron DW.** Cofactors in male-female sexual transmission of human immunodeficiency virus type 1. J Infect Dis 1991;163:233–239.

44 **Anderson RM.** Mathematical and statistical studies of the epidemiology of HIV-1. AIDS 1989;3:333–346.

45 **Donnelly C, Leisenring W, Kanki P, et al.** Comparison of transmission rates of HIV-1 and HIV-2 in a cohort of prostitutes in Senegal. Bull Math Biol 1993;55:731–743.

46 **Poulson AG, Kvinesdal BB, Aaby P, et al.** Lack of evidence of vertical transmission of HIV-2 in a sample of the general population in Bissau. J Acquir Immune Defic Syndr 1992;5:25–30.

47 **Matheron S, Courpotin C, Simon F, et al.** Vertical transmission of HIV-2. Lancet 1990; 335:1103–1104.

48 **Gayle HD, Gnaore E, Adjrlolo G, et al.** HIV-1 and HIV-2 infection in children in Abidjan, Cote d'Ivoire. J Acquir Immune Defic Syndr 1992;5:513–517.

49 **Andreasson PA, Dias F, Naucler A, et al.** A prospective study of vertical transmission of HIV-2 in Bissau, Guinea-Bissau. AIDS 1993; 7:989–993.

50 **The HIV Infection in Newborns French Collaborative Study Group.** Comparison of vertical human immunodeficiency virus type 2 and human immunodeficiency virus type 1 transmission in the French prospective cohort. Pediatr Infect Dis J 1994;13:502–506.

51 **Quinn TC.** Population migration and the spread of types 1 and 2 human immunodeficiency viruses. Proc Natl Acad Sci USA 1994; 91:2407–2414.

52 **Ancelle R, Bletry O, Baglin AC, et al.** Long incubation period for HIV-2 infection. Lancet 1987;1:688–689.

53 **Dufoort G, Courouce A-M, Ancelle-Park R, Bletry O.** No clinical signs 14 years after HIV-2 transmission after blood transfusion. Lancet 1988;2:510.

54 **Romieu I, Marlink R, Kanki P, et al.** HIV-2 link to AIDS in West Africa. J Acquir Immune Defic Syndr 1990;3:220–230.

55 **Marlink RG, Ricard D, M'Boup S, et al.** Clinical, hematologic, and immunologic cross-sectional evaluation of individuals exposed to human immunodeficiency virus type-2 (HIV-2). AIDS Res Hum Retroviruses 1988;4:137–148.

56 **Le Guenno BM, Barabe P, Griffet PA, et al.** HIV-2 and HIV-1 AIDS cases in Senegal: clinical patterns and immunological perturbations. J Acquir Immune Defic Syndr 1991; 4:421–427.

57 **Whittle H, Morris J, Todd J, et al.** HIV-2-infected patients survive longer than HIV-1 infected patients. AIDS 1994;8:1617–1620.

58 **Biggar RJ.** AIDS incubation in 1891 HIV seroconverters from different exposure groups. International Registry of Seroconverters. AIDS 1990;4:1059–1066.

59 Centers for Disease Control and Prevention. Revision of CDC Surveillance case definition for the Acquired Immunodeficiency syndrome. MMWR 1987, 36:Supplement MMWR 1986;35:334.

60 **Simon F, Matheron S, Tamalet C, et al.** Cellular and plasma viral load in patients infected with HIV-2. AIDS 1993;7:1411–1417.

61 **Rouzioux C, Puel J, Agut H, et al.** Comparative assessment of quantitative HIV viraemia assays. AIDS 1992;6:373–377.

62 **Berry N, Ariyoshi K, Jobe O, et al.** HIV type 2 proviral load measured by quantitative polymerase chain reaction correlates with

CD4+ lymphopenia in HIV type 2-infected individuals. AIDS Res Hum Retroviruses 1994;10:1031–1037.

63 **Cao Y, Qin L, Zhang L, et al.** Virologic and immunologic characterization of long-term survivors of human immunodeficiency virus type 1 infection. N Engl J Med 1995; 332:201–208.

64 **Tristem M, Marshall C, Karpas A, Hill F.** Evolution of primate lentiviruses: evidence from vpx and vpr. EMBO J 1992;11:3405–3412.

65 **Marcon L, Michaels F, Hattori N, et al.** Dispensable role of the human immunodeficiency virus type 2 Vpx protein in viral replication. J Virol 1991;65:3938–3942.

66 **Kappes JC, Conway JA, Lee SW, et al.** Human immunodeficiency virus type 2 vpx protein augments viral infectivity. Virology 1991;184:197–209.

67 **Johnson PR, Hirsch VM.** Genetic variation in simian immunodeficiency viruses in nonhuman primates. AIDS Res Human Retroviruses 1992;8:367–372.

68 **Cullen BR, Garrett ED.** A comparison of regulatory features in primate lentiviruses. AIDS Res Hum Retroviruses 1992;8:387–393.

69 **Garcia JA, Gaynor RB.** Regulatory mechanisms involved in control of HIV-1 gene expression. AIDS 1994;8(suppl 1):S3–S17.

70 **Markovitz DM.** Infection with the human immunodeficiency virus type 2. Ann Intern Med 1993;118:211–218.

71 **Hannibal MC, Markovitz DM, Nabel GJ.** Multiple cis-acting elements in the human immunodeficiency virus type 2 enhancer mediate the response to T-cell receptor stimulation by antigen in a T-cell hybridoma line. Blood 1994;83:1839–1846.

72 **Hannibal MC, Markovitz DM, Clark N, Nabel GJ.** Differential activation of human immunodeficiency virus type 1 and 2 transcription by specific T-cell activation signals. J Virol 1993;67:5035–5040.

73 **Hilfinger JM, Clark N, Smith M, et al.** Differential regulation of the human immunodeficiency virus type 2 enhancer in monocytes at various stages of differentiation. J Virol 1993;67:4448–4453.

74 **Whitcomb JM, Hughes SH.** The sequence of human immunodeficiency virus type 2 circle junction suggests that integration protein cleaves the ends of linear DNA asymmetrically. J Virol 1991;65:3906–3910.

75 **Talbott R, Kraus G, Looney D, Wong-Staal F.** Mapping the determinants of human immunodeficiency virus 2 for infectivity, replication efficiency, and cytopathicity. Proc Natl Acad Sci USA 1993;90:4226–4230.

76 **Barnett SW, Quiroga M, Werner A, et al.** Distinguishing features of an infectious molecular clone of the highly divergent and noncytopathic human immunodeficiency virus type 2 UC1 strain. J Virol 1993;67:1006–1014.

77 **Hoxie JA, Brass LF, Pletcher CH, et al.** Cytopathic variants of an attenuated isolate of human immunodeficiency virus type 2 exhibit increased affinity for CD4. J Virol 1991; 65:5096–5101.

78 **Chollet-Martin S, Simon F, Matheron S, et al.** Comparison of plasma cytokine levels in African patients with HIV-1 and HIV-2 infection. AIDS 1994;8:879–884.

79 **Rowland-Jones S, Sutton J, Dong T, et al.** HIV-specific cytotoxic T-cells in HIV-exposed but uninfected Gambian women. Nature Medicine 1995;1:59–64.

80 **Leonard G, Chaput A, Courgnaud V, et al.** Characterization of dual HIV-1 and HIV-2 serological profiles by polymerase chain reaction. AIDS 1993;7:1185–1189.

81 **Ness PM, Nass CC.** Blood donor testing for HIV-I/II and HTLV-I/II. Arch Pathol Lab Med 1994;118:337–341. Review.

82 **Felsenstein J.** Confidence limits on phylogenies: an approach using the bootstrap. Evolution 1985;39:783–791.

83 **Higgins DG, Sharp PM.** Fast and sensitive multiple sequence alignments on a microcomputer. Comp Appl Biosci 1989;5:151–153.

84 **Kimura M.** The neutral theory of molecular evolution. Cambridge: Cambridge University Press, 1983.

85 **Saitou N, Nei M.** The neighbor-joining method: a new method for reconstructing phylogenetic trees. Mol Biol Evol 1987;4: 406–425.

86 **Higgins DG, Bleasby AJ, Fuchs R.** CLUSTAL V: improved software for multiple sequence alignment. Comp Appl Biosci 1992;8:189–191.

Community-Acquired Pneumonia

DANIEL M. MUSHER
STEVEN J. SPINDEL

Pneumonia is an infection of the lungs in which proliferation of microorganisms in the alveoli stimulates an inflammatory response or otherwise damages lung tissues. In bacterial pneumonia, infection begins in one area and extends via the pores of Kohn tending to involve a segment or a lobe; in many nonbacterial pneumonias, infective organisms spread via the bronchial tree, causing multiple areas of involvement. When the filling of alveoli with infective organisms, plasma constituents, pneumocytes, and white blood cells—nearly exclusively polymorphonuclear leukocytes (PMN) in bacterial pneumonia with a greater proportion of lymphocytes and macrophages in infection due to other microorganisms—is extensive enough to be detected radiographically, pneumonia is said to be present.

PATHOGENESIS

Within this definition, a broad spectrum of abnormalities can actually be detected. For example, common bacterial pathogens such as *Streptococcus pneumoniae* and *Haemophilus influenzae* vigorously activate complement via classic and alternative pathways; in the case of these organisms, which are not noted for production of exotoxins, the pneumonia is largely a result of the intense inflammatory response generated by the host. In contrast, pneumonia caused by *Pneumocystis carinii* may cause relatively little inflammation, and the radiographic abnormalities reflects the filling of alveoli by profuse numbers of organisms and proteinaceous fluid. Infection by *Staphylococcus aureus* or gram-negative bacilli, such as *Klebsiella*, *Enterobacter*, and *Pseudomonas* species, tends to cause small abscesses (0.5 to 1.0 cm) that may coalesce to form one or more larger ones. Large abscesses (2.5 cm), generally single cavities, are regularly caused by the synergistic action of microaerophilic and anaerobic bacteria of the mouth. Tuberculous and fungal infections characteristically cavitate as well, probably as a result of forming large granulomas that outgrow their blood supply.

Microorganisms other than bacteria cause pneumonia by different pathogenetic mechanisms. *Chlamydia psittaci* and influenza virus, for example, are taken into, and damage, epithelial cells by a process resembling receptor-mediated endocytosis. Another chlamydia, *C. trachomatis*, is taken up by a mechanism that more closely resembles phagocytosis, a process that may actually favor this obligate intracellular pathogen which is unable to replicate outside of cells. Mycoplasmas attach to epithelial cells of the respiratory tract and then damage them, first by eliminating ciliary action and then causing the cells to slough. A common sequence for many of these nonbacterial pathogenic microorganisms is to replicate and progressively disrupt superficial cell layers. This interferes with normal clearance mechanisms, thus leading to an accumulation of sloughed cells and organisms in alveolar spaces.

These differences in pathogenesis are associated with clinical differences that may be relevant for medical diagnosis. The presence of an inflammatory exudate, as seen in bacterial pneumonia, leads to a cough productive of prominent purulent secretions that have a characteristic microscopic appearance showing bacteria and PMNs on Gram stain. In contrast, viral, chlamydial, and mycoplasmal pneumonias tend to be associated with sparse secretions; only small amounts of sputum are characteristically produced, with few inflammatory cells and, of course, no detectable bacteria.

EPIDEMIOLOGY

Pneumonia remains a major cause of hospitalization, one of the most frequent serious complications of hospitalization, and a common cause of death both in advanced and developing countries. Based on results of careful study in a large prepaid medical group in Seattle, the yearly incidence of pneumonia due to all causes in the population at large is about 1 per 100 (1). Lower respiratory infection is said to account for 6 million outpatient visits in the United States each year (2). In the preantibiotic era, bacteremic lobar pneumonia, caused by *S. pneumoniae* in 95% of cases, occurred in 1 of 100 persons in the population per year and caused about 8% of all deaths (3). The incidence of pneumococcal pneumonia in recent years is one tenth to one hundredth that number (Figure 5.1 [3,4]). To a large extent, the difference reflects the efficacy of antimicrobial therapy in treating conditions that might have represented—or might have progressed to—pneumonia, although other factors are also involved because the incidence was declining even before the discovery of antibiotics.

Pneumonia due to all causes is far more frequent in infants and toddlers and persons over the age of 60 years than in older children or young adults (Figure 5.2 [5]); this is especially true of pneumonia that requires hospitalization. The death rate from bacteremic pneumococcal pneumonia increases with age, exceeding 50% in the elderly (Figure 5.3 [6]). Persons who have underlying lung

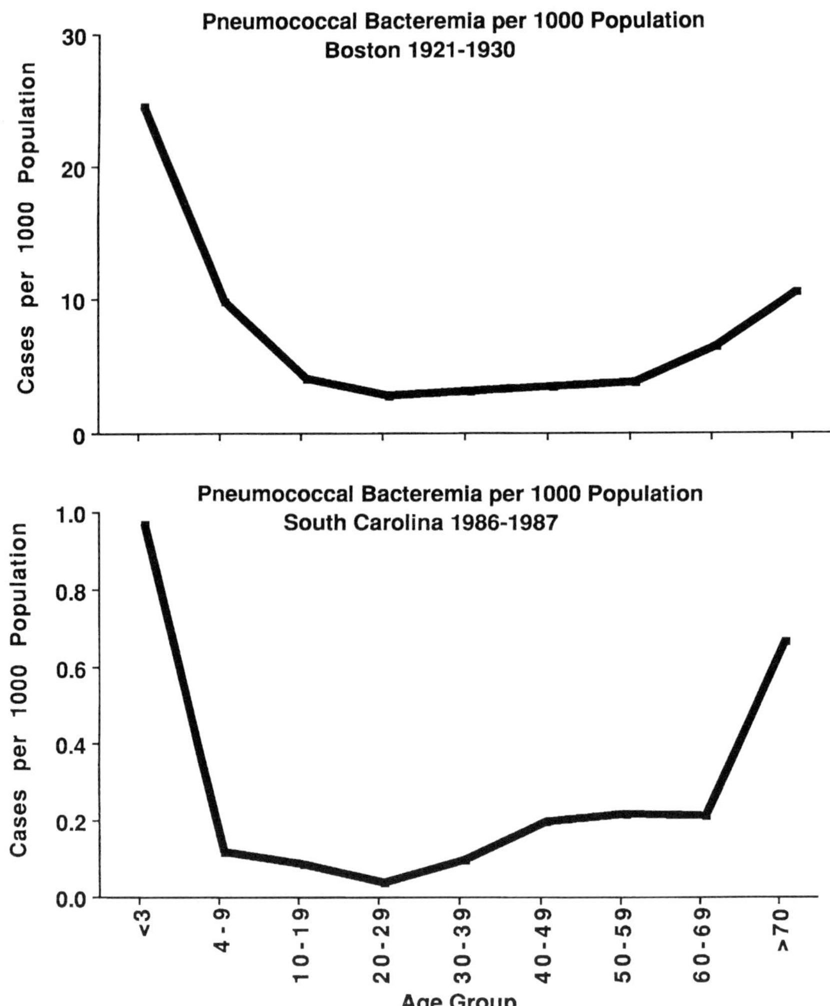

Figure 5.1. The incidence of bacteremic pneumococcal pneumonia is shown for each age group in the preantibiotic era (top, reference 3) and the postantibiotic era (bottom, reference 4). It is interesting to note the remarkable similarity in the shape of the curves, although the scale of the vertical axis is much greater in the top figure, indicating that the actual numbers of cases per 100,000 population was 10 to 100 times greater in the preantibiotic era.

disease, such as asthma, chronic bronchitis, or chronic obstructive pulmonary disease, are far more susceptible than the normal population. Similarly, alcoholics, malnourished individuals, and those with disease of the heart, liver, or kidneys are more susceptible. Conditions characterized by poor immunoglobulin (IgG) responses, including human immunodeficiency virus (HIV) infection, lymphoma, myeloma, and common variable immunodeficiency, cause greatly

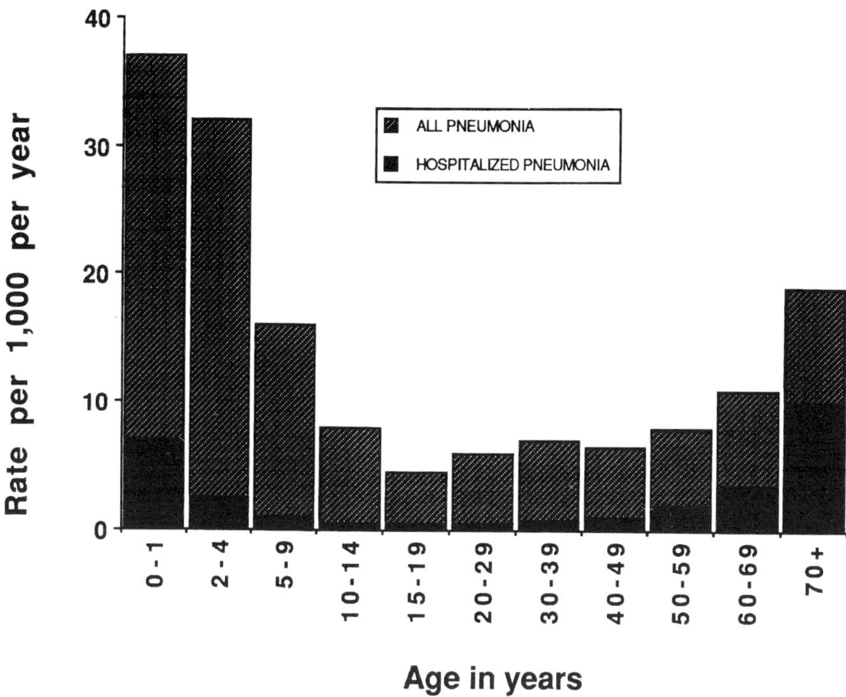

Figure 5.2. All cases of pneumonia in a large prepaid health plan in Seattle, Washington indicates that most pneumonias of all causes and, especially, pneumonias that are judged serious enough to require hospitalization occur in very young children and older adults. Reproduced with permission from Foy HM. Clin Infect Dis 1993;17(suppl):S37–46.

increased susceptibility to common bacterial pneumonias. Tuberculosis and fungal infections are more likely to occur in individuals whose cellular immune mechanisms are diminished, either by glucocorticosteroid therapy or by diseases such as HIV infection or Hodgkin's disease. Pneumonia caused by mycoplasmas tends to occur in family clusters, and Legionella pneumonia can often be traced to an environmental source. During outbreaks, influenza virus may cause pneumonia in anyone, especially those with underlying diseases of heart or lungs; infants, elderly persons, and pregnant women also have especially increased susceptibility.

ETIOLOGY

It should be clear, from the foregoing remarks, that the etiology of community-acquired pneumonia is remarkably diverse, a fact that cannot be overemphasized as health care providers evaluate patients with symptoms and physical findings that suggest the diagnosis. The extensive literature on causes of com-

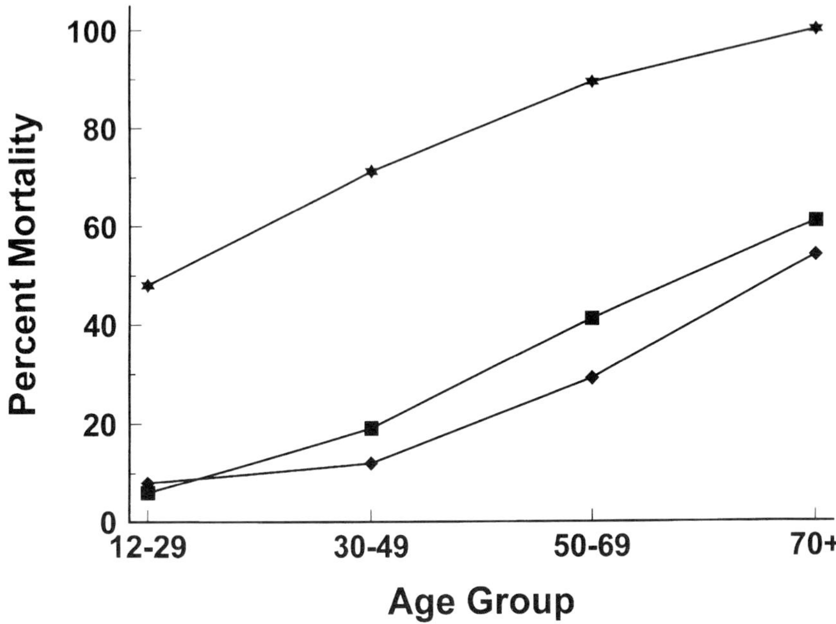

Figure 5.3. Mortality from bacteremic pneumococcal pneumonia by age from preantibiotic and modern eras. ☆, data from Boston, 1929 to 1935; ■, Chicago, 1967 to 1970; ◆, Brooklyn, 1952 to 1962. Reproduced with permission from Watson DA et al. Clin Infect Dis 1993;17:913–924.

munity-acquired pneumonia reveals remarkable inconsistencies that can be largely explained in two ways. First (and more shall be said of this in the section on diagnosis) is reliance on bad data. Studies of pneumonia, even in hospitalized adults, have rarely been based on carefully obtained sputum samples, with exclusion of persons who received prior antibiotics and careful attempts to find nonbacterial causes by appropriate cultures and serologic studies. Second is the important phenomenon of observer bias. In accordance with the parable of the blind men and the elephant, each practitioner is biased by the source of his or her patients. At a University of Washington student health clinic (7), *Chlamydia pneumoniae* was an important cause of community-acquired pneumonia, whereas Mycoplasma and *Coxiella burnetii* were the most frequent causes at an Air Force base in Laredo, Texas (8). Geriatricians in East Johnson, Tennessee (9), emphasized the importance of *S. pneumoniae, H. influenzae* and *Moraxella (Branhamella) catarrhalis*, along with *Enterobacteriaceae* and *S. aureus*. In Pittsburgh, the pneumococcus and *Legionella* predominate among the identified agents, but most pneumonias are of undetermined cause (10). With better diagnostic techniques, some of these differences will diminish; others will certainly remain. Even within each microcosm, there are important variations. At Laredo Air Force Base, Q fever was seasonal, and pneumonia in a retired military officer was more likely to be bacterial than in a younger person on active duty. Similarly, differences might be expected among emeritus professors and undergraduate students at a university health clinic.

Our own part of the proverbial elephant is a hospital-based practice at a Veterans Affairs Medical Center that provides care for an enormous number of persons, nearly all male and mainly of middle and advanced age. Because most pneumonias do occur in older adults and the incidence is greater in men than women, it is not unreasonable to emphasize our experience, although one cannot generalize it to all medical practices. *S. pneumoniae* (reviewed extensively in reference 11) is the most common cause of community-acquired bacteremic pneumonia. Our 1000-bed Veterans Hospital admits 25 to 30 patients with bacteremic pneumococcal pneumonia and, therefore, can be presumed to admit a total of 125 cases of pneumococcal pneumonia each year, with a midwinter peak and a striking decrease in incidence in summer months (12). *H. influenzae* (13) is the second most common cause and is found throughout the year, perhaps equalling the pneumococcus in frequency in late spring, summer, and early autumn. *Moraxella catarrhalis* is third, well behind *Haemophilus* and pneumococcus.

S. aureus causes pneumonia by one of two routes (14), aerogenous or hematogenous. In aerogenous *S. aureus* pneumonia, organisms are inhaled or aspirated directly into the lungs where they proliferate and cause disease. This condition most often occurs in persons who have both damaged local defense mechanisms such as laryngectomy or bronchogenic carcinoma together with one or more generalized defects in immunity, for example, caused by glucocorticosteroid therapy, malnutrition, or metastatic malignancy. Hematogenous *S. aureus* pneumonia results from infection in the bloodstream, as seen with intravenous drug users or persons on hemodialysis who have infected shunts. Our hospital may admit five such persons each year. Gram-negative rods such as *Klebsiella*, *Acinetobacter*, or *Pseudomonas* are responsible for no more than a few cases of community-acquired pneumonia each year, virtually always occurring in severely immunocompromised patients (e.g., neutropenic persons or those taking glucocorticosteroids for severe chronic obstructive pulmonary disease). The column in Table 5.1 (discussed in detail under "Diagnosis") that shows data from Gram-stained smears obtained in the late 1960s continues to reflect our experience. The 25% of cases in which no diagnosis could be made were probably due to organisms that could not be recognized, such as *Chlamydiae* and Mycoplasma, as well as viruses such as influenza and parainfluenza.

The problem with diagnosing nonbacterial pneumonia in our hospital is that cultures for many other kinds of organisms are usually not done, a fact that derives, in part, from economic circumstances (cultures of viruses or *Chlamydiae* require tissue cultures and are sent out at a high cost) and from the disincentive to request them because of the time it has usually taken to report the results. Contributing to the problem is the failure to aggressively obtain a good sputum specimen, examine it microscopically, and think rigorously about causes of pneumonia when bacteria are not visualized. Because every sputum culture, in

Table 5.1. One Hundred Consecutive Admissions for Pneumonia: Primary Pathogen by Sputum Gram Stain and Culture

Organism	*Gram stain*	*Culture*
Pneumococcus	52	42
Haemophilus	15	14
Pneumococcus + *Haemophilus*	1	1
Moraxella catarrhalis	3	3
Staphylococcus aureus	2	5
Gram-negative bacilli	2	22
Cannot determine/normal flora	25	25
Total	100	100

These data were derived from a large public hospital experience in the late 1960s and continue to reflect the experience at the Houston Veterans Affairs Medical Center in the 1990s. The senior author of the present chapter (D.M.M.) has lost the reference and would be most grateful for the correct attribution.

the way in which the sample is obtained, yields bacterial growth, the report of "normal flora" (which is the only one the laboratory can reasonably make) may hide the fact that a nonbacterial agent is responsible. In winter months, we see patients who are presumed to have viral pneumonia, especially during an influenza outbreak; influenza, or respiratory syncytial parainfluenza viruses are likely to be responsible. Some patients, whose Gram-stained smear of sputum shows many inflammatory cells without bacteria, are thought to have *Mycoplasma*, *Chlamydia*, or *Legionella* pneumonia and respond well to treatment with tetracyclines or a macrolide. For reasons that remain unclear, *Legionella* is only rarely implicated as a cause of pneumonia in Houston, although it is more commonly the cause in other cities.

This list of causes of a syndrome consistent with pneumonia is only partial. Patients do not come to the doctor with a diagnosis (such as pneumonia) but rather with symptoms. If fever, cough, intermittent sputum production, and/or oxygen desaturation are the hallmark of pneumonia, then patients with many other kinds of conditions may have this constellation of abnormalities as well (Table 5.2). Lung cancer, tuberculosis, and *P. carinii* are common causes for the syndrome of pneumonia at our hospital, and patients who are subsequently proven to have these diseases are often diagnosed with pneumonia at the time the admitting history, physical examination, laboratory data and chest radiographs have been completed. The same is true for congestive heart failure with fever from another site, pulmonary infarction, noninfectious alveolitis, and, in some parts of the country, acute histoplasmosis or coccidioidomycosis. The breadth of this list of potential causes for a pneumonia-like syndrome is sufficiently great that no physician, in our opinion, should ever be *content* with "empiric therapy for pneumonia" even though that may be the best that can be done in some proportion of cases.

Table 5.2. Causes of a Pneumonia Syndrome Leading to Hospitalization of Adult Men at the Veterans Affairs Medical Center, Houston, Texas

Common	*Less Common*
Streptococcus pneumoniae	*Moraxella catarrhalis*
Haemophilus influenzae	*Staphylococcus aureus*
Lung cancer	*Legionella* spp.
Pneumocystis carinii	Influenza virus
Mycobacterium tuberculosis	*Klebsiella pneumoniae*
	Mixed microaerophilic and anaerobic flora
	Pseudomonas aeruginosa
	Chlamydia pneumoniae
	Mycoplasma pneumoniae
	Histoplasma capsulatum
	Coccidioides immitis
	Pulmonary infarction
	Respiratory distress syndrome
	Desquamative alveolitis, Hamman-Rich syndrome, etc.

SYMPTOMS OF COMMUNITY-ACQUIRED PNEUMONIA

Fever and cough are the most common presenting symptoms, but one or both may be absent in elderly persons who may simply not "feel themselves" or "look right" to those who know them. Sputum production is commonly present in men with bacterial pneumonia but less regularly so in women. Many physicians, ourselves included, have the opinion that nonbacterial pneumonias, such as those due to Mycoplasma or viruses, are associated with little or no sputum production because they tend to disrupt bronchial and bronchiolar epithelium but cause little inflammation. However, some studies have shown extensive overlap in symptoms among groups of patients with these different conditions (15–17).

In perhaps 10% to 15% of cases, the onset of pneumococcal pneumonia may follow a distinctive hyperacute pattern in which there is a single episode of shaking chills lasting for 5 to 15 minutes, followed by sustained fever and the subsequent development of a cough. Unfortunately, this clinical appearance is termed "classic," although the meaning of this term tends to be unclear, even to those doctors who use it. In most sporadic cases of bacterial pneumonia, some underlying condition has undergone a distinct but less acute deterioration. For example, in a patient who smokes and has chronic bronchitis, the production of sputum may increase, with the sputum becoming yellow or green and thicker than usual; a fever may appear, becoming progressively higher within 24 to 48 hours. If a viral upper respiratory illness is the predisposing factor, the patient may have felt unwell for several days, with coryza or a nonproductive cough and low-grade fever; at the time of onset of bacterial pneumonia, however, the temperature rises to 102 to 103°F and cough and sputum production appear. In any subjects, but especially elderly ones, bacterial pneumonia may present not with these characteristic findings but rather with dehydration, confusion, general clinical deterioration, hypothermia, and/or shock.

Acute presentations are more common in pneumonia caused by *S. pneumoniae*, *H. influenzae* type b, or *Streptococcus pyogenes*. Pneumonia due to nontypable *H. influenzae* or *M. catarrhalis* presents less acutely and almost always in patients who have underlying chronic bronchitis; on average, symptoms progress for 5 to 7 days before patients seek medical attention. Anaerobic bacterial pneumonia or lung abscess generally causes fever and foul-smelling sputum that last for weeks and is accompanied by weight loss of 10 lb or more. The delay in diagnosis is probably related in part to the low level of health consciousness among persons who develop this condition. Mycoplasmal pneumonia causes a dry hacking cough and fever that are likely to persist for days to weeks before the patient seeks medical attention; the history reveals a similar condition in a family member in one-third of cases. Q fever produces similar symptoms but is almost always associated with headache and fever and has both regional and seasonal associations, not to mention, in some instances, occupational ones. Influenza virus pneumonia may be as acute in onset as that due to the pneumococcus, but other symptoms of influenza are also present, and an outbreak in the community is likely.

Other symptoms may be seen with bacterial pneumonia. Chest pain that makes breathing painful results from extension of the pneumonia to the visceral pleura and raises concern about empyema, the accumulation of bacteria, and inflammatory products in the pleural space. Constant coughing, especially in mycoplasmal pneumonia, causes chest pain that may suddenly worsen if a costal ligament is torn or a rib is actually broken. Shortness of breath (as opposed to tachypnea) is unexpected in pneumonia, although it may occur in patients with chronic pulmonary disease. Headache is seen in a small proportion of patients with bacterial pneumonia and raises concern about concurrent meningitis; in contrast, headache is regularly present in Q fever and, to a lesser extent, in mycoplasmal pneumonia.

PHYSICAL FINDINGS

Patients with bacterial pneumonia appear ill. The experienced examiner learns to recognize a grayish color and anxious appearance, which is somewhat different from the general appearance of patients with viral or mycoplasmal pneumonia or even tuberculosis. In bacterial pneumonia, the temperature usually exceeds 101.5°F, the pulse 90, and the respiratory rate 20 per minute. The absence of fever and, especially, hypothermia are associated with greatly increased morbidity and mortality. The skin is normal, although herpes labialis may appear in a small percentage of cases.

In the absence of complications, other physical abnormalities of bacterial pneumonia are confined to the chest. Respiratory excursion may be diminished on the affected side because of pain. Dullness to percussion is said to be present in about two thirds of cases. Crackling sounds are heard on careful auscultation in nearly all cases, but in patients who have abnormal physical findings because of chronic bronchitis, it may be difficult to be certain that such sounds signify the presence of pneumonia. Bronchial or tubular breath sounds may be heard if consolidation is present. Flatness to percussion at the lung base and inability to detect the expected degree of diaphragmatic motion based on the patient's respiratory excursion suggest the presence of pleural fluid. The finding of a heart murmur raises concern about endocarditis, a rare but serious complication. Confusion or neck stiffness should lead to immediate consideration of meningitis. In viral and mycoplasmal pneumonia, the crackling sounds may be present or absent, and the physical examination may be entirely normal. Often this diagnosis is made only when the chest roentgenogram reveals an infiltrate.

RADIOGRAPHIC FINDINGS

In the majority of cases in which the diagnosis of pneumonia is made, even that due to *S. pneumoniae*, chest radiographs reveal an area of infiltration involving less than a full segment of the lung (18). A homogeneous consolidation involving a full segment or lobe is detected in a greater proportion of bacteremic pneumococcal cases. The very small cavities that characterize gram-negative bacillary pneumonias may be recognized on radiography, but pneumonia due to any cause in a patient with centrilobular emphysema may cause a similar picture. Hematogenous pneumonia caused by *S. aureus* is manifested by discrete round lesions, 1 to 3 cm in diameter, often with cavitation. As noted above, mixed anaerobic bacteria act synergistically to produce a large lung abscess, usually single and ≥2.5 cm, which can also be seen but only rarely, in pneumonia caused by *S. pneumoniae*, especially type 3. Despite numerous articles that have claimed to show distinctive radiographic abnormalities for individual etiologic agents, it is our opinion that nearly all bacterial infections, including legionellosis, cause similar radiographic abnormalities. Except in cases of anaerobic lung abscess or hematogenous staphylococcal pneumonia, little help in suggesting a specific etiologic agent is provided by radiographic appearance alone. Infiltrates that are confined to the posterior segment of an upper lobe are more likely to be due to reactivation tuberculosis or fungal infection, especially if they are cavitary. However, bacterial pneumonia can occur in this area, and mycobacteria or fungi can cause infiltrates without cavitation in other parts of the lung, most frequently in the initial stage of infection. Lung cancer, especially bronchoalveolar carcinoma, is readily confused with pneumonia and may, in turn, be mimicked by infection due to *Nocardia*.

Viral, mycoplasmal, and rickettsial infection do not generally cause segmental consolidation. Rather, a pattern of patchy, often multifocal, involvement is seen, although rapidly progressive diffuse interstitial involvement may rarely occur with severe influenza virus pneumonia as well as with desquamative interstitial pneumonia, Hamman-Rich disease, and related syndromes.

Fulminating infection of any kind can culminate in acute respiratory distress syndrome.

LABORATORY FINDINGS

The majority of patients with bacterial pneumonia has a white blood cell (WBC) count greater than 13,000/mm^3, although in one quarter of cases, the WBC count is within normal limits. A WBC count less than 5000/mm^3 in the face of overwhelming bacterial infection is thought to reflect the accumulation of all available WBCs at the infected site; this grave prognostic factor (19) is generally seen in the presence of factors such as ethanol ingestion or malnutrition, which might directly suppress bone marrow responsiveness. A normal or low WBC count might also be seen in far more benign conditions such as viral or mycoplasmal pneumonia, as well as in tuberculosis. Elevation of the serum bilirubin to levels not exceeding 3 mg/dl is seen in bacterial pneumonia. Lactic dehydrogenase may be elevated to extremely high levels in pneumonia due to *P. carinii*.

DIAGNOSIS

General Approach, Bacterial Pneumonia

When a segment of lung is involved by a bacterial infectious process, several hundred milliliters of pus may well be present Under this circumstance, it should not be difficult to obtain a sputum sample that reflects the presence of the infective agent. Ideally, obtaining a sputum specimen should be the obligation of the physician, who recognizes its importance, rather than ancillary personnel, who may not. Microscopic examination after Gram staining should reveal areas with many WBC and no epithelial cells (the presence of epithelial cells serves as a marker for salivary contamination). Large numbers of bacteria, usually 10^7 to 10^8 viable bacteria per ml sputum, are present in bacterial pneumonia if antibiotic therapy has not been given; they are readily visible and numerous, greater than 10 bacteria for each PMN. In nonbacterial pneumonia, inflammatory cells are present but without bacteria, although the reliability of this finding is limited by the relative absence of a distinct inflammatory exudate. Microscopic examination of a good specimen is both sensitive and specific (20,21) because the examiner focuses on areas of the slide that show inflammatory cells. When a specimen is cultured, some admixture of saliva and sputum is spread on the surface of the agar, and the bacteriologist cannot distinguish between the portion from the oral cavity and that from the bronchial tree. Culture may be less sensitive, because pneumococcal colonies may not be distinguishable from those of viridans streptococci, and less specific, because small numbers of gram-negative bacilli or *S. aureus* present in the mouth are readily identified and reported (see Table 5.1). In the 1970s, when great emphasis was being placed on transtracheal aspiration, a small series of cases showed that a carefully obtained sputum sample could provide results identical to those obtained by transtracheal aspirate or bronchoscopy (22).

When a specimen cannot be obtained by coughing, further steps should be considered. Nasotracheal suction may provide a specimen of sufficient quality for making a diagnosis, although contamination with squamous cells is often a problem. The unpleasantness and potential complications of bronchoscopy or transtracheal aspiration should be evaluated very carefully in light of the possible effect they might have on therapy. The more clinically ill the patient, the more important it is to establish a specific etiologic diagnosis; the a priori exclusion of a patient because he or she is "too sick" is not acceptable because in such a case there is also the least possible margin for error.

Blood Cultures

Blood cultures yield a causative agent in about 20% of adult patients who are hospitalized for bacterial pneumonia. The precise percentage varies from one organism to another, being somewhat higher in pneumococcal pneumonia, lower in pneumonia caused by nontypable *H. influenzae*, and almost unheard of in that due to *M. catarrhalis*. Bacteremic pneumococcal pneumonia has been shown repeatedly to be associated with substantially greater morbidity and mortality. It is always worthwhile to try to culture the blood. Positive cultures serve a dual purpose, both providing a more certain diagnosis and warning the physician to be even more vigilant in the search for complications.

Newer Techniques

Even if microscopic examination and culture of sputum reliably identify the etiologic agent of pneumonia in most cases, these tests miss the diagnosis in a substantial minority. As a result, other diagnostic studies have been developed, most of which suffer from one or more of the following problems. 1) A diagnosis cannot be made unless a sputum of very good quality is obtained (in which case the Gram stain and culture would provide the same answer). This is also true of coagglutination tests for bacterial antigen in sputum. 2) As a corollary of the preceding, an extremely sensitive test, such as the polymerase chain reaction, may detect genetic material from a specific microorganism, but colonization is not readily distinguished from infection. 3) A diagnosis can be made using special techniques, such as counterimmunoelectrophoresis, which, for example, detects pneumococcal polysaccharide in the urine but which requires special equipment and supplies. An advantage to this type of technique is that antigen may persist and be detected after antibiotics have been given. 4) A diagnosis can be made retrospectively, based on serologic response, but the results are sometimes questionable in that the response may be nonspecific and results become available too late to assist the clinician. Examples of such serologic responses include the emergence of antibody to surface antigens of infect-

straightforward compared with treatment of pneumococial pneumonia. These organisms have remained susceptible to amoxicillin and clavulanic acid, tetracyclines, and advanced macrolides (azithromycin may be preferred to clarithromycin) (30), as well as to the quinolones and third-generation cephalosporins. Patients with pneumonia due to *S. aureus* or gram-negative bacilli will presumably always be hospitalized, and treatment will be tailored based on antibiotic susceptibility data. Pneumonia or lung abscess caused by mixed microaerophilic and anaerobic bacteria is treated with a β-lactam (e.g., amoxicillin) antibiotic and a β-lactamase inhibitor; metronidazole is an inferior choice because it has no effect against typical facultative bacteria that might also be present. Legionella remains susceptible to the macrolides, tetracyclines, quinolones, and TMP/SMX.

Viral pneumonia has become increasingly treatable, with amantadine and rimantidine being effective in the first few days of influenza virus A infection and ribavirin showing efficacy for respiratory syncytial virus infections. The problem of multiple drug resistance in *M. tuberculosis* has attracted a great degree of attention in the past few years. An older person who has not been exposed to an active case is often regarded as having reactivation; unless the person has emigrated to the United States from an area where drug resistance has long been recognized (e.g., southeast Asia), it is likely that the Mycobacterium will be drug susceptible. In contrast, more recent immigrants or persons exposed to them have a much higher rate of drug resistance as do HIV-infected persons in most major cities in the United States. An extraordinary rate of multidrug resistance has been observed in New York City; as a result five- or six-drug empiric therapy is often used in initial therapy for patients who may have acquired infection by exposure in the inner city. Infection due to other infecting organisms, such as *Histoplasma capsulatum* or *Coccidioides immitis*, are treated in endemic areas by physicians who know precisely what drugs are active or, elsewhere, by infectious disease specialists.

The differential diagnosis of a pulmonary infiltrate includes many other illnesses, and each of these should be considered briefly even in the seemingly obvious cases of pneumonia. A cancer may obstruct the bronchus, as may a foreign body. Failure to defervesce in response to specific treatment in a susceptible host should suggest one of these possibilities. Pulmonary embolus with infarction produces a picture of pneumonia with sputum that contains WBCs and red blood cells but few or no bacteria. Septic emboli may reflect another focus of infection, for example, right-sided endocarditis, infection of a vascular shunt, or disease in the abdomen or pelvis. In aspiration of gastric contents, pneumonia results from the presence of acid; in theory, antibiotic treatment is not indicated, although most physicians reason that the stomach is not sterile and an antibiotic should be given. Intrabronchial hemorrhage may cause pulmonary infiltrates. Vasculitis may cause cavitary lesions or infiltrates. Pulmonary edema and respiratory distress syndrome may be indistinguishable from pneumonia; establishing the diagnosis is especially problematic in an intensive care setting.

PREVENTION

Influenza vaccine has finally come into its own. Community-wide efforts ranging from advertisements on radio and television to mass vaccinations in shopping centers have created a sense of commitment and a knowledge base that leads many Americans in high-risk groups to receive this vaccine every autumn. Even if the epidemic strain is related to the vaccine, vaccination does not guarantee against becoming infected, especially among those at greatest risk (e.g., persons in nursing homes), but it greatly reduces the incidence of serious influenza virus infection, especially in healthier younger adults.

In contrast, pneumococcal vaccination is much less well accepted. The efficacy of this preventive measure is not questioned in otherwise healthy young adults and adults of all ages in an epidemic setting. However, the incidence of pneumococcal pneumonia in such persons is very low, and vaccination of this group of persons has not been recommended. In older adults who have underlying diseases and, therefore, are in greatest need of the vaccine, a beneficial effect has been far more difficult to demonstrate. The VA Cooperative Study (31), a prospective placebo-controlled trial involving 2500 older men with the underlying conditions for which pneumococcal vaccination is most strongly recommended, failed to show any benefit, and recent meta-analyses (32,33) of the few properly designed prospective studies that have been done in such persons have reached the same conclusion; however, we participated in a presentation of the opposing view (34). A case-controlled study in Connecticut (Table 5.7 [35]) appeared to show distinct benefit from pneumococcal vaccine. Protection was more striking and long lasting in younger adults and declined with advancing age such that only a modest degree of protection was seen for up to 3 years (and none beyond that time) in the very elderly.

In the absence of vaccination, most adults lack antibody to the majority of commonly infecting serotypes of *S. pneumoniae* (36). Vaccination stimulates production of specific IgG that generally remains measurable for at least 6 years in middle-aged and older adults but may decline more rapidly in the very

Table 5.7. Protective Efficacy of Pneumococcal Vaccine Against Vaccine Serotypes: A Case Control Study*

Age (yr)	*Number of Case/Control Pairs*	*Years Since Vaccination*		
		<3	*3–5*	*>5*
		(Percent Protective éfficacy)		
<55	125	93	89	85
55–64	149	88	82	75
65–74	213	80	71	58
75–84	188	67	53	32
≥85	138	46	22	0

*Shapiro et al. (32).

elderly. Responses in older adults who have serious underlying disease, such as chronic obstructive pulmonary disease on treatment with glucocorticosteroids, have not been measured using the current assay. Predictably, HIV-infected persons exhibit poor antibody responses as their CD4 cells decrease. On balance, we believe that there should be increasingly aggressive use of pneumococcal vaccine, even though its efficacy may be limited in those who need it the most. Although distinctly more uncomfortable at the injection site than influenza vaccine, no other adverse reactions have been documented. With multidrug resistant pneumococci rapidly increasing in prevalence, it seems reasonable to use the only preventive means we have at our disposal, namely, pneumococcal vaccination.

Vaccines for nontypable *H. influenzae*, the second most common bacterial cause of pneumonia, are currently under study in infants and toddlers with a view to preventing otitis media. The potential problem with such vaccines in adults is that ample bactericidal antibody is already present in persons who are hospitalized for *Haemophilus* pneumonia (12). However, opsonizing antibody does increase during infection, so it may be possible to observe benefit from stimulation of the immune system.

CONCLUSIONS

Acute pneumonia is a syndrome with many possible causes; in any individual case, the causative organism is related, at least in part, to the background and epidemiologic features of the patient. The majority of cases of community-acquired pneumonia that lead to hospitalization of adults occur in middle-aged and older men, often in the presence of an underlying condition such as lung disease, cigarette smoking, alcoholism, malnutrition, or diabetes. The causative agents in such cases are most often *S. pneumoniae* and *H. influenzae*; other organisms including *M. catarrhalis*, influenza and parainfluenza viruses, Legionella sp., *C. pneumoniae*, and Mycoplasma may also be responsible. Tuberculosis, fungal disease, infection due to anaerobic, *P. carinii* pneumonia, and lung cancer usually cause a more subacute pneumonia syndrome but may present acutely.

Treatment of pneumonia is, of course, dependent on the causative agent. A proper appreciation for the multiple causes should preclude a generic empiric approach to first-line therapy, especially with increasing resistance of pneumococci to most available antimicrobial agents. Unfortunately, reliance on empiricism seems to have the effect of removing the impetus to establish the correct etiologic diagnosis. In most cases, the physician, by dint of patience, explanation, and effort, can obtain a valid sputum specimen that allows specific diagnosis to be made and specific therapy to be given. When such effort is not undertaken, the physician becomes reactive rather than proactive, responding to changing circumstances such as incomplete or slow improvement with therapy drug allergy, and complications without really knowing what therapy is needed. When an effort is made and no specimen can be obtained, empiric therapy in accord with guidelines becomes a necessary fallback position, but the all-too-common error is the adherence to guidelines for empiric therapy as if they provided optimal care. Although they provide good care in general, they may be inappropriate for the treatment of an individual patient.

REFERENCES

1 **Foy HM, Cooney MK, et al.** Rates of pneumonia during influenza epidemics in Seattle, 1964 to 1975. JAMA 1979;241:253–258.

2 **Schroeder SA.** Current medical diagnosis. Lange Publishers, 1990.

3 **Heffron R.** Pneumonia: with special reference to pneumococcus lobar pneumonia. A Commonwealth Fund Book. (Copyright 1939). The Commonwealth Fund. Cambridge, MA: Reprinted by Harvard University Press, 1979.

4 **Breiman RF, Spika JS, Navarro VJ, et al.** Pneumococcal bacteremia in Charleston County, South Carolina: a decade later. Arch Intern Med 1990;150:1401–1405.

5 **Foy HM.** Infections caused by *Mycoplasma pneumoniae* and possible carrier state in different populations of patients. Clin Infect Dis 1993;17(suppl):S37–46.

6 **Mufson MA:** *Streptococcus pneumoniae*. In: Mandell GL, Douglas RG Jr, Bennett JE, eds. *Principles and Practice of Infectious Diseases*. 3rd ed. New York: Churchill Livingstone, 1990.

7 **Grayston JT, Kuo CC, Wang SP, Altman J.** *Chlamydia psittaci strain*, TWAR, isolated in acute respiratory tract infections. N Engl J Med 1986;315:161–168.

8 **Musher DM.** Q fever. a common treatable cause of non-bacterial pneumonia. JAMA 1968;204:863–866.

9 **Verghese A, Berk SL.** Bacterial pneumonia in the elderly. Medicine (Baltimore) 1983;62: 271–285.

10 **Fang G, Fine M, Orloff J, et al.** New and emerging etiologies for community-acquired pneumonia with implications for therapy: a prospective multicenter study of 359 cases. Medicine (Baltimore) 1990;69:307–316.

11 **Musher DM.** *Streptococcus pneumoniae*. In: Mandell GL, Douglass RG Jr, Bennett JE (eds). *Principles and Practice of Infectious Diseases*. 4th ed. New York: Churchill Livingston, 1994:2732–2737.

12 **Musher DM, Glezen WP, Rodriguez-Barradas M, Nahm WK, Wright CE.** Invasive pneumococcal disease and the association with season, atmospheric temperature and isolation of respiratory viruses. Clin Infect Dis. In press, 1996.

13 **Musher DM, Kubitschek KR, Crennan J, Baughn RE.** Pneumonia and acute febrile tracheobronchitis due to *Haemophilus influenzae*. Ann Intern Med 1983;99:444–450.

14 **Musher DM, McKenzie SO.** Infections due to *Staphylococcus aureus*. Medicine (Baltimore) 1977;56:383–409.

15 **Helms CM, Viner JP, Sturm RH, et al.** Comparative features of pneumococcal, mycoplasmal, and Legionnaires' disease pneumonias. Ann Intern Med 1979;90:543–547.

16 **Yu VL, Kroboth RJ, Shonnard J, et al.** Legionnaires' disease: New clinical perspective from a prospective pneumonia study. Am J Med 1982;73:357.

17 **Luby JP.** Southwestern internal medicine conference: pneumonias in adults due to Mycoplasma, Chamydiae, and viruses. Am J Med Sci 1987;30:45–63.

18 **Ort S, Ryan RL, Barden G, D'Esposo N.** Pneumococcal pneumonia in hospitalized patients. JAMA 1983;249:214–218.

19 **Hook EW III, Horton CA, Schaberg DR.** Failure of intensive care unit support to influence mortality from pneumococcal bacteremia. JAMA 1983;249:1055–1057.

20 **Rein MF, Gwaltney JM Jr, O'Brien WM, et al.** Accuracy, of Gram's stain in identifying pneumococci in sputum. JAMA 1978;239: 2671–2673.

21 **Boerner DF, Zwadyk P.** The value of the sputum Gram's stain in community-acquired pneumonia. JAMA 1981;247:642–645.

22 **Thorsteinsson SB, Musher DM, Fagan T.** The diagnostic value of sputum cultures in acute pneumonia. JAMA 1975;233:894–895.

23 **Kerula Y, Leinonen M, Koskela M, Mãkelã PH.** The aetiology of pneumonia. Applica-

tion of bacterial serology and basic laboratory methods. J Infect 1987;14:21–30.

24 **Feldman C, Kallenbach JM, Levy H, et al.** Community-acquired pneumonia of diverse aetiology: prognostic features in patients admitted to an intensive care unit and a "severity of illness" score. Intensive Care Med 1989;15:302–307.

25 **Franklin C, Henrickson K, Weil MH.** Reduced mortality of pneumococcal bacteremia after early intensive care. J Intensive Care Med 1992;6:307–312.

26 **American Thoracic Society, Medical Section of the American Lung Association.** Guidelines for the initial management of adults with community-acquired pneumonia: diagnosis, assessment of severity, and initial antimicrobial therapy. Am Rev Respir Dis 1993;148:1418–1426.

27 **Centers for Disease Control and Prevention.** Drug-resistant *Streptococcus pneumoniae*—Kentucky and Tennessee, 1993. MMWR 1994;43:23–25.

28 **Gross ME, Giron KP, Septimus JD, et al.** Antimicrobial activity of beta-lactam antibiotics and gentamicin against penicillin-susceptible and penicillin-resistant pneumococci. Antimicrob Agents Chemother (in press).

29 **Giron KP, Gross ME, Musher DM, Williams TW Jr, Tharappel RA:** In vitro antimicrobial effect against Streptococcus pneumoniae of adding rifampin to penicillin, ceftriaxone or l-ofloxacin. Antimicrob Agents Chemother, in press, December 1995.

30 **Fass RJ.** Erythromycin, clarithromycin and azithromycin: use of frequency distribution curves, scattergrams, and regression analyses to compare in vitro activities and describe cross-resistance. Antimicrob Agents Chemother 1993;37:2080–2086.

31 **Simberkoff MS.** Efficacy of pneumococcal vaccine in high risk patients: results of a Veterans Administration cooperative study. N Engl J Med 1986;315:1318–1329.

32 **Hirschmann JV, Lipsky BA.** The pneumococcal vaccine after 15 years of use. Arch Intern Med 1994;154:373–377.

33 **Fine MJ, Smith MA, Carson CA, et al.** Efficacy of pneumococcal vaccination in adults. A meta-analysis of randomized controlled trials. Arch Intern Med 1994;154:2666–2667.

34 **Fedson DS, Shapiro ED, LaForce FM, et al.** Pneumococcal vaccine after 15 years of use: another review. Arch Intern Med 1994; 154:2531–2535.

35 **Shapiro ED, Berg AT, Austrian R, et al.** The protective efficacy of polyvalent pneumococcal polysaccharide vaccine. N Engl J Med 1991;325:1453–1460.

36 **Musher DM, Groover J, Rowland J et al.** Antibody to capsular polysaccharides of *Streptococcus pneumoniae*: prevalence, persistence and response to revaccination. Clin Infect Dis 1993;17:66–73.

Infections of the Eyelid, Lacrimal System, Conjunctiva, and Cornea

MARLENE DURAND
ANTHONY ADAMIS
ANN SULLIVAN BAKER

Internists and pediatricians are frequently the first physicians to see and treat patients with infections of the anterior eye (e.g., conjunctivitis), eyelids (e.g., hordeolum), or lacrimal system (e.g., dacryocystitis). Thus, they need to know both the optimal management of these infections and when to refer these patients to an ophthalmologist. Infectious disease specialists often work closely with ophthalmologists in diagnosing and treating the more difficult anterior eye infections, such as hyperacute conjunctivitis or keratitis (infection of the cornea). They also may be asked to choose an antibiotic for treatment of acute dacryocystitis or dacryoadenitis, or to evaluate possible infectious etiologies of chronic dacryoadenitis.

Familiarity with ocular anatomy is essential in understanding these infections, and a brief description or diagram of the pertinent anatomy precedes the discussion of each topic in this chapter.

EYELID INFECTIONS (BLEPHARITIS)

Blepharitis refers to any infection of the eyelid, although the term is often used to mean marginal blepharitis or infection of the lid margins.

Anatomy

The cross-sectional anatomy of the eyelid is shown in Figure 6.1. The dense fibrous tarsal plate forms the "skeleton" of the lid. In this plate run the sebaceous *meibomian* (or tarsal) glands (Figure 6.2). These may be seen in the inverted lid as faint parallel vertical lines that end at the lid margin. Smaller glands, both sebaceous (glands of Zeis) and sweat glands (glands of Möll), are found adjacent to eyelash follicles.

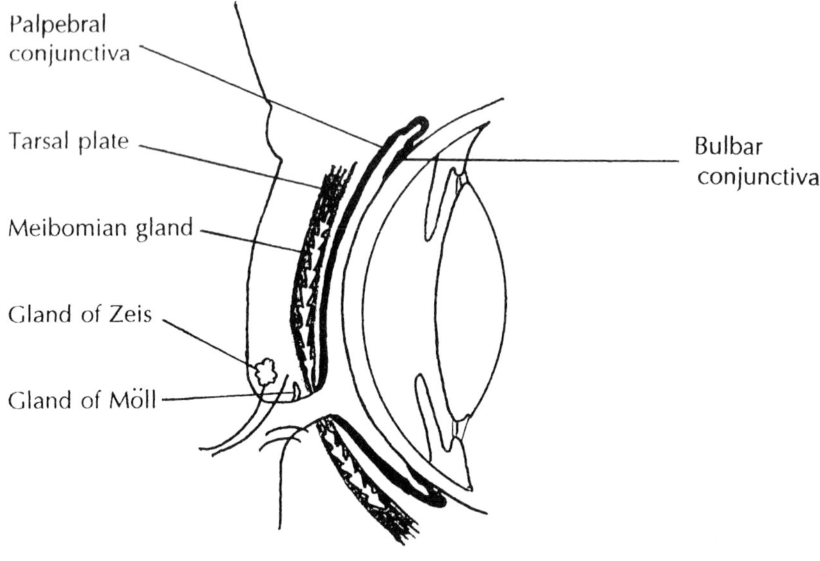

Figure 6.1. Sagittal section of the lids and anterior eye.

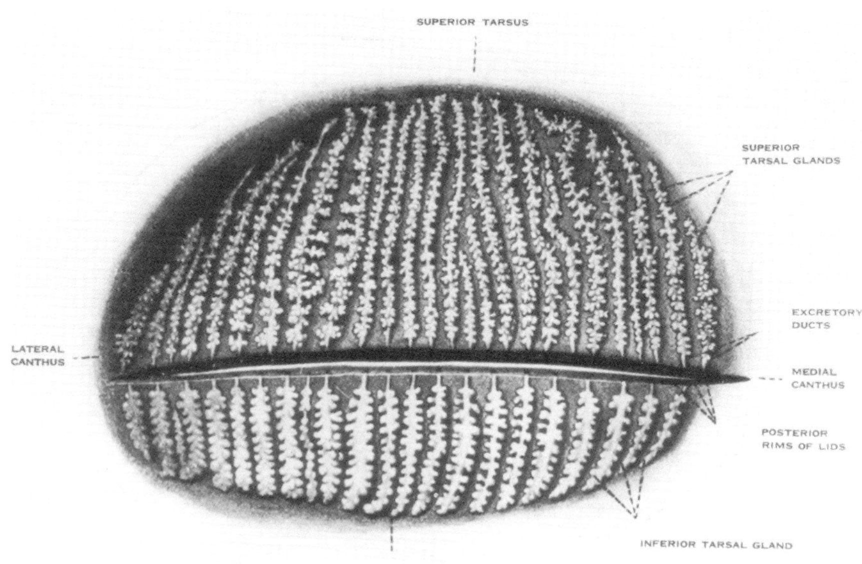

Figure 6.2. The meibomian (tarsal) glands of the eyelids. (Reproduced with permission from Warwick R. Eugene Wolff's anatomy of the eye and orbit. Philadelphia: WB Saunders, 1976.)

Marginal Blepharitis

This is chronic, with acute exacerbations recurring over years. It is often associated with seborrheic dermatitis and rosacea. The etiology is thought to be excessive secretions of the meibomian glands of the lids. Traditionally, *Staphylococcus aureus* was believed to play an important role in blepharitis. Studies have shown that *S. aureus* colonizes normal lids as often as lids with blepharitis (1) but that the latter has a heavier growth of *S. aureus* or "normal flora" (*S. epidermidis* and *Propionibacterium acnes*) (1). The main symptoms are burning and itching of the lid margins, which show redness, scaling, crusting, telangiectatic vessels, and, in severe cases, destruction of lash follicles and tiny ulcerations.

Treatment for acute exacerbations includes gentle scrubbing of the lids with a warm washcloth and application of bacitracin or erythromycin ointment to the base of the lashes 2 to 4 times daily for the first 2 weeks, tapering to once nightly over the next few weeks. For severe cases, it may be helpful to add a topical steroid (e.g., prednisolone acetate 0.125%) and oral tetracycline (250 mg four times a day) or minocycline (50 mg twice a day) for the first 2 weeks, then tapering the antibiotic to once daily for several weeks. Patients with recurrent exacerbations often have associated rosacea. These patients should wash scalp, lashes, and eyebrows twice weekly with a lather of baby shampoo, wash the lids twice daily to remove scales, apply bacitracin or erythromycin ointment nightly, and, in severe cases, take a maintenance dose of tetracycline (250 mg orally every day).

Hordeolum

This is an infection of a sebaceous gland of the lid. If a meibomian gland is infected, an internal hordeolum results; if a gland of Zeis is infected, an external hordeolum (stye) results. A stye points to the lash margin. The main pathogen is *S. aureus*. Treatment consists of frequent (every 4 to 6 hours) warm compresses and topical bacitracin or erythromycin ointment at night. Incision and drainage is indicated if this treatment fails.

Chalazion

This is a sterile granulomatous reaction to inspissated sebum in a "plugged" meibomian gland. An acute chalazion is a painful red swelling that points to the inside of the lid; this may become a chronic painless nodule. Most resolve within a month, but recurrences are common if there is underlying chronic blepharitis. Patients with a recurrent or persistent chalazion should have eyelid scrapings or biopsy to rule out sebaceous cell carcinoma (2), a rare but lethal malignancy.

Treatment of the acute lesions is the same as for internal hordeola. Treatment of any underlying blepharitis will help prevent recurrences. Chronic lesions may be treated with intralesional steroids (3) or may require surgical excision (4).

INFECTIONS OF THE LACRIMAL SYSTEM

Infections of the lacrimal system include dacryoadenitis, canaliculitis, and dacryocystitis.

Anatomy

The lacrimal gland is located beneath the upper outer rim of the orbit (Figure 6.3). It produces tears that flow across the eye and drain via canaliculi into the lacrimal sac and then into the nose below the inferior turbinate.

Dacryoadenitis

Dacryoadenitis is an inflammation of the lacrimal gland. An uncommon condition, it may be acute or chronic. Acute dacryoadenitis presents with a red, hot, tender swelling of the lateral part of the upper eyelid. It may progress to orbital

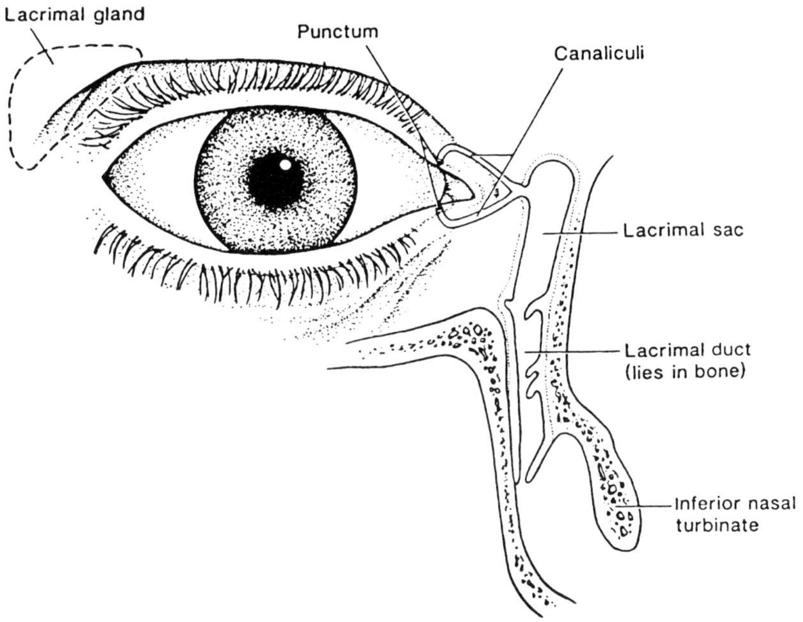

Figure 6.3. The lacrimal system. (Adapted with permission from Barza M, Baum J. Ocular infections. Med Clin North Am 1983;67:131–152.)

cellulitis. Most cases are due to *S. aureus*, although some may be caused by streptococci or, rarely, *Neisseria gonorrhoeae* (5). Viruses that include mumps, Epstein-Barr virus, cytomegalovirus, coxsackievirus, echoviruses, and varicella-zoster virus may cause a nonsuppurative acute dacryoadenitis. A case due to cysticercosis has also been described (6).

Chronic dacryoadenitis presents with painless swelling of the gland and may be due to an autoimmune condition, such as Sjögren's syndrome, sarcoidosis (7), or idiopathic inflammatory pseudotumor (8,9). Infectious causes include tuberculosis, syphilis, leprosy, and schistosomiasis (10). Tumors cause about 50% of lacrimal gland swellings (8); bony destruction on computed tomography scanning suggests neoplasm (11).

Canaliculitis

This is usually a chronic infection almost always due to *Actinomyces israelii*. Other causes include *Propionibacterium* species, *Nocardia*, *Fusobacterium*, and *Bacteroides* (12). Canaliculitis presents with a swollen "pouting" punctum, nasal conjunctival redness, and excessive tearing (epiphora). With *Actinomyces* infection, yellow "sulphur granules" may be expressed from the canaliculi with pressure near the medial canthus. Gram stain of the material reveals delicate gram-positive branching filaments; the actinomyces will grow on cultures incubated anaerobically. Expression of the material, probing through the punctum by an ophthalmologist, and irrigating with penicillin drops is usually curative.

Dacryocystitis

Inflammation of the lacrimal sac is the most common infection of the lacrimal system. Acute disease affects all ages, and patients present with pain, redness, discharge, and swelling in the nasal corner of the eye, as well as epiphora (Figure 6.4). Infants frequently have tear duct obstruction with epiphora, and acute dacryocystitis occurs in 3% of such infants (13). At any age, orbital cellulitis may occur as a complication. The most common causes of acute dacryocystitis are *S. aureus* and *Streptococcus pyogenes*, with *Streptococcus pneumoniae* an important cause in infants and *Haemophilus influenzae* in children. Gram-negative organisms, including *Pasteurella multocida* (14), *Proteus* (15), and *Pseudomonas* (16) have been described as etiologies, and, in one study, gram-negative bacteria caused 7 of 12 cases in adults (16). Good bacteriologic data are lacking, however, as most studies include cultures taken after empiric therapy was started (17).

Empiric antimicrobial treatment of acute disease in adults should consist of an antistaphylococcal antibiotic, such as nafcillin or dicloxacillin (in mild cases). In children, an antibiotic active against both *S. aureus* and *H. influenzae*, such as cefuroxime, should be used. Surgical drainage by an ophthalmologist may be necessary. In infants, probing of the nasolacrimal duct is usually curative; the

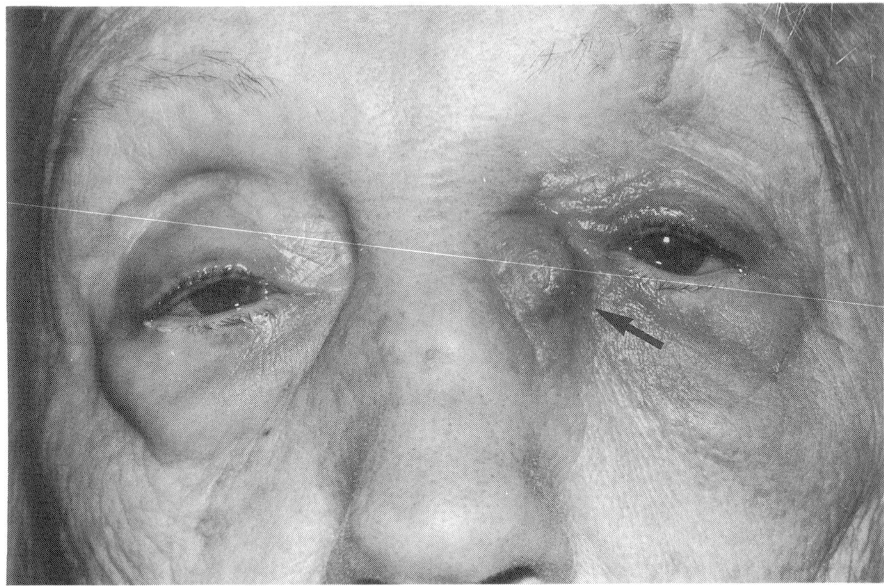

Figure 6.4. Acute dacryocystitis: inflammation of the lacrimal sac (*arrow*). (Courtesy of P. Rubin, MD).

need for systemic antibiotics is controversial (13,18), although bacteremia after probing has been reported (19).

In chronic dacryocystitis, epiphora and a painless swelling may be the only findings. The most common bacterial etiology of chronic dacryocystitis is unknown, as organisms cultured from the nasolacrimal sac at the time of surgery, such as *Staphylococcus epidermidis* (47%) and *S. aureus* (27%) (20), may be colonizers rather than pathogens. Adults usually require dacryocystorhinostomy for cure; empiric tobramycin or bacitracin irrigation is often given.

CONJUNCTIVITIS

Infectious conjunctivitis is the most common ocular infection seen by primary care physicians and must be distinguished from other more serious causes of "red eye."

Anatomy

The conjunctiva (see Figure 6.1) is a translucent, vascularized, mucous membrane that covers the anterior sclera (bulbar conjunctiva) and reflects over the inside of the eyelids (palpebral conjunctiva). It meets the corneal epithelium at the limbus (corneal/scleral border). The conjunctiva adds mucus to the tear film that lubricates the eye.

Signs and Symptoms

Patients usually complain of itching or burning discomfort but not of eye pain. Symptoms usually start in one eye and then become bilateral. Deep eye pain, visual impairment, and photophobia suggest more serious eye infections such as keratitis.

Dilation of the conjunctival blood vessels and the resulting redness of the eye is greater at the periphery than at the limbus, in contrast to keratitis. Fine papillae (<0.5 mm), each with a central blood vessel, may give the palpebral conjunctiva a velvety appearance. Follicles are larger (1 to 2 mm), lack a central vascular core, and give the palpebral conjunctiva a pebbly appearance. Follicles are characteristic of viral and occasionally chlamydial infection: papillae are nonspecific. Conjunctival discharge is thin and watery in viral infections and purulent in those due to bacteria.

Viral Conjunctivitis

Adenovirus is the most common cause of viral conjunctivitis in developed countries.

Pharyngoconjunctival fever This is characterized by fever, sore throat, and conjunctivitis and is caused by adenovirus types 3 and 7. It is highly contagious and may be transmitted in poorly chlorinated swimming pools (21).

Epidemic Keratoconjunctivitis This is usually caused by adenovirus type 8 (22), but other serotypes have been reported. Because of corneal involvement, symptoms of eye pain and photophobia may be present. Symptoms in the second eye may be delayed and less severe. Preauricular adenopathy is often present. Corneal findings consist of either punctate epithelial defects or subepithelial infiltrates (23). The virus is extremely contagious and can remain infectious on equipment, door knobs, and other fomites for up to 2 months (24). Epidemics originating in ophthalmology offices are well documented (25), and rooms and equipment exposed to infected patients should be sterilized with sodium hypochlorite solution. Treatment is supportive, and patients should be followed by a cornea specialist. Patients should be advised that they may be contagious (by touching anything) for 2 weeks after the onset of symptoms and should stay home from work or school. Symptoms may persist for 6 weeks or more if keratitis is severe.

Acute Hemorrhagic Conjunctivitis This form of conjunctivitis has been reported in epidemics caused by enterovirus type 70 and coxsackievirus A24 (26–28). This illness is characterized by a short incubation period (8 to 48 hours), bilateral follicular conjunctivitis, bulbar conjunctival hemorrhages, and a short (5 to 7 days) course.

Herpes Simplex Virus This may cause a follicular conjunctivitis at the time of primary infection if vesicles involve the eyelids, but it usually produces a concomitant keratitis (see below).

Molluscum Contagiosum This is caused by an unidentified pox virus, is common in human immunodeficiency virus- (HIV) infected patients. The umbilicated lesions are particularly common on the eyelids (29) and may cause a chronic follicular conjunctivitis (30).

Bacterial Conjunctivitis

Depending on the pace of disease progression, bacterial conjunctivitis may be classified as hyperacute, acute, or chronic.

Hyperacute Conjunctivitis Hyperacute conjunctivitis usually caused by *Neisseria gonorrhoeae* and rarely by *N. meningitidis*, is characterized by copious purulent discharge, marked chemosis (conjunctival edema), lid swelling, and preauricular adenopathy. Gonococcal conjunctivitis is seen in neonates (see "Ophthalmia neonatorum" below) and in sexually active adults. It is rare, causing only 4 of 700 cases of acute conjunctivitis in one report (31). In one of the largest series (21 cases), bilateral involvement (38%) and keratitis (64% of eyes) were common (32). Keratitis is usually mild, but may progress to perforation within 24 hours if inadequately treated (33).

After cultures are taken, therapy should be given immediately if the Gram stain is positive. Treatment of adult gonococcal conjunctivitis involves use of a single 1-gm dose of IM or IV ceftriaxone (34). Saline eyedrops may be used to clear the exudate; the value of adding penicillin eyedrops is unknown. In highly penicillin-allergic patients, single doses of oral ciprofloxacin (500 mg) or ofloxacin (400 mg) will treat most cases of genital or pharyngeal gonorrhoeae and would presumably treat conjunctivitis as well, although data are lacking. Patients also should be cultured and treated for possible chlamydial infection.

Meningococcal conjunctivitis may mimic gonococcal disease and is followed by systemic meningococcal illness in nearly 20% (35). Treatment is with systemic penicillin.

Acute Conjunctivitis This form of conjunctivitis is associated with a mucopurulent discharge and is most commonly caused by *S. aureus*, *S. pneumoniae* (31), and, in children, *H. influenzae* (36,37). Epidemics of *S. pneumoniae* conjunctivitis have been described (38). *H. influenzae* biogroup *aegyptius* has caused epidemic conjunctivitis in warm humid climates and also causes conjunctivitis as part of Brazilian purpuric fever (39). Other gram-negative bacteria are rare causes of conjunctivitis, but a nosocomial outbreak of *Pseudomonas* conjunctivitis has been reported (40). *Moraxella catarrhalis* may also cause acute conjunctivitis, at times in outbreaks (41,42).

It has been recommended that children with *H. influenzae* conjunctivitis be treated with oral as well as topical antibiotics to avoid the conjunctivitis-otitis media syndrome (43). Other types of bacterial conjunctivitis need only be treated topically with antibiotic drops (every 2 to 4 hours) or ointment (every 4 to 6 hours), usually for 7 to 10 days. Table 6.1 lists some commercially available preparations. For infections due to gram-positive bacteria or for empiric therapy of mild cases, bacitracin or erythromycin ointments are useful; for infections due to gram-negative bacteria, ciprofloxacin, gentamicin, or tobramycin drops are used. For empiric therapy of cases of moderate severity, sulfonamides are frequently used (44), although combinations of bacitracin/polymyxin B and trimethoprim/polymyxin B also provide broad-spectrum coverage.

About 10% of patients with early Lyme disease have conjunctivitis (45,46). Patients with classic cat-scratch disease have a unilateral follicular conjunctivitis (47) associated with adenopathy (Parinaud's syndrome). Both of these illnesses are treated with systemic antibiotics.

Chronic Conjunctivitis Chronic conjunctivitis may be divided into two types: follicular and nonfollicular. Nonfollicular chronic conjunctivitis is usually caused by *S. aureus* and *Moraxella lacunata* and may be associated with chronic blepharitis. If blepharitis is present, treatment should include lid hygiene as well as topical antibiotics. Anaerobes rarely cause chronic conjunctivitis, and a response to oral metronidazole plus amoxicillin has been described (48).

Table 6.1. Some Commercially Available Antibiotic Eyedrops and Ophthalmic Ointments

Antibiotic	*Trade Name**	*Concentration*
Bacitracin (o)	AK-TRACIN	500 units/gm
Ciprofloxacin (s)	Ciloxan	0.3%
Erythromycin (o)	—	0.5%
Gentamicin (o,s)	Genoptic, Gentacidin	0.3%
Sulfacetamide sodium (o)	AK-SULF, Cetamide	10%
Sulfacetamide sodium (s)	Ocu-Sul-10, -15, -30	10%, 15%, 30%
Sulfisoxazole dioloamine (s)	Gantrisin	4%
Tetracycline (o,s)	Achromycin	1%
Tobramycin (o,s)	Tobrex	0.3%
Combinations		
Bacitracin, polymyxin B (o)	Polysporin	—
Neomycin, polymyxin B, plus bacitracin (o) or gramicidin (s)	Neosporin	—
Trimethoprim, polymyxin B (s)	Polytrim	—

*The trade name list is not all-inclusive. In addition, most of these antibiotics are also available as generic preparations.
o, ointment available; s, solution (eyedrops) available.

Follicular chronic conjunctivitis is primarily caused by *Chlamydia trachomatis*. This organism causes two distinct ocular syndromes: trachoma, caused by serotypes A to C, and inclusion conjunctivitis, caused by types D to K.

Trachoma is a leading cause of blindness in parts of Africa, the Middle East, and northern India, where many children acquire the infection by age 2 years (49). The prevalence of active disease closely correlates with the availability of water for personal hygiene and with the standard of living (50). Although the initial infection may heal spontaneously, repeated reinfections lead progressively to chronic conjunctivitis, corneal vascularization, scarring, and scar retraction.

Inclusion conjunctivitis occurs in neonates (see "Ophthalmia neonatorum" below) and sexually active adults. Adult inclusion conjunctivitis occurs in about 1 in 300 patients with genital chlamydial infections (51). It is a bilateral conjunctivitis, with minimal discharge, characterized by follicles on the conjunctiva lining the lower lid; in trachoma, follicles are found under the upper lid. Unlike trachoma, scarring of the cornea does not typically occur, although untreated adult inclusion conjunctivitis may last for months to years (52).

Diagnosis of either trachoma or inclusion conjunctivitis is by isolation of chlamydia in tissue culture, demonstration of chlamydial antigen by direct fluorescent monoclonal antibody stain or by enzyme immunoassay (53) (e.g. MicroTrak, Syva Corp., Palo Alto, CA; Chlamydiazyme, Abbott Laboratories, N. Chicago, IL), or by nucleic acid hybridization technique (e.g. Gen-Probe PACE 2, Gen-Probe Inc, San Diego, CA). These methods are more sensitive than Giemsa stain, which shows basophilic inclusion bodies in conjunctival cell cytoplasm.

An oral tetracycline (e.g., doxycycline 100 mg twice daily) or erythromycin (500 mg four times a day) for 2 weeks will treat adult inclusion conjunctivitis: sexual partners should also be examined and treated for chlamydial infection. Single-dose azithromycin will treat genital chlamydia infection, but its efficacy in treating conjunctival disease is unknown. A tetracycline or erythromycin orally for 2 weeks will also treat sporadic cases of trachoma. Treatment of cases in endemic areas is difficult because of the high likelihood of reinfection; economic development and improved sanitation and hygiene are needed to eliminate disease.

Ophthalmia Neonatorum

This process refers to any conjunctival inflammation, infectious or not, occurring during the first month of life. Gonococci are the most serious cause, and chlamydiae, the most common infectious cause (54). The usual time of onset of symptoms varies somewhat between these etiologic agents, gonococci causing ophthalmia earlier than chlamydia (days 2 to 5 vs. days 5 to 14), for example, but there is sufficient overlap in timing and clinical appearance that smears and cultures of the exudate should be obtained in all cases.

Silver nitrate prophylaxis reduced the incidence of gonococcal ophthalmia neonatorum from 10% to 0.3% after its introduction in 1881. Before this, ophthalmia neonatorum was the leading cause of blindness in European children (55). All currently used types of prophylaxis—silver nitrate, erythromycin, tetracycline, and, recently, 2.5% povidone-iodine (56)—are equally effective in preventing gonococcal ophthalmia neonatorum. All are relatively poor at preventing chlamydial disease, with a breakthrough incidence of 15% in infants born to infected women (57). A recent study suggests that povidone-iodine may be superior to silver nitrate or erythromycin in preventing chlamydial ophthalmia (56).

C. trachomatis types D to K cause inclusion conjunctivitis in neonates, as in adults. Newborns lack conjunctival lymphoid tissue, however, and thus do not develop the characteristic follicles of adult disease. Diagnostic features are the same as for adult inclusion conjunctivitis (see above). Treatment with oral erythromycin (50 mg/kg/d) for 10 to 14 days is effective and also eradicates the nasopharyngeal carrier state.

Gonococcal conjunctivitis is an ophthalmic emergency, because if untreated, it may progress to keratitis with perforation and blindness. Definative diagnosis is by culture, but therapy should be started immediately if Gram stain shows gram-negative intracellular diplococci, as this finding is highly sensitive and specific (58). A single dose of ceftriaxone (25 to 50 mg/kg IM or IV, maximum 125 mg) provides effective treatment of gonococcal ophthalmia neonatorum (59), but we recommend continuing this therapy for at least 72 hours to ensure that cerebrospinal fluid and blood cultures are negative. In infants with hyperbilirubinemia, cefotaxime may be substituted for ceftriaxone. Topical antibiotics are not necessary, although saline lavage will help clear exudate.

Other bacterial causes of ophthalmia neonatorum include *S. aureus*, *H. influenzae*, and *S. pneumoniae*. Conjunctivitis due to either of the latter two has been associated with an obstructed lacrimal duct (54).

Herpes simplex virus type 2 may cause a bilateral conjunctivitis in the newborn and may precede or follow dissemination (see "Viral keratitis" below).

Chemical conjunctivitis is a common reaction to topical prophylaxis, occurring in 10% to 14% of infants (56). There is typically a watery discharge within 24 hours of prophylaxis that resolves without treatment in 24 to 48 hours.

INFECTIOUS KERATITIS (INFECTION OF THE CORNEA)

Keratitis means inflammation of the cornea and has both infectious and noninfectious etiologies. Infectious etiologies usually produce corneal ulcers, and these may result in loss of vision by either progression to perforation and endophthalmitis or by corneal scarring. An ophthalmologist must be involved in the care of any patient with keratitis.

Anatomy

The cornea is only about 0.5 mm thick but supports the most powerful refracting surface of the eye, that is, the air-tear film surface. Including this surface, it accounts for almost three fourths of the total refractive power of the eye (60).

The cornea is avascular, although inflammatory cells may migrate into it, but has a rich supply of sensory nerve fibers (cranial nerve V). The five-cell-thick corneal epithelium is continuous with the conjunctiva near the *limbus* (cornea/sclera border) and serves as a barrier to infection. Breaks in this barrier are usually due to past surgery, trauma, contact lenses, or abrasions resulting from "dry eyes." These breaks allow microbial invasion of the corneal stroma, which may result in a corneal ulcer.

Signs and Symptoms

The patient with infectious keratitis usually presents with a unilateral red eye and complains of eye pain, photophobia, tearing, and blurred vision. There is no fever, and the white blood count is typically normal. Clouding of the cornea may be apparent from direct inspection with a bright light. Fluorescein staining may reveal the ulcer, although small ulcerations may only be seen with a slit lamp. There may be a visible layer of pus in the anterior chamber (*hypopyon*; Figure 6.5); this is usually a sterile inflammatory response.

The pace of progression of the defect depends on the etiology: an ulcer due to *Pseudomonas* may progress to perforation in 24 to 48 hours, whereas an ulcer due to *Acanthamoeba* typically progresses over weeks.

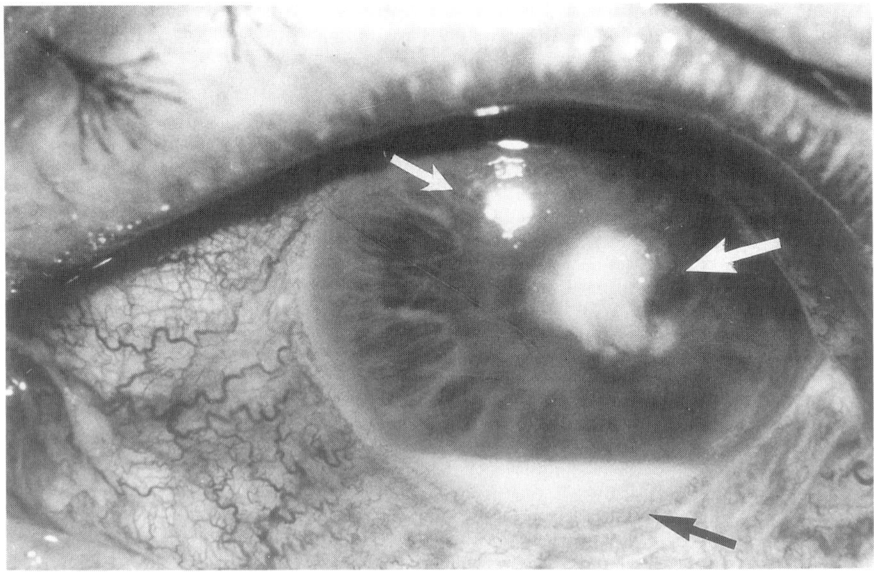

Figure 6.5. Bacterial keratitis (*large arrow*) due to *Streptococcus pneumoniae*. Note hypopyon (*black arrow*), a layering of pus in the anterior chamber. *Small arrow* points to reflection artifact. (Courtesy of Wagoner, MD.)

Viral Keratitis

Herpes Simplex Herpes simplex virus (HSV) is the most common cause of infectious keratitis in the United States, with an estimated 500,000 cases occurring each year (61). Except in neonates, the first episode of ocular HSV is not usually due to primary infection with HSV (*primary ocular HSV*). Rather, it is most often due to reactivation of HSV, latent in the trigeminal ganglion, that was acquired during an earlier subclinical primary ocular or orofacial infection (62). Most ocular HSV infections in adults are caused by HSV-1, whereas 70% to 80% of neonatal infections are due to HSV-2 (62,63).

About 15% to 20% of neonates born with HSV infection have ocular involvement (63,64). This is most often a conjunctivitis, frequently associated with a keratitis comprised of diffuse microdendrites, serpiginous epithelial defects, or punctate lesions (61,65). Other complications of neonatal HSV infection include necrotizing chorioretinitis, optic neuritis, and cataracts (66). Because of the high association between neonatal HSV ocular and systemic infection, infants should have a full evaluation. Treatment consists of both intravenous acyclovir and topical antiviral ophthalmic drops (67). About 40% will eventually have less than 20/200 visual acuity (67).

Primary ocular HSV in the nonneonate may be asymptomatic, and some patients with no history of ocular herpes may have HSV in the tear film (68). Approximately 75% of patients with overt ocular disease have herpetic vesicles on the eyelid (63), and this may be accompanied by a follicular conjunctivitis. About 60% develop keratitis (61), and this tends to be more superficial than that of recurrent disease.

Most initial episodes of ocular HSV infection are due to reactivation of latent virus rather than primary infection, as noted above. This "reactivation" disease is characterized by an epithelial keratitis caused by viral replication within the epithelial cells of the cornea. Initially, there may be punctate epithelial lesions, but within 1 to 2 days these coalesce to form the classic dendritic ulcer of HSV (Figure 6.6). There may be one or several dendritic ulcers, and those within 2 mm of the limbus are more resistant to therapy than central ulcers (61). Each ulcer has linear branches that end in globular "terminal bulbs"; these bulbs distinguish them from herpes zoster dendrites (69).

Diagnosis, usually suggested by clinical appearance, may be confirmed by culturing a swab of the cornea for HSV before starting topical antivirals.

Epithelial keratitis resolves without sequelae in 40% of patients with no treatment (usually in 2 to 3 weeks) (70), in 70% with debridement of involved epithelium, and in 90% to 95% who also receive topical antiviral agents (61). Treatment is therefore local epithelial debridement by an ophthalmologist plus topical antiviral drops. The latter include trifluridine (Viroptic i gtt (one drop) every 2 hours while awake), idoxuridine (Herplex i gtt (one drop) every 1 hour), or vidarabine (Vira-A ointment 5id (5 times dailey)) for 2 to 3 weeks. Trifluridine may be the most active of the three (71,72). Topical 3% acyclovir ophthalmic ointment also appears to be highly effective but is not yet available

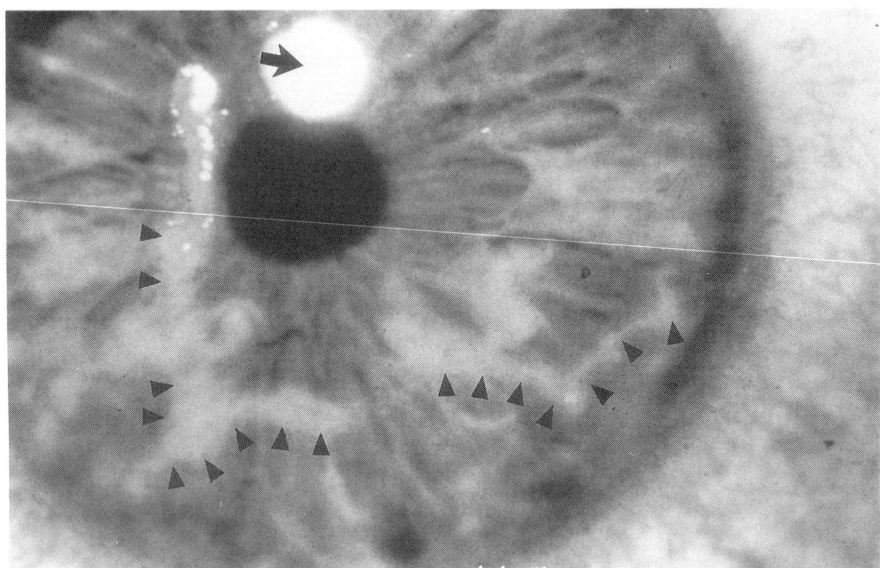

Figure 6.6. Herpes simplex dendritic keratitis. Dendrites stained with fluorescein and outlined here with *small arrows*. *Large arrow* points to reflection artifact. (Reproduced with permission from Pavan-Langston D. Diagnosis and management of Herpes simplex ocular infection. International Opthalmal Clinics 1975.)

in the United States (73). Use of topical steroids may cause progression to large "geographic" epithelial ulcers and are contraindicated in the absence of stromal autoimmune disease (74) (see below).

One third of patients with an initial episode of ocular HSV have recurrent disease within the subsequent 2 years (75). These recurrences are similar to the first episode but carry a greater risk of stromal involvement. Stromal involvement may lead to corneal scarring, nonhealing trophic ulcer, or stromal keratitis or disciform edema. The last category is thought to be an immune reaction to viral antigen and usually responds to topical steroids, concomitant with "prophylactic" antiviral drops. Oral acyclovir may be effective in treating stromal keratitis (76), and this is currently the subject of a multicenter study (77).

Varicella-Zoster Varicella-zoster virus (VZV) causes two ocular conditions, namely, ocular varicella and herpes zoster ophthalmicus. The first is rare. Vesicles may appear on the eyelids in chickenpox, but vesicular lesions on the conjunctiva are uncommon and usually appear at the corneal limbus (78). A dendritic keratitis involving the corneal epithelium may develop during acute varicella or weeks to months afterward (79). Unlike HSV dendrites, varicella dendrites lack terminal bulbs (80). Lesions may be treated with topical antivirals but probably resolve spontaneously (78).

Herpes zoster ophthalmicus is defined as involvement of the ophthalmic division of the trigeminal nerve by herpes zoster and occurs in about 9% to 16% of all cases of zoster (81). Vesicles on the tip of the nose signify involvement of the nasociliary branch of cranial nerve V and are said to make corneal involvement more likely, although this has been questioned (82).

Corneal involvement, usually with associated corneal hypesthesia, occurs in almost two thirds of patients with herpes zoster ophthalmicus (81,83). The three most common forms of keratitis are epithelial, stromal, and neurotrophic. Epithelial keratitis occurs in about 50% of patients (82), usually around the time of the rash, and consists of punctate or dendritic lesions. Stromal keratitis may follow epithelial lesions by several weeks and is thought to be immune mediated. Neurotrophic keratitis, caused by corneal anesthesia, develops in 25% of patients and may lead to corneal "melting" (progressive ulceration).

Treatment for herpes zoster ophthalmicus is oral acyclovir (800 mg 5id, 5 times daily) for 10 days. This decreases the incidence and severity of ophthalmic complications (84). The value of topical antiviral agents is unclear. Topical steroids are indicated for treatment of the immune-mediated stromal infiltrates and, unlike HSV keratitis, do not seem to cause progression of epithelial disease (85,86).

Bacterial Keratitis

Patients with bacterial corneal ulcers usually present with pain, decreased vision, and conjunctival injection. The conjunctiva is more injected around the limbus than the periphery, unlike conjunctivitis. Larger ulcers appear as gray-white well-defined lesions (see Figure 6.5).

Although some bacteria, such a *N. gonorrhoeae*, can penetrate an intact corneal epithelium, most require breaks in this five-cell-thick barrier to invade the corneal stroma. Contact lens wear can cause such breaks and is a major risk factor for development of corneal ulcers (87,88). Soft contact lenses worn overnight carry an especially high risk—10 to 15 times higher than the risk with daily-wear lenses (89). A recent article emphasizes that it is this overnight wear, for as little as one to three nights, that is the major risk factor rather than lens type; one half to three quarters of cases of contact lens-related keratitis could be prevented by eliminating overnight wear (90). Other risk factors for corneal ulcers (and epithelial defects) include trauma (e.g., corneal abrasion), previous corneal graft (penetrating keratoplasty) (91), chronic corneal disease (e.g., bullous keratitis) (92), dry eyes, exposure keratitis (e.g., in comatose patients), absence of normal corneal sensation (neurotrophic keratitis), and topical steroid use. Contaminated ocular solutions (93), lens cases, eyedroppers (94), and mascara (95) may be sources of pathogens for some cases of keratitis.

Many different bacteria can cause corneal ulcers. In one recent study, gram-positive organisms caused about 75% and gram-negative organisms 25% of culture-positive cases (96). Most common were coagulase-negative staphylococci (29%), *S. aureus* (17%), *P. aeruginosa* (12%), *S. pneumoniae* (7%), and viridans streptococci (7%). *P. aeruginosa* is the most common etiology of corneal ulcers associated with contact lens use (97–99). Gram-negative bacilli, including *Pseudomonas* species, are common causes of corneal ulcers in comatose patients in an intensive care unit (100).

When bacterial keratitis is suspected, the patient should be seen by an ophthalmologist on an emergency basis. Viewing the cornea with a slit-lamp, the ophthalmologist should apply a topical anaesthetic and scrape the corneal ulcer with a Kimura spatula or a number 15 Bard-Parker blade, directly planting the scrapings as rows of "C" streaks onto agar. Additional scrapings can be placed on slides for Gram and fungal stains. A moistened calcium alginate applicator can also be swabbed on the ulcer and placed in thioglycolate broth.

The patient should be admitted to the hospital for frequent topical antibiotic drops. A loading dose (1 qtt one drop every 1 min × 5) is followed by one drop every 15 to 30 minutes around the clock for the first day or two and then tapering (e.g., every 30 minutes while awake and every 2 hours while asleep) and as the ulcer improves. Intravenous antibiotics are indicated only for impending perforation or for extension of the ulcer into the sclera (as may occur with *Pseudomonas* ulcers). Topical steroids should not be used.

Almost all antibiotic drops used for treating keratitis must be made up by the hospital pharmacy, as they are more concentrated than commercially available ones (Table 6.2). Initial empiric topical therapy should be broad spectrum, such as either vancomycin or cefazolin drops, plus either tobramycin or ciprofloxacin drops. Ciprofloxacin drops alone have been used and have a reported success rate (about 90%) equal to that of most standard regimens (96). However, we prefer combination regimens because of ciprofloxacin's potentially inadequate coverage of gram-positive organisms and reports of cases of keratitis resistant to treatment with ciprofloxacin (101). Once culture results are known, therapy should be directed against the specific pathogen (Table 6.3). As many as one quarter of cases of presumed bacterial keratitis will be culture negative (96), and many will respond to topical antibiotic therapy. However, failure to respond to therapy warrants repeat corneal scraping or biopsy for culture (102). These must include cultures for fungi, mycobacteria, and *Acanthamoeba*, as well as aerobes and anaerobes.

Interstitial (Stromal) Keratitis This is a nonulcerative and nonsuppurative inflammation of the cornea and has numerous infectious and noninfectious etiologies. Common infectious causes are herpes simplex and syphilis, whereas Cogan's syndrome and sarcoidosis are common autoimmune causes. About 90% of syphilitic interstitial keratitis cases are due to congenital syphilis and 10% percent to acquired syphilis (103). The incidence of neurosyphilis and ocular syphilis may be higher in HIV-infected patients than in others infected with syphilis (104,105), and HIV testing should be considered in all patients with ocular syphilis. Other causes of interstitial keratitis include leprosy (106), tuberculosis (107,108), and Lyme disease (109,110).

Table 6.2. Concentration of Fortified Topical Antibiotic Solutions (eyedrops) Used to Treat Bacterial Corneal Ulcers (keratitis)

Antibiotic[a]	*Concentration*
Amikacin	20 mg/ml
Bacitracin	10,000 units/ml
Cefazolin	33, 50, or 133 mg/ml
Chloramphenical[b]	5 mg/ml (0.5%)[c]
Clindamycin	20 mg/ml
Ciprofloxacin[b]	3 mg/ml (0.3%)
Gentamicin	14 mg/ml
Penicillin G	100,000 units/ml
Sulfacetamide[b]	10%, 15%, 30%
Sulfisoxazole[b]	4%
Ticarcillin	6 mg/ml
Tobramycin	14 mg/ml
Vancomycin	14 or 25 mg/ml

[a] Start with a loading dose of 1 drop per minute for 5 min and then one drop every 30 min.

[b] Available commercially at this concentration. All others must be made up by the hospital pharmacist.

[c] Concentrations may be expressed either as mg/ml or as percent (10 mg/ml equals 1%).

Table 6.3. Suggested Therapeutic Regimen for Bacterial Corneal Ulcers

Etiology	*Topical Drop (every 30 min)*	*Systemic (IV)*
Empiric therapy	Cefazolin or vancomycin plus Ciprofloxacin or tobramycin	If spread into sclera
S. aureus	Cefazolin or vancomycin	
S. pyogenes	Cefazolin or vancomycin	
Viridans streptococci	Cefazolin or vancomycin	
S. pneumoniae	Cefazolin or vancomycin	
N. gonorrhoeae	Penicillin or saline wash	Ceftriazone or penicillin
Pseudomonas	Ciprofloxacin or ticarcillin plus tobramycin	Ceftazidime; or ticarcillin, plus tobramycin (if no improvement after 24 hr topical therapy)
Moraxella	Gentamicin	
Nocardia	Sulfacetamide	

Fungal Keratitis

Fungi cause less than 2% of infectious corneal ulcers (111). Many different fungi have been reported as etiologic agents of keratitis, but *Aspergillus, Fusarium,* and *Candida* predominate. The predominant type is climate specific, with *Fusarium* the most common species in southern climates and Candida in the north (112). Filamentous fungi are more likely pathogens after trauma to the cornea with vegetable matter, for example, in farm workers. Recently, several cases of filamentous fungal keratitis resulted from use of nylon lawn trimmers (113). Yeasts are more likely pathogens in patients on chronic treatment with topical steroid drops or who have abnormal corneas (e.g., in the presence of keratoconjunctivitis sicca).

Unlike bacterial keratitis, fungal keratitis is usually indolent. The typical appearance of a corneal ulcer due to filamentous fungi like *Aspergillus or Fusarium* is a gray-white stromal infiltrate with feathery borders, a raised appearance, and surrounding satellite lesions (Figure 6.7). In contrast, a Candida corneal ulcer often lacks a feathery border and may mimic a bacterial ulcer

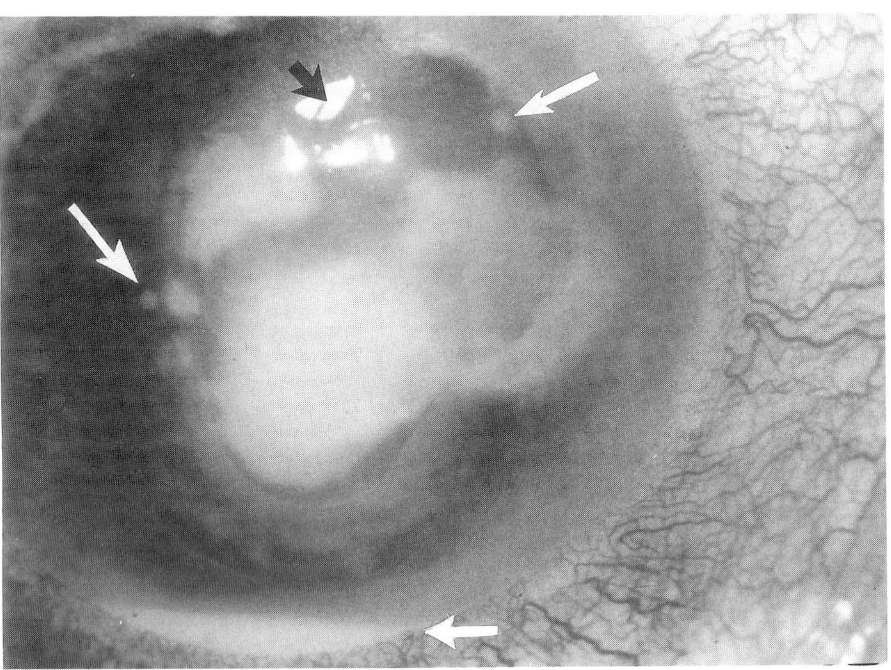

Figure 6.7. Fungal keratitis due to *Fusarium*. Note satellite lesions (*large arrows*) and small hypopyon (*small arrow*). Black arrow points to reflection artifact. (Reproduced with permission from Mandel ER, Wagoner MD. Atlas of corneal disease. Philadelphia: WB Saunders, 1989.)

(114). As with bacterial ulcers, fungal ulcers may be accompanied by a sterile hypopyon.

Diagnosis may be difficult. If initial cultures are negative, repeat corneal scrapings or biopsy for calcofluor smear and fungal culture is indicated. Biopsy specimens should be divided with the pathology laboratory, where special fungal stains (e.g., periodic acid-Schiff and Gomori methenamine silver) should be requested.

Therapy may also be difficult (112,115). Natamycin, a polyene, is the only topical antifungal agent approved by the U.S. Food and Drug Administration. It is especially useful for treating *Fusarium* infections. Topical solutions of other antifungal agents, such as amphotericin, must be made by the hospital pharmacy, usually from the intravenous solution. Recommended therapy is listed in Table 6.4. Drops should be given hourly around the clock for the first several days and then slowly tapered. Prolonged therapy (3 months) has been recommended, especially for keratitis due to filamentous fungi (116). Topical miconazole has been used for over a decade to treat keratomycosis (117), but experience with the newer azoles is more limited (118). Topical or oral ketoconazole and fluconazole produce high corneal and aqueous levels in rabbits (119–121) (oral fluconazole > ketoconazole) (121), and topical fluconazole successfully treats candida keratitis in rabbits (122). We now consider adding oral fluconazole (400 to 800 mg every day) to standard topical therapy (see Table 6.4) when treating candida keratitis, carefully monitoring liver function tests while on fluconazole. Itraconazole is the only azole active against *Aspergillus*, but intraocular concentrations are low after oral administration in the rabbit model (121), and its usefulness in treating keratomycosis is unknown (123).

Parasitic Keratitis

Acanthamoeba Acanthamoeba is a rare cause of keratitis, but the most common cause of parasitic keratitis in the United States. The first case was diagnosed in 1973 (124), and most cases have been reported in the literature

Table 6.4. Topical Treatment of Fungal Corneal Ulcers

Organism	*Drug*	*Topical Concentration*
*Candida**	Amphotericin	1.5 or 3 mg/ml (0.15 or 0.3%)
	Flucytosine	10 mg/ml
Aspergillus	Amphotericin	1.5 or 3 mg/ml
Fusarium	Natamycin	5%

*We add oral fluconazole (400 to 800 mg every day) for severe cases of candida keratitis.

over the past 10 years (125). Contact lens wear, especially with soft lenses, is the most important risk factor, accounting for 85% to 89% of cases (125,126). These patients are significantly more likely than controls to use homemade saline lens solutions rather than commercial preparations (127). Many contact lens cases from affected patients (128) and some from asymptomatic patients (129,130) are contaminated with *Acanthamoeba* as well as with bacteria, and the bacteria may provide a nutrient medium for the amoebae. Other risk factors for *Acanthamoeba* keratitis are corneal trauma and exposure to contaminated water.

Like keratomycosis, *Acanthamoeba* keratitis is usually chronic, often relentlessly progressing over weeks to months in a patient being treated for presumed herpes simplex keratitis or less frequently for presumed "culture-negative" bacterial keratitis. Features of *Acanthamoeba* keratitis include pain out of proportion to clinical findings (131); infiltrates along corneal nerves, almost pathognomonic in early cases (132,133); a ring corneal infiltrate (134), classic in late cases (Figure 6.8); and absence of neovascularization in the cornea despite the presence of chronic keratitis (135). The disease is usually unilateral, but cases of bilateral keratitis have been described (136).

Diagnosis can be difficult and requires special stains and cultures. A slide with corneal scrapings should be examined for cysts under the fluorescent microscope using the calcofluor white stain (137). Cultures of corneal scrapings or biopsy material should be plated on a nonnutrient agar that has an overlay of *Escherichia coli*. If the material cannot be directly plated, the material should

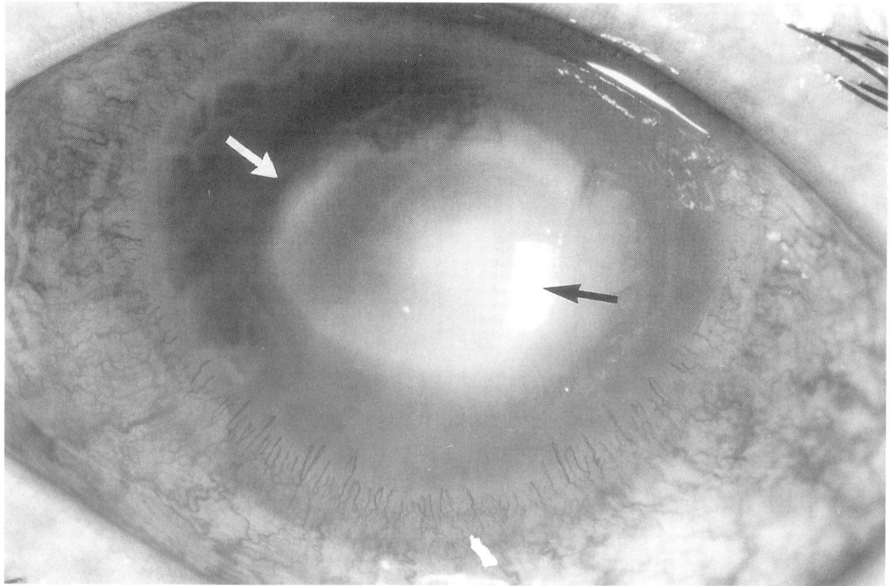

Figure 6.8. *Acanthamoeba* keratitis with classic ring infiltrate (*white arrow*). *Black arrow* points to reflection artifact. (Courtesy of A. Adamis, MD).

be placed in Page's saline for transport. Modifications of this technique to improve yield have been described (138,139). The organisms will often grow within 48 hours, and cysts and amoebae may be seen by viewing the agar plate under a light microscope. Cultures of lens cases and solutions may also be helpful. Recently, a new instrument, the tandem scanning confocal microscope, allowed *in vivo* visualizaton of highly reflective ovoid organisms consistent with *Acanthamoeba* in corneas of several patients subsequently proven to have *Acanthamoeba* keratitis (140,141), but it is too early to assess the value of this tool.

Early diagnosis is especially important in *Acanthamoeba* keratitis, and a medical cure rate of 88% has been reported (126), but this is higher than in most centers. *Acanthamoeba* is resistant to most medications, and clinical correlation with *in vitro* sensitivity testing may be poor (142). Treatment for advanced cases is very difficult. A corneal graft (penetrating keratoplasty) may be necessary but should be delayed if possible until the eye is no longer inflamed, as graft survival is otherwise poor (143). Medical treatment has been successful using hourly triple therapy with topical Brolene solution (propamidine isethionate 0.1%), Neosporin (neomycin-polymyxin-gramicidin), and miconazole 1%, as well as dibromopropamidine isethionate 0.15% ointment at night (144). Oral ketoconazole is sometimes added. Brolene is commercially available in the United Kingdom (Rhone-Poulenc Rorer, Dagenham, England) but not in the United States. Recently the disinfectant Baquacil (polyhexamethylene biguanide) has shown marked cysticidal activity, low toxicity, and clinical efficacy (145), and a Brolene plus Baquacil regimen has become first-line therapy at Moorfields Eye Hospital in London over the past 5 years (126). Concurrent bacterial infection should be considered in all patients with *Acanthamoeba* keratitis who fail therapy (126).

Other Parasitic Corneal Diseases Onchocerciasis is a major cause of blindness worldwide. The microfilariae of *Onchocerca volvulus* may invade the cornea and provoke an inflammatory response; repeated infections may lead to a sclerosing keratitis. Ivermectin is used for treatment of onchocerciasis (146).

Microsporidia have caused epithelial keratitis or keratoconjunctivitis in patients with acquired immunodeficiency syndrome (147–149). Medical treatment is usually unsuccessful, although two reports describe three patients whose keratitis gradually improved or resolved while they were receiving a prolonged course of oral fluconazole or itraconazole for cryptococcal meningitis (149,150).

REFERENCES

1 **Groden LR, Murphy B, Rodnite J, Genvert GI.** Lid flora in blepharitis. Cornea 1991;10:50–53.

2 **Raskin EM, Speaker MG, Laibson PR.** Blepharitis. Infect Dis Clin North Am 1992;6:777–787.

3 **Pizzarello LD, Jakobiec FA, Hofeldt AJ, et al.** Intralesional corticosteroid therapy of chalazia. Am J Ophthalmol 1978;85:818–821.

4 **Goldberg RA, Shorr N.** "Vertical slat" chalazion excision. Ophthalmic Surg 1992;23:120–122.

5 **Boruchoff SA, Boruchoff SE.** Infections of the lacrimal system. Infect Dis Clin North Am 1992;6:925–932.

6 **Sen DK.** Acute suppurative dacryoadenitis caused by a *Cysticercus cellulosa*. J Pediatr Ophthalmol Strabismus 1982;19:100–102.

7 **Nowinski T, Flanagan J, Ruchman M.** Lacrimal gland enlargement in familial sarcoidosis. Ophthalmology 1983;90:909–913.

8 **Sutula FC.** Tumors of the lacrimal gland and sac. In: Albert DM, Jacobiec FA, eds. Principles and practice of ophthalmology. Philadelphia: WB Saunders, 1994:1952–1967.

9 **Duke-Elder S, MacFaul P.** The ocular adnexa. In: System of ophthalmology. St. Louis: CV Mosby, 1974:638–672.

10 **Jakobiec FA, Gess L, Zimmerman LE.** Granulomatous dacryoadenitis caused by *Schistosoma haematobium*. Arch Ophthalmol 1977;95:278–280.

11 **Jakobiec FA, Yeo JH, Trokel SL, et al.** Combined clinical and computed tomographic diagnosis of primary lacrimal fossa lesions. Am J Ophthalmol 1982; 94:785–807.

12 **Bartley GB.** Acquired lacrimal drainage obstruction: an etiologic classification system, case reports, and a review of the literature. Part 1. Ophthalmic Plast Reconstruct Surg 1992;8:237–242.

13 **Pollard ZF.** Treatment of acute dacryocystitis in neonates. J Pediatr Ophthalmol Strabismus 1991;28:341–343.

14 **Meyer DR, Wobig JL.** Acute dacryocystitis caused by *Pasteurella multocida*. Am J Ophthalmol 1990;110:444–445.

15 **Evans AR, Strong JD, Buck AC.** Combined anaerobic and coliform infection in acute dacryocystitis. J Pediatr Ophthalmol Strabismus 1991;28:292.

16 **Cahill KV, Burns JA.** Management of acute dacryocystitis in adults. Ophthalmic Plast Reconstruct Surg 1993;9:38–41.

17 **Coden DJ, Hornblass A, Haas BD.** Clinical bacteriology of dacryocystitis in adults. Ophthalmic Plast Reconstruct Surg 1993;9:125–131.

18 **Katz NNK.** Treatment of acute dacryocystitis in neonates: discussion. J Pediatr Ophthalmol Strabismus 1991; 28:343.

19 **Gordon RA, Schaeffer A, Sood S.** Bacteremia following nasolacrimal duct probing. Ophthalmology 1990;97(suppl): 149.

20 **Blicker JA, Buffam FV.** Lacrimal sac, conjunctival, and nasal culture results in dacryocystorhinostomy patients. Ophthalmic Plast Reconstr Surg 1993;9:43–46.

21 Outbreak of pharyngoconjunctival fever at a summer camp. North Carolina, 1991. Infect Control Hosp Epidemiol 1992;13:499–500.

22 **Murrah WF.** Epidemic keratoconjunctivitis. Ann Ophthalmol 1988;20:36–38.

23 **Dawson CR, Hanna L, Wood TR, et al.** Adenovirus type 8 keratoconjunctivitis. III. Epidemiologic, clinical, and microbiologic features. Am J Ophthalmol 1970;69:473.

24 **Syed NA, Hyndiuk RA.** Infectious conjunctivitis. Infect Dis Clin North Am 1992;6:789–805.

25 **Dawson CR, Darrell D.** Infections due to adenovirus type 8 in the United States. I. An outbreak of epidemic keratoconjuncitivitis originating in physician's office. N Engl J Med 1963;268:1031–1034.

26 **Communicable Disease Surveillance Centre.** Acute hemorrhagic conjunctivitis. Br Med J 1982;284:833–834.

27 **Christopher S, Theogaraj S, Godbole S, John TJ.** An epidemic of acute hemorrhagic conjunctivitis due to coxsackievirus A24. J Infect Dis 1982;146:16–19.

28 **Hatch MH, Malison MD, Palmer EL.** Isolation of enterovirus 70 from patients with acute hemorrhagic conjunctivitis in Key West, Florida. N Engl J Med 1981;305:1648–1649. Letter.

29 **Berger TG.** Dermatologic care in the AIDS patient. In: Sande MA, Volberding PA, eds. The medical management of AIDS. 3rd ed. Philadelphia: WB Saunders, 1992:145–160.

30 **Kohn SR.** Molluscum contagiosum in patients with acquired immune deficiency syndrome. Arch Ophthalmol 1987;105:458. Letter.

31 **Stenson S, Newman R, Fedukowicz H.** Laboratory studies in acute conjunctivitis. Arch Ophthalmol 1982;100:1275–1277.

32 **Wan WL, Farkas GC, May WN, Robin JB.** The clinical characteristics and course of adult gonococcal conjunctivitis. Am J Ophthalmol 1986;102:575–583.

33 **Ullman S, Roussell TJ, Culbertson WW, et al.** *Neisseria gonorrhoeae* keratoconjunctivitis. Ophthalmology 1987;94:525–531.

34 **Centers for Disease Control and Prevention.** 1993 sexually transmitted diseases treatment guidelines. MMWR 1993;42:60.

35 **Barquet N, Gasser I, Domingo P, et al.** Primary meningococcal conjunctivitis: report of 21 patients and review. Rev Infect Dis 1990;12:838–847.

36 **Trottier S, Stenberg K, VonRosen IA, et al.** *Haemophilus influenzae* causing conjunctivitis in day-care children. Pediatr Infect Dis J 1991;10:578–584.

37 **Weiss A, Brinser JH, Nazar-Stewart V.** Acute conjunctivitis in childhood. J Pediatr 1993;122:10–14.

38 **Shayegani M, Parsons LM, Gibbons WE Jr, et al.** Characterization of non-typeable *Streptococcus pneumoniae*-like organisms isolated from outbreaks of conjunctivitis. J Clin Microbiol 1982;16:8.

39 **Harrison LH, da Silva GA, Pittman M, et al.** Epidemiology and clinical spectrum of Brazilian purpuric fever. Brazilian purpuric fever study group. J Clin Microbiol 1989;27:599–604.

40 **King S, Devi SP, Mindroff C, et al.** Nosocomial *Pseudomonas aeruginosa* conjunctivitis in a pediatric hospital. Infect Control Hosp Epidemiol 1988;9:77–80.

41 **Romberger JA, Wald ER, Wright PF.** *Branhamella catarrhalis* conjunctivitis. South Med J 1987;80:926–928.

42 **Schwartz B, Harrison LH, Motter JS, et al.** Investigation of an outbreak of Moraxella conjunctivitis at a Navajo boarding school. Am J Ophthalmol 1988;107:341–347.

43 **Bodor FF.** Systemic antibiotics for the treatment of the conjunctivitis-otitis media syndrome. Pediatr Infect Dis J 1989;8:287–290.

44 **Ellis PP.** Commonly used eye medications. In: Baughan D, Asbury T, Riordan-Eva P, eds. General ophthalmology. 13 ed. Norwalk: Appleton & Lange, 1992:63–77.

45 **Steere AC, Bartenhagen NH, Craft JE, et al.** The early clinical manifestations of Lyme disease. Ann Intern Med 1983;99:76.

46 **Flach AJ, Lavoie PE.** Episcleritis, conjunctivitis and keratitis as ocular manifestations of Lyme disease. Ophthalmology 1990;97:973–975.

47 **Wear DJ, Malaty RH, Zimmerman LE, et al.** Cat-scratch disease bacilli in the conjunctiva of patients with Parinaud's oculoglandular syndrome. Ophthalmology 1985;92:1282–1287.

48 **van Winkelhoff AJ, Abbas F, Pavicic MJ, et al.** Chronic conjunctivitis caused by oral anaerobes and effectively treated with systemic metronidazole plus amoxicillin. J Clin Microbiol 1991;29:723–725.

49 **Schachter J. Chlamydial infections.** First of 3 parts. N Engl J Med 1978;298:428–435.

50 **Schwab L, Whitfield R, Ross-Degnan DR, et al.** The epidemiology of trachoma in rural Kenya: variation in prevalence with lifestyle and environment. Ophthalmology 1995;102:475–482.

51 **Schwab IR, Dawson CR.** Conjunctiva. In: Vaughan D, Asbury T, Riordan-Eva P, eds. General ophthalmology. 13th ed. Norwalk: Appleton & Lange, 1992:96–124.

52 **Adamis AP, Schein OD.** *Chlamydia* and *Acanthamoeba* infection of the eye. In: Albert DM, Jakobiec FA, eds. Principles and practice of ophthalmology. Philadelphia: WB Saunders, 1994:179–190.

53 **Rapoza PA, Quinn TC, Kiessling LA, et al.** Assessment of neonatal conjunctivitis with a direct immunofluorescent monoclonal antibody stain for *Chlamydia*. JAMA 1986; 255:3369–3373.

54 **Sandstrom KI, Bell TA, Chandler JW, et al.** Microbial causes of neonatal conjunctivitis. J Pediatr 1984;105:706–711.

55 **Laga M, Meheus A, Piot P.** Epidemiology and control of gonococcal ophthalmia neonatorum. Bull World Health Organ 1989;67:471–477.

56 **Isenberg SJ, Apt L, Wood M.** A controlled trial of povidone-iodine as prophylaxis against ophthalmia neonatorum. N Engl J Med 1995;332:562–566.

57 **Hammerschlag MR, Cummings C, Roblin PM, et al.** Efficacy of neonatal ocular prophylaxis for the prevention of chlamydial and gonococcal conjunctivitis. N Engl J Med 1989;320:769–772.

58 **Winceslaus J, Goh BT, Dunlop EMC, et al.** Diagnosis of ophthalmia neonatorum. Br Med J 1987;295:1377–1379.

59 **Laga M, Naamara W, Brunham RC, et al.** Single dose therapy of gonococcal ophthalmia neonatorum with ceftriaxone. N Engl J Med 1986;315:1382–1385.

60 **Buckley RJ.** The cornea. In: Miller S, ed. Clinical ophthalmology. Bristol: Wright, 1987:129.

61 **Pavan-Langston D.** Viral disease of the cornea and external eye. In: Albert DM, Jakobiec FA, eds. Principles and practice of ophthalmology. Philadelphia: WB Saunders, 1994:117–161.

62 **Mader TH, Stulting RD.** Viral keratitis. Infect Dis Clin North Am 1992;6:831–849.

63 **O'Brien TP, Green WR.** Keratitis. In: Mandell GL, Bennett JE, Dolin R, eds.

Mandell, Douglas and Bennett's principles and practice of infectious diseases. 4th ed. New York: Churchill Livingstone, 1995: 1110–1120.

64 **Nahmias AJ, Visintine AM, Caldwell DR, Wilson LA.** Eye infections with herpes simplex viruses in neonates. Surv Ophthalmol 1976;21:100–105.

65 **Hutchinson DS, Smith RE, Haughton PB.** Congenital herpetic keratitis. Arch Ophthalmol 1975;93:70–73.

66 **el Azazi M, Gunilla M, Forsgren M.** Late ophthalmologic manifestations of neonatal herpes simplex virus infection. Am J Ophthalmol 1990;109:1–7.

67 **Binder PS.** A review of the treatment of ocular herpes simplex infections in the neonate and immunocompromised host. Cornea 1985;3:178–182.

68 **Kaye SB, Madan N, Dowd TC, et al.** Ocular herpes virus shedding. Br J Ophthalmol 1990;74:114–116.

69 **Pavan-Langston D.** Herpetic infections. In: Smolin G, Thoft RA, eds. The cornea. 3rd ed. Boston: Little, Brown, 1994:183–215.

70 **Gunderson T.** Herpes corneae. Arch Ophthalmol 1936;15:225–249.

71 **Medical Letter.** Trifluridine (Viroptic) for herpetic keratitis. Med Lett Drugs Ther 1980;22:46–48.

72 **Medical Letter.** Drugs for viral infections. Med Lett Drugs Ther 1990;32:73.

73 **Coster DJ, Wilhelmus KR, Michaud R, Jones BR.** A comparison of acyclovir and idoxuridine as treatment for ulcerative herpetic keratitis. Br J Ophthalmol 1980; 64:763–765.

74 **Williams HP, Falcon MG, Jones BR.** Corticosteroids in the management of herpetic eye disease. Trans Ophthalmol Soc UK 1977;97:341–344.

75 **Shuster JJ, Kaufman HE, Nesburn AB.** Statistical analysis of the rate of recurrence of herpes virus ocular epithelial disease. Am J Ophthalmol 1981;91:328–331.

76 **Schwab IR.** Oral acyclovir in the management of herpes simplex ocular infections. Ophthalmology 1988;95:423–430.

77 **Dawson C.** The herpetic eye disease study (HEDS). Arch Ophthalmol 1990;108:191–192. Editorial.

78 **Wilson F II.** Varicella and herpes zoster ophthalmicus. In: Tabbara K, Hyndiuk R, eds. Ocular infections. Boston: Little, Brown, 1986:369.

79 **deFreitas D, Sato EH, Kelly L, Pavan-Langston D.** Delayed onset of varicella keratitis. Cornea 1992;11:471–474.

80 **Pavan-Langston D, Dunkel E.** Herpes zoster ophthalmicus. Compr Ther 1988; 15:3.

81 **Ragozzino M, Melton M, Kerland L, et al.** Population-based study of herpes zoster and its sequelae. Medicine (Baltimore) 1982;61:310.

82 **Womack LW, Liesegang TJ.** Complications of herpes zoster ophthalmicus. Arch Ophthalmol 1983;101:42–45.

83 **Liesegang TJ.** Corneal complications from herpes zoster ophthalmicus. Ophthalmology 1985;92:316–24.

84 **Cobo LM, Foulks GN, Liesegang T, et al.** Oral acyclovir in the treatment of acute herpes zoster ophthalmicus. Ophthalmology 1986;93:763–770.

85 **Bergaust B, Westby RK.** Zoster ophthalmicus: local treatment with cortisone. Acta Ophthalmol 1967;45:787–793.

86 **Piebenga LW, Laibson PR.** Dendritic lesions in herpes zoster ophthalmicus. Arch Ophthalmol 1973;90:268–270.

87 **Cohen EJ, Laibson PR, Arentson JJ, Clemons CS.** Corneal ulcers associated with cosmetic extended wear soft contact lenses. Ophthalmology 1987;94:109–114.

88 **Poggio EC, Glynn RJ, Schein OD, et al.** The incidence of ulcerative keratitis among users of daily-wear and extended wear soft contact lenses. N Engl J Med 1989;321:779.

89 **Schein OD, Glynn RJ, Poggio EC, et al.** The relative risk of ulcerative keratitis among users of daily-wear and extended-wear soft contact lenses: a case-control study. N Engl J Med 1989;321:773.

90 **Schein OD, Buehler PO, Stamler JF, et al.** The impact of overnight wear on the risk of contact lens-associated ulcertive keratitis. Arch Ophthalmol 1994;112:186–190.

91 **Fong LP, Ormerod LD, Kenyon KR, Foster CS.** Microbial keratitis complicating penetrating keratoplasty. Ophthalmology 1988;95:1269–1275.

92 **Musch DC, Sugar A, Meyer RF.** Demographic and predisposing factors in corneal ulceration. Arch Ophthalmol 1983;101: 1545–1548.

93 **Schein OD, Hibberd PL, Starck T, et al.** Microbial contamination of in-use ocular medications. Arch Ophthalmol 1992;110:82–85.

94 **Templeton WC, Eiferman RA, Snyder JW, et al.** Serratia keratitis transmitted by contaminated eyedroppers. Am J Ophthalmol 1982;93:723–726.

95 **Wilson LA, Ahern DG.** *Pseudomonas*-induced corneal ulcers associated with contaminated eye mascaras. Am J Ophthalmol 1977;84:112–119.

96 **Leibowitz HM.** Clinical evaluation of ciprofloxacin 0.3% ophthalmic solution for the treatment of bacterial keratitis. Am J Ophthalmol 1991;112:34S–47S.

97 **Schein OD, Ormerod LD, Barraquer E, et al.** Microbiology of contact lenses-related keratitis. Cornea 1990;8:281–285.

98 **Alfonso E, Mandelbaum S, Fox MJ, Forster RK.** Ulcerative keratitis associated with contact lens wear. Am J Ophthalmol 1986;101:429–433.

99 **Aswad MI, John T, Barza M, Baum J.** Bacterial adherance to extended wear soft contact lenses. Ophthalmology 1990;97: 296–302.

100 **Hutton WL, Sexton RR.** Atypical *Pseudomonas* corneal ulcers in semi-comatose patients. Am J Ophthalmol 1972;73:37–39.

101 **Snyder ME, Katz HR.** Ciprofloxacin-resistant bacterial keratitis. Am J Ophthalmol 1992;114:336–338.

102 **Ficker L, Kirkness C, McCartney A, Seal D.** Microbial keratitis—the false negative. Eye 1991;5:549–559.

103 **Raizman MB, Whitcup SM.** Syphilitic keratitis. Ophthalmol Clin North Am 1994;7:591–595.

104 **Passo MS, Rosenbaum JT.** Ocular syphilis in patients with human immunodeficiency virus infection. Am J Ophthalmol 1988; 106:1–6.

105 **Tramont EC.** Syphilis in the AIDS era. N Engl J Med 1987;316:1600–1601. Editorial.

106 **Schwab IR, Ostler HB, Dawson CR.** Hansen's disease of the eye (ocular leprosy). In: Tasman WT, Jaeger EA, eds. Duane's clinical ophthalmology vol. 5. 1994:1–9.

107 **Donahue HC.** Ophthalmologic experience in a tuberculosis sanitorium. Am J Ophthalmol 1967;64:742–748.

108 **Helm CJ, Holland GN.** Ocular tuberculosis. Surv Ophthalmol 1993;38:229–256.

109 **Baum J, Barza M, Weinstein P, et al.** Bilateral kratitis as a manifestation of Lyme disease. Am J Ophthalmol 1988;105:75–77.

110 **Carpenetti SR, Sulewski ME, Ringel DM.** Lyme disease related keratitis. Ann Ophthalmol 1995;27:101–106.

111 **Foster CS.** Fungal keratitis. In: Albert DM, Jakobiec FA, eds. Principles and practice of ophthalmology. Philadelphia: WB Saunders, 1994:171–179.

112 **O'Day DM.** Selection of appropriate antifungal therapy. Cornea 1987;6:238–245.

113 **Clinch TE, Robinson MJ, Barron BA, et al.** Fungal keratitis from nylon lawn trimmers. Am J Ophthalmol 1992;114:437–440.

114 **O'Brien TP, Green WR.** Keratitis. In: Mandell GL, Bennett JE, Dolin R, eds. Principles and practice of infectious diseases. 4th ed. New York: Churchill Livingstone, 1995:1110–1120.

115 **Johns KJ, O'Day DM.** Pharmacologic management of keratomycoses. Surv Ophthalmol 1988;33:178–188.

116 **Foster CS.** Fungal keratitis. Infect Dis Clin North Am 1992;6:851–857.

117 **Foster CS.** Miconazole therapy for keratomycosis. Am J Ophthalmol 1981; 91:622–629.

118 **Rosa RH, Miller D, Alfonso EC.** The changing spectrum of fungal keratitis in south Florida. Ophthalmology 1994;101: 1005–1013.

119 **Park SS, D'Amico DJ, Paton B, Baker AS.** Treatment of exogenous *Candida* endophthalmitis in rabbits with oral fluconazole. Antimicrobial Agents Chemother 1995;39:958–963.

120 **Hemady RK, Chu W, Foster CS.** Intraocular penetration of ketoconazole in rabbits. Cornea 1992;11:329–333.

121 **Savani DV, Perfecti JR, Cobo LM, Durack DT.** Penetration of new azole compounds into the eye and efficacy in experimental candida endophthalmitis. Antimicrob Agents Chemother 1987;31:6–10.

122 **Behrens-Baumann W, Klinge B, Ruchel R.** Topical fluconazole for experimental candida keratitis in rabbits. Br J Ophthalmol 1990;74:40–43.

123 **Thomas PA, Abraham BJ, Kalavathy CM, et al.** Oral itraconazole therapy for mycotic keratitis. Mycoses 1988;31:271–279.

124 **Nagington J, Watson PG, Playfair TJ, et al.** Amoebic infection of the eye. Lancet 1974;2:1537–1540.

125 **Stehr-Green JK, Bailey TM, Visvesvara GS.** The epidemiology of *Acanthamoeba* keratitis in the United States. Am J Ophthalmol 1989;107:331–336.

126 **Bacon AS, Frazer DG, Dart JKG, et al.** A review of 72 consecutive cases of *Acanthamoeba* keratitis, 1984–1992. Eye 1993;7:719–725.

127 **Stehr-Green JK, Bailey TM, Brandt FH, et al.** *Acanthamoeba* keratitis in soft contact lens wearers. A case-control study. JAMA 1987;258:57–60.

128 **Donzis PB, Mondino BJ, Weissman BA, Bruckner DA.** Microbial analysis of contact lens care systems contaminated with *Acanthamoeba*. Am J Ophthalmol 1989; 108:53–56.

129 **Larkin DFP, Kilvington S, Easty DL.** Contamination of contact lens storage cases by *Acanthamoeba* and bacteria. Br J Ophthalmol 1990;74:133–135.

130 **Devonshire P, Munro FA, Abernethy C, Clark BJ.** Microbial contamination of contact lens cases in the west of Scotland. Br J Ophthalmol 1993;77:41–45.

131 **Bardy SE, Cohen EJ.** *Acanthamoeba* keratitis. Ophthalmol Clin North Am 1990;3:537–544.

132 **Moore MB, McCulley JP, Kaufman HE, Robin JB.** Radial keratoneuritis as a presenting sign in *Acanthamoeba* keratitis. Ophthalmology 1986;93:1310–1315.

133 **Feist RM, Sugar J, Tessler H.** Radial keratoneuritis in *Pseudomonas* keratitis. Arch Ophthalmol 1991;109:774–775. Letter.

134 **Theodore FH, Jakobiec FA, Juechter KB, et al.** The diagnostic value of a ring infiltrate in *Acanthamoebic* keratitis. Ophthalmology 1985;92:1471–1479.

135 **Cohen EJ, Buchanan HW, Laughrea PA, et al.** Diagnosis and management of *Acanthamoeba* keratitis. Am J Ophthalmol 1985;100:389–395.

136 **Sculley RE, Mark EJ, McNeely BU.** Case 10–1985: case records of the Massachusetts General Hospital. N Engl J Med 1984; 312:634–641.

137 **Wilhelmus KR, Osato MS, Font RL, et al.** Rapid diagnosis of *Acanthamoeba* keratitis using calcofluor white. Arch Ophthalmol 1986;104:1309–1312.

138 **Gradus MS, Keenig SB, Hyundiuk RA, DeCarlo J.** Filter-culture technique using amoeba saline transport medium for the noninvasive diagnosis of *Acanthamoeba* keratitis. Am J Clin Pathol 1980;92:682.

139 **Bottone EJ, Qureshi MN, Asbell PA.** A simplified method for demonstration and isolation of *Acanthamoeba* organisms from corneal scrapings and lens care systems. Am J Ophthalmol 1992;113:214–215.

140 **Auran JD, Starr MB, Koester CJ, LaBombardi VJ.** In vivo scanning slit confocal microscopy of *Acanthamoeba* keratitis: a case report. Cornea 1994;13:183–185.

141 **Winchester K, Mathers WD, Sutphin JE, Daley TE.** Diagnosis of *Acanthamoeba* keratitis in vivo with confocal microscopy. Cornea 1995;14:10–17.

142 **Elder MJ, Kilvington S, Dart JKG.** A clinicopathologic study of in vitro sensitivity testing and *Acanthamoeba* keratitis. Invest Ophthalmol Vis Sci 1994;35:1059–1064.

143 **Ficker LA, Kirkness C, Wright P.** Prognosis for keratoplasty in *Acanthamoeba* keratitis. Ophthalmology 1993;100:105–110.

144 **Berger ST, Mondino BJ, Hoft RH, et al.** Successful medical management of *Acanthamoeba* keratitis. Am J Ophthalmol 1990;110:395–403.

145 **Larkin DFP, Kilvington S, Dart JKG.** Treatment of *Acanthamoeba* keratitis with polyhexamethylene biguanide. Ophthalmology 1992;99:185–191.

146 **White AT, Newland HS, Taylor HR, et al.** Controlled trial and dose-finding study of ivermectin for treatment of onchocerciasis. J Infect Dis 1987;156:463–470.

147 **Friedberg DN, Stenson SM, Orenstein JM, et al.** Microsporidial keratoconjunctivitis in acquired immunodeficiency syndrome. Arch Ophthalmol 1990;108:504–508.

148 **Didier ES, Didier PJ, Friedberg DN, et al.** Isolation and characterization of a new human microsporidian, *Encephalitozoon hellem* (n.sp.), from three AIDS patients with keratoconjunctivitis. J Infect Dis 1991;163:617–621.

149 Microsporidian keratoconjunctivitis in patients with AIDS. MMWR 1990;39:188–189.

150 **Yee RW, Tio FO, Martinez JA, et al.** Resolution of microsporidial epithelial keratopathy in a patient with AIDS. Ophthalmology 1991;98:196–201.

Novel Plasmid-mediated β-Lactamases in Enterobacteriaceae: Emerging Problems for New β-Lactam Antibiotics

KENNETH S. THOMSON
ANDREA M. PREVAN
CHRISTINE C. SANDERS

The production of β-lactamase has always been the primary mechanism of resistance to β-lactam antibiotics among gram-negative pathogens. To circumvent this very important mechanism of resistance, the pharmaceutical industry has developed numerous β-lactam agents that have been chemically modified to resist the action of β-lactamases. In addition, combinations containing a β-lactamase inhibitor and a β-lactamase labile drug have been developed. Both approaches have been moderately successful in providing clinically useful agents for the treatment of infections due to β-lactamase–producing gram-negative bacteria. However, both approaches have also been met with new forms of microbial resistance. This has occurred primarily in areas where the new agents have been overused or used injudiciously.

Microbial responses among the Enterobacteriaceae to the newer β-lactamase stable drugs have included the emergence of mutant forms of older plasmid-mediated β-lactamases. These mutant β-lactamases are capable of hydrolyzing not only the same penicillins and older cephalosporins as their parental enzymes but also the newer cephalosporins and aztreonam. In addition, resistance to β-lactamase stable drugs has arisen among strains of certain Enterobacteriaceae via the acquisition of plasmids containing the normally chromosomally encoded AmpC β-lactamase found in *Enterobacter*, *Serratia*, or *Pseudomonas aeruginosa*. Acquisition of these plasmid-mediated AmpC β-lactamases confers resistance to virtually all classes of β-lactam drugs except the carbapenems. Resistance to β-lactamase inhibitor/β-lactam drug combinations has arisen via multiple mechanisms. One increasingly important mechanism involves the production of inhibitor-insensitive forms of the older plasmid-mediated TEM-1 β-lactamase.

Because novel forms of plasmid-mediated β-lactamases have been a very important avenue for the development of resistance to newer β-lactam agents among the Enterobacteriaceae, this review focuses on problems caused by these enzymes. It includes a description of the derivation of the enzymes, their epidemiology, impact on therapy, and implications for infection control.

BACKGROUND

Historically, it has been common to classify the β-lactamases of gram-negative bacteria into groups based on the location of the gene encoding the enzyme (1,2). Two major groups of enzymes arose from such classification schemes: the plasmid-mediated β-lactamases, whose genes were encoded by extrachromosomal DNA and thus were capable of independent spread among bacteria, and the chromosomally-mediated β-lactamases, whose genes were encoded by chromosomal DNA and thus were a predictable trait of the genus or species in which they were found (Table 7.1). This type of classification scheme had its advantages in that it also tended to separate the enzymes along several additional lines as well. This classification separated the mode of enzymatic expression. Plasmid-mediated enzymes in gram-negative bacteria are constitutively expressed, whereas chromosomal β-lactamases are often inducible. It also separated the enzymes in terms of their susceptibility to β-lactamase inhibitors. Most plasmid-mediated enzymes are susceptible to inhibitors, whereas most chromosomal β-lactamases are not. It also tended to separate the species of the Enterobacteriaceae into two groups based on the types of enzymes most commonly found within the species. Plasmid-mediated enzymes were most common in *Escherichia coli*, *Proteus mirabilis*, and *Klebsiella pneumoniae*, whereas chromosomal β-lactamases were characteristic of *Klebsiella oxytoca*, species of *Enterobacter* and *Serratia*, *Citrobacter freundii*, and the indole-positive Proteae (see Table 7.1).

With the advent of molecular techniques for classifying enzymes and the recognition that genes encoding β-lactamases could move between chromosomal and plasmid DNA, classification of β-lactamases on more sophisticated bases became popular (3) (Table 7.2). In these schemes, the older plasmid-mediated β-lactamases are grouped together with the chromosomal β-lactamases of *K. oxytoca* and *Proteus vulgaris* (group 2) as most of these enzymes

Table 7.1. Older Classification of β-Lactamases of Enterobacteriaceae by Location of Gene Encoding the Enzyme

Characteristic	*Plasmid-Mediated*	*Chromosomal*
Expression	Constitutive	Often inducible
Sensitivity to β-lactamase inhibitors	Yes	Often no
Species commonly possessing enzymes	*E. coli, K. pneumoniae, P. mirabilis*	*Enterobacter, Citrobacter, Serratia,* indole-positive proteae
Examples of enzymes	TEM-1, TEM-2, SHV-1, OXA-1	AmpC, K1

SOURCE: Richmond MH, Sykes RB. The β-lactamases of gram-negative bacteria and their possible physiological role. Adv Microbial Physiol 1973;9:31–88; and Sykes RB, Matthew M. The β-lactamases of gram-negative bacteria. J Antimicrob Chemother 1976;2:115–157.

Table 7.2. Newer Classification of β-Lactamases of Enterobacteriaceae Using Molecular and Biochemical Bases

Characteristic	*Group*			
	1	*2*	*3*	*4*
Primary substrates	Cephalosporins	Pen and/or cephalosporins	Most β-lactamases	Pens
Susceptible to β-lactamase inhibitors	No	Yes	No	No
Examples of enzymes found among Enterobacteriaceae	Amp C	TEM-1, TEM-2, SHV-1, ESBLs, IRTs, K1	Metallo-β-lactamase in *S. marcescens*	SAR-2

SOURCE: Bush K, Jacoby GA, Medeiros AA. A functional classification scheme for β-lactamases and its correlation with molecular structure. Antimicrob Agents Chemother 1995;39:1211–1233.

share similar sequences and are intrinsically susceptible to β-lactamase inhibitors. The inducible chromosomally mediated β-lactamases of *Enterobacter*, *Serratia*, and *P. aeruginosa* are grouped together (group 1) because of the similarity of their sequences and their intrinsic resistance to β-lactamase inhibitors. The more recently described metallo-β-lactamases capable of hydrolyzing carbapenems and the intrinsically β-lactamase inhibitor-insensitive penicillinases occupy distinct groups as well (groups 3 and 4, respectively) (Table 7.2).

INHIBITOR-RESISTANT TEM DERIVATIVES

The most commonly encountered β-lactamases in isolates of *E. coli* and *K. pneumoniae* are the plasmid-mediated TEM-1, TEM-2, and SHV-1 enzymes (4,5). These are responsible for most of the ampicillin resistance that occurs in *E. coli* and the penicillin-cephalothin resistance of many *K. pneumoniae*. Most strains of these two species that produce TEM-1, TEM-2, or SHV-1 β-lactamases were sensitive to β-lactamase inhibitor/β-lactam drug combinations when these drugs were first introduced into clinical use, because these enzymes are highly susceptible to inhibition by clavulanate, sulbactam, or tazobactam.

However, resistant strains are now being seen. Most of this resistance is due to the hyperproduction of TEM-1, TEM-2, or SHV-1 β-lactamases. Although still highly sensitive to inhibition, the very high levels of these enzymes within the periplasmic space of the gram-negative bacterium provide resistance to inhibitor/drug combinations. This occurs because it is not possible to achieve periplasmic levels of inhibitor sufficient to inactivate enough β-lactamase to restore susceptibility to the companion enzyme-labile drug (5,6).

A second less commonly encountered mechanism of resistance to inhibitor/drug combinations involves the appearance of derivatives of TEM-1 β-lactamase that are insusceptible to β-lactamase inhibitors. In 1992, Thomson and Amyes (7) reported a clinical isolate of *E. coli* in which amino acid substitutions in the TEM-1 β-lactamase reduced the susceptibility of the enzyme to the β-lactamase inhibitors. Since then, clinical isolates of *E. coli* recovered from patients in Europe and the United States have been found that produce the same or similar inhibitor-resistant TEM-1 (IRT) β-lactamases (8–11). To date, at least 10 different IRTs have been reported, and each has shown reduced susceptibility to clavulanate, sulbactam, and/or tazobactam (8–12). Whether the greater susceptibility to inhibition by tazobactam of some of these IRTs is of clinical significance has not been determined.

There have been few studies that have examined the prevalence of IRTs among clinical isolates of *E. coli*. Early studies suggest that IRTs are rare, but data are evolving that suggest they may be on the increase. The detection of IRTs in geographically diverse countries such as Scotland, France, Spain, Greece, and the United States also suggests that IRTs may be more common than suspected. This is supported by a French study conducted over a six-month period in 1993 in which 417 (14%) of 2972 urinary isolates of *E. coli* were found to be resistant to amoxicillin/clavulanate (10). Among these amoxicillin/clavulanate-resistant isolates, IRT production was inferred if resistance to amoxicillin/clavulanate was accompanied by susceptibility to cephalothin. This phenotype differed from that associated with resistance to amoxicillin/clavulanate due to hyperproduction of TEM-1, TEM-2, or SHV-1, a mechanism of resistance that usually also causes resistance to cephalothin. Using these criteria, the percent of amoxicillin/clavulanate-resistant isolates that produced IRTs was 28% from hospitalized patients and 45% from outpatients. The diversity of IRTs that have appeared in a relatively short period suggests that they have emerged independently because of antibiotic selective pressure (12) caused by the frequent use of clavulanate-containing combinations in hospitals and in general practice (9,10).

EXTENDED-SPECTRUM β-LACTAMASES

After the introduction of the expanded spectrum cephalosporins into general clinical use in the late 1970s, rapid emergence of resistance to these agents was observed among isolates of *Enterobacter*, *P. aeruginosa*, and other gram-negative bacilli that characteristically produce inducible chromosomally-mediated β-lactamases. Such resistance was generally not observed among those species of Enterobacteriaceae that did not possess such enzymes. However, by the mid 1980s, resistance to expanded-spectrum cephalosporins and aztreonam began to appear among *E. coli* and *K. pneumoniae*. This resistance was found to be due to the appearance of mutant forms of TEM-1, TEM-2, and SHV-1 β-lactamases that were capable of hydrolyzing the newer cephalosporins and aztreonam (13,14). Because these mutant β-lactamases hydrolyzed new substrates in addition to the same drugs as their parental enzymes, they were named extended-spectrum β-lactamases (ESBLs).

ESBLs are mutant enzymes derived primarily from amino acid substitutions in TEM-1, TEM-2, and SHV-1 β-lactamases (13,15). To date, there have been over 20 derivatives of TEM-1 or TEM-2 described (numbered TEM-3 and higher) and 6 derivatives of SHV-1 described (numbered SHV-2 and higher) (3,14–17). These amino acid substitutions have occurred in areas of the enzyme near the active site that allow the β-lactamase to accommodate the bulkier side chains of the newer cephalosporins and aztreonam (14,15). Like their parental enzymes, ESBLs are highly susceptible to β-lactamase inhibitors. However, many strains of ESBL-producing Enterobacteriaceae may be resistant to inhibitor/drug combinations because of the high levels of enzyme produced or to the simultaneous presence of the parental enzyme that helps to protect the ESBL from inhibition. Therefore, organisms possessing ESBLs are often resistant to all penicillins, most inhibitor/drug combinations, cephalosporins, and aztreonam. Among the β-lactam antibiotics, the carbapenems and cephamycins are the only classes predictably active against ESBL-producing strains. Because most ESBLs are encoded by genes located on very large plasmids, these plasmids often carry genes for resistance to other antimicrobial agents as well. Resistance to aminoglycosides, trimethoprim, sulfonamides, tetracyclines, and chloramphenicol may also be encoded by additional genes on these large plasmids (13,18,19). Thus, very broad antibiotic resistance extending to multiple antibiotic classes is a frequent characteristic of ESBL-producing organisms. The predominant ESBL-producing organisms are *E. coli* and *K. pneumoniae* (13). However, ESBLs have been found on occasion in *K. oxytoca*, *K. ozaenae*, *Serratia marcescens*, species of *Enterobacter*, *Salmonella*, *Proteus*, *Citrobacter*, and *Morganella morganii* (4,14,15).

Although ESBL-producing Enterobacteriaceae were first reported in Europe in 1983 and 1984, ESBLs have now been found in Enterobacteriaceae recovered from patients in all continents except Antarctica (13,14). The occurrence of the different ESBLs varies widely. Some ESBLs are more prevalent in Europe (TEM-3), others are more prevalent in the United States (TEM-10, TEM-12, and TEM-26), and others have appeared virtually worldwide (SHV-5). The true prevalence of ESBL-producing Enterobacteriaceae is currently unknown. In routine susceptibility tests, many strains that produce ESBLs may appear sensitive to newer cephalosporins and aztreonam. Thus, any attempt to use resistance to these agents as an indicator of the prevalence of ESBLs in isolates of *E. coli* or *K. pneumoniae* will grossly underestimate the true prevalence of ESBLs. In studies that used special tests to actually detect ESBLs among isolates of Enterobacteriaceae, prevalence has ranged from less than 1% to as high as 74% of isolates examined (4). From the data available, it is clear that there are "hot spots" for ESBL-producing Enterobacteriaceae. Such organisms are becoming increasingly common in certain hospitals, especially among isolates recovered from patients in intensive care units, whereas in other hospitals it appears that ESBL-producing Enterobacteriaceae have not yet arrived (4,20).

Not surprisingly, ESBL-producing organisms are often found in areas of the hospital where antibiotic use is heavy and the patient's condition critical. Various risk factors have been implicated in the selection and spread of ESBL-producing strains. These include antibiotic exposure, especially exposure to ceftazidime; recent surgery; instrumentation; admission to an intensive care unit; prolonged hospital stay; and admission to a nursing home (21,22). The problem of antibiotic exposure and the issue of restricting the use of drugs that can select ESBL-producing organisms is complex because such strains are frequently resistant to multiple classes of antibiotics. Thus, any one of several antibiotics can act to maintain ESBLs in a bacterial population once they have arrived.

Heavy use of ceftazidime has been particularly implicated in nosocomial outbreaks in the United States (21,23–26). In an outbreak of TEM-12 and TEM-26 producing Enterobacteriaceae in a Massachusetts chronic care facility, 15 of 29 patients involved had received ceftazidime during the prior month (25). Another outbreak involving 432 TEM-26 producing isolates from 155 patients over a 2-year period at a New York general hospital occurred after a 2-year period in which ceftazidime use increased by 600% (24). In a third outbreak at Stanford University Medical Center in California, 14 TEM-26–producing isolates were isolated from 13 pediatric oncology patients who received ceftazidime as empiric therapy for fever and neutropenia (23). In each outbreak, the number of ESBL-producing Enterobacteriaceae isolated at the institution decreased markedly when restrictions were placed on ceftazidime use with complete eradication of these organisms being achieved in the smallest outbreak (23–25).

The standard modalities of infection control should be used to contain the spread of ESBL-producing organisms within hospitals. However, the most difficult task facing clinical microbiologists, infectious disease specialists, and infection control practitioners is the reliable detection of ESBL-producing organisms. As mentioned previously, many ESBL-producing *E. coli* and *K. pneumoniae* do not appear resistant to newer cephalosporins or aztreonam in routine susceptibility tests. However, it is very clear that these drugs are usually unsuccessful in treating infections due to ESBL-producing Enterobacteriaceae unless the infection is confined to the urinary tract (23,24). Therefore, the laboratory must find a more accurate procedure for detecting ESBL-producing Enterobacteriaceae than merely looking for resistance in routine susceptibility tests.

The most reliable approach to detection of ESBL-producing Enterobacteriaceae is the use of special tests that are designed to indicate the presence of a clavulanate-sensitive enzyme capable of hydrolyzing one of the newer cephalosporins and/or aztreonam. Unfortunately, all of these tests have limitations that prevent their immediate adoption by the routine clinical laboratory. The most widely used test is the double disk test of Jarlier et al (19) in which a disk containing clavulanate is placed on an inoculated plate 30 mm from disks containing cefotaxime, ceftriaxone, ceftazidime, and/or aztreonam (Figure 7.1). Clavulanate-susceptible ESBL production is indicated by enhancement of the zone of inhibition between the clavulanate-containing disk and one or more of the test drugs. Although this is a generally reliable test that uses materials already available to the laboratory for performance of standard disk diffusion tests, there are several limitations (27–29). Against some strains, the standard disk spacing of 30 mm is either too large or too small to allow interpretation of results. Thus, the test must be repeated using a more appropriate spacing. Secondly, interpretation of the test is highly subjective and requires experience on the part of the technician before reliable results are generated. A commercially manufactured test for the detection of ESBLs, the Vitek ESBL Test (bioMérieux Vitek, St, Louis, MO), is highly reliable for detection of ESBLs in *E. coli*, *K. pneumoniae*, and *K. oxytoca* (30,31). It has not been proven to be reliable in tests with other species of Enterobacteriaceae and is unlikely to be reliable in tests with those species that characteristically produce an inducible chromosomally-mediated β-lactamase. However, this is not a major disadvantage because the great majority of strains producing ESBLs are either *E. coli* or *Klebsiella* spp. The major drawback is that only laboratories using the Vitek System can use this new test. Other commercial systems are currently under developement.

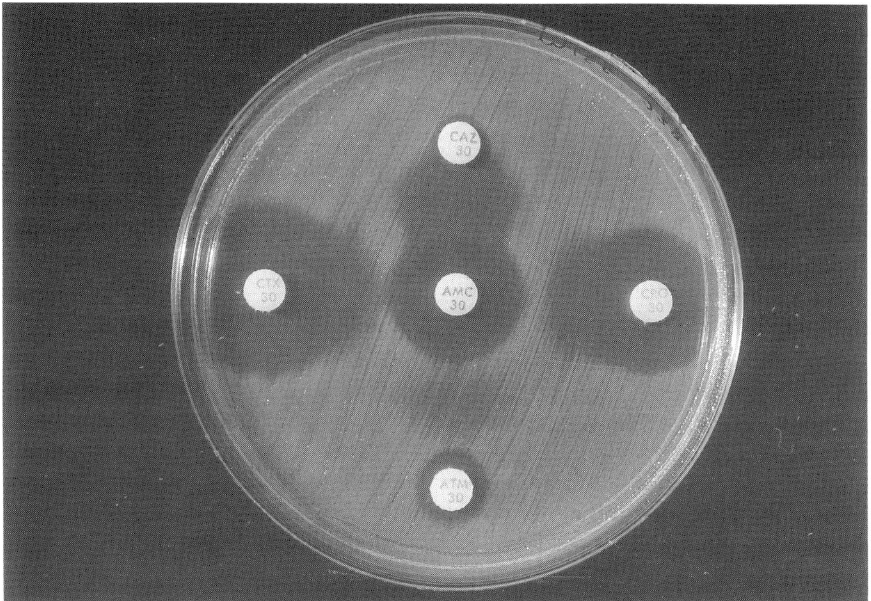

Figure 7.1. Double disk test with an isolate of *E. coli* that produces the TEM-10 β-lactamase. Disks containing ceftazidime (CAZ), cefotaxime (CTX), aztreonam (ATM), and ceftriaxone (CRO) are located around an amoxicillin/clavulanate disk (AMC). Extended spectrum β-lactamase production is indicated by extended inhibition zones where the clavulanate potentiated the activity of ceftazidime, cefotaxime and ceftriaxone, and a lens of inhibition of growth between the aztreonam and amoxicillin/clavulanate disks.

Because of the lack of a simple reliable test for the detection of ESBLs that can be added to routine testing without considerable cost, many laboratories have devised ways of screening Enterobacteriaceae for ESBLs (Table 7.3). Certainly, any *E. coli*, *Klebsiella* spp., or *P. mirabilis* that displays resistance or intermediate susceptibility to any of the extended spectrum cephalosporins or aztreonam should be assumed to possess an ESBL. To enhance detection of such strains, routine susceptibility tests should include at least cefotaxime, ceftazidime, and aztreonam because ESBL-producing Enterobacteriaceae are most likely to show diminished susceptibility to one of these agents. With such strains, resistance to all cephalosporins and aztreonam should be assumed regardless of results of susceptibility tests.

The major problem faced by laboratories is how to handle those strains that do not show resistance or intermediate susceptibility to any of the extended spectrum cephalosporins or aztreonam in routine susceptibility tests. One solution to this problem is to subject all such strains to a special test for the detection of ESBLs. This is probably not an economical approach because most of these tests would be negative. A second approach is possible for those laboratories that routinely use disk diffusion or a susceptibility test that generates a true

Table 7.3. Flow chart for screening Enterobacteriaceae* for the presence of ESBLs

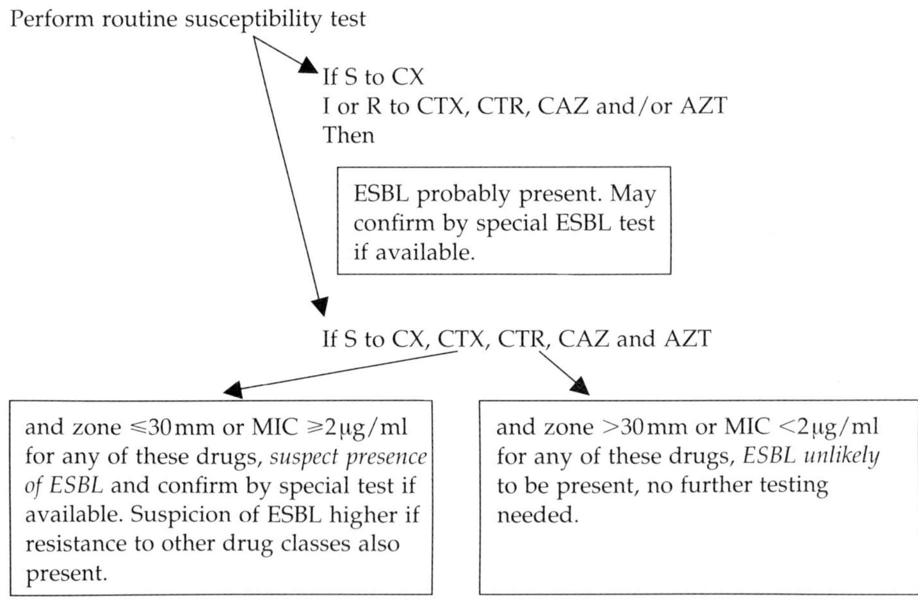

*Includes only those species that do not characteristically produce an inducible chromosomally mediated β-lactamase.
S, susceptible; I, intermediate; R, resistant; CTX, cefotaxime; CAZ, ceftazidime; CTR; ceftriaxone; AZT, aztreonam; CX, cefoxitin.

minimum inhibitory concentration (MIC); this excludes laboratories using breakpoint methods. If MICs are at least 2 μg/ml or if zone sizes are no more than 30 mm or less for one or more extended spectrum cephalosporins or aztreonam, there should be a high degree of suspicion that an ESBL may be present. The index of suspicion should go even higher if the strain is resistant to aminoglycosides, sulfonamides, trimethoprim, and/or chloramphenicol. As before, the greatest reliability of this approach will be attained if cefotaxime, ceftazidime, and aztreonam are included in the tests. These strains could then be subjected to a special test for ESBLs. In laboratories lacking any special tests, a warning should accompany results of susceptibility tests that the profile of the strain strongly suggests the presence of an ESBL and the physician may wish to avoid use of expanded-spectrum cephalosporins or aztreonam in therapy.

In addition to identifying ESBL-producing organisms within the hospital, infection-control personnel should identify patients who are admitted already colonized or infected with an ESBL-producing Enterobacteriaceae. Such patients would include those transferred from another acute care hospital, patients with multiple previous admissions to the hospital, and patients from chronic care facilities or nursing homes. In Chicago, where TEM-10–producing *K. pneumoniae* are now endemic, a recent survey showed that 75% of the ceftazidime-resistant *Klebsiella* isolates at the Michael Reese Hospital were recovered from patients admitted from nursing homes (21). Many of these isolates represented asymptomatic rectal colonization.

Once an ESBL-producing Enterobacteriaceae has been identified as the etiologic agent of infection, selection of appropriate therapy may be complex. As mentioned previously, ESBL-producing organisms may be resistant to multiple classes of antimicrobial agents. Those drugs with the most reliable activity include the new fluoroquinolones, imipenem, and the cephamycins. It should be noted, however, that resistance to the fluoroquinolones has been seen in some ESBL-producing Enterobacteriaceae and resistance to cefoxitin has emerged during therapy with this drug (32). For some strains, an aminoglycoside may also be used in therapy because not all ESBL-producing Enterobacteriaceae are resistant to all aminoglycosides. This is especially true for strains recovered in the United States (23–25). Although most ESBL-producing Enterobacteriaceae are resistant to ampicillin/sulbactam and ticarcillin/clavulanate, many appear susceptible to piperacillin/tazobactam. The clinical utility of this inhibitor/drug combination, however, has yet to be established.

The efficacy of expanded-spectrum cephalosporins in treatment of infections due to ESBL-producing Enterobacteriaceae remains unresolved. Clearly, there are numerous examples of failures of these drugs. However, there are some successes (23,24,33–35). The type of infection can play an important role in the success of therapy. In a urinary tract infection, where achievable drug levels are high, a cephalosporin with an MIC for the infecting strain that is high in the sensitive range could be used in treatment. Conversely, the same drug would not be appropriate therapy for infections such as pneumonia, meningitis, endocarditis, and bone and soft tissue infections where adequate drug levels are not attainable. Indeed, failure of cephalosporin therapy in an infection caused by an Enterobacteriaceae reported to be sensitive to the drug in routine susceptibility tests has often been the first indicator that the infecting strain produced an ESBL (19,24,34).

AmpC DERIVATIVES

The most frequently encountered chromosomally-encoded β-lactamase is the inducible AmpC cephalosporinase that is characteristically found in *Enterobacter*, *C. freundii*, certain indole-positive Proteae, *Serratia*, and *P. aeruginosa* (4). This enzyme has a significantly different substrate profile from the ESBLs in that it hydrolyzes penicillins, cephalosporins, monobactams, and cephamycins. It also differs from ESBLS in that it is intrinsically resistant to the β-lactamase inhibitors. Production of high levels of this β-lactamase thus produces resistance to all of the currently available penicillins, inhibitor/ drug combinations, cephalosporins, cephamycins, and monobactams. Only imipenem is active against such strains.

In the late 1980s, 11 isolates of *K. pneumoniae* that were resistant to cefoxitin in addition to penicillins, cephalosporins, and aztreonam were recovered from patients at the Miriam Hospital in Providence, Rhode Island (36). Analysis of these strains revealed the presence of a plasmid-mediated β-lactamase (MIR-1) most similar to the chromosomal AmpC β-lactamase of *E. cloacae* (36). Unlike the inducible expression of this enzyme in its usual *Enterobacter* parent, this plasmid-mediated derivative was constitutively expressed at a very high level. In each of the 11 patients carrying these isolates, acquisition was thought to be nosocomial. They had either prolonged or multiple hospitalizations, and nine had undergone at least one surgical procedure. The sources of the cultures were wounds, urines, and sputa. Ten of the isolates caused infection. Eight of the patients had received prior cephalosporin therapy, but only two received cefoxitin.

In addition to this first U.S. report of a plasmid-mediated derivative of the AmpC β-lactamase (36), eight other derivatives (CMY-1, CMY-2, BIL-1, MOX-1, FOX-1, LAT-1, ATH-1, and an unnamed enzyme) have been detected in isolates of *K. pneumoniae* and *E. coli* (37–44). Organisms possessing such enzymes have been recovered from patients in North America, South America, Europe, and Asia. Molecular analyses suggest diverse origins of the enzymes with likely sources being the chromosomal genes of *E. cloacae*, *C. freundii*, and *P. aeruginosa* (36,38,40,42,45,46). Seven of these were found in *K. pneumoniae*. BIL-1, reported in 1992 (39), is the only AmpC derivative to have been found in *E. coli* and is thought to have originated from *C. freundii*. The isolate was cultured from a patient with burns over 35% of his body who had been transferred to London from Pakistan. Actual samples were taken by swab from raw areas of skin and from biopsy specimen. This case clearly illustrates the potential for widespread dissemination of these enzymes. In all cases involving organisms that produced AmpC derivatives, imipenem was the only reliable β-lactam drug available.

The prevalence of these plasmid-mediated derivatives of the AmpC β-lactamase is not as great as that of the ESBLs. However, therapeutic options for treatment of infections caused by organisms producing these enzymes are even more limited. Among the β-lactam family of drugs, only imipenem is uniformly active against strains producing these AmpC β-lactamases.

CONCLUSIONS

These new plasmid-mediated β-lactamases in Enterobacteriaceae present special challenges to infectious disease clinicians, microbiologists, and infection control practitioners. Clearly, methods to identify the presence of strains possessing such enzymes must be developed in the laboratory so that their detection and containment can be realized. Clinically relevant resistance mediated by these new enzymes needs to be identified so that inappropriate therapy can be avoided. Most importantly, factors leading to the selection, maintenance, and spread of strains producing these new enzymes need to be identified and, where possible, eliminated from the hospital environment. Many of the problems caused by these new plasmid-mediated β-lactamases have arisen because of the overuse of newer cephalosporins, cephamycins, and inhibitor/drug combinations, especially in certain patient populations. If these problems are to be minimized and future problems prevented, it is important that these antimicrobial agents be used judiciously.

REFERENCES

1 **Richmond MH, Sykes RB.** The β-lactamases of gram-negative bacteria and their possible physiological role. Adv Microbiol Physiol 1973;9:31–88.

2 **Sykes RB, Matthew M.** The β-lactamases of gram-negative bacteria. J Antimicrob Chemother 1976;2:115–157.

3 **Bush K, Jacoby GA, Medeiros AA.** A functional classification scheme for β-lactamases and its correlation with molecular structure. Antimicrob Agents Chemother 1995;39: 1211–1233.

4 **Sanders CC, Sanders WE Jr.** β-Lactam resistance in gram-negative bacteria: global trends and clinical impact. Clin Infect Dis 1992;15:824–839.

5 **Sanders CC, Iaconis JP, Bodey GP, Samonis G.** Resistance to ticarcillin-potassium clavulanate among clinical isolates of the family Enterobacteriaceae: role of PSE-1 β-lactamase and high levels of TEM-1 and SHV-1 and problems with false susceptibility in disk diffusion tests. Antimicrob Agents Chemother 1988;32:1365–1369.

6 **Thomson KS, Weber DA, Sanders CC, Sanders WE Jr.** β-Lactamase production in members of the family Enterobacteriaceae and resistance of β-lactam-enzyme inhibitor combinations. Antimicrob Agents Chemother 1990;34:622–627.

7 **Thomson CJ, Amyes SBG.** TRC-1: emergence of a clavulanic acid-resistant TEM β-lactamase in a clinical strain. FEMS Microbiol Lett 1992;91:113–117.

8 **Vedel G, Belaaouaj A, Gilly L, et al.** Clinical isolates of *Escherichia coli* producing TRI β-lactamases: novel TEM-enzymes conferring resistance to β-lactamase inhibi-

tors. J Antimicrob Chemother 1992;30:449–462.

9 **Blazquez J, Baquero M, Canton R, et al.** Characterization of a new TEM-type β-lactamase resistant to clavulanate, sulbactam, and tazobactam in a clinical isolate of *Escherichia coli.* Antimicrob Agents Chemother 1993;37:2059–2063.

10 **Henquell C, Sirot D, Chanal C, et al.** Frequency of inhibitor-resistant TEM β-lactamases in *Escherichia coli* isolates from urinary tract infections in France. J Antimicrob Chemother 1994;34:707–714.

11 **Thomson CJ, Thomson KS, Sanders CC, Amyes SGB.** TEM β-lactamase resistant to clavulanic acid (TRC-1) first emerged in Texas. Presented at the 94th General Meeting of the American Society for Microbiology, Las Vegas, 1994.

12 **Henquell C, Chanal C, Sirot D, et al.** Molecular characterization of nine different types of mutants among 107 inhibitor-resistant TEM β-lactamases from clinical isolates of *Escherichia coli.* Antimicrob Agents Chemother 1995;39:427–430.

13 **Philippon A, Labia R, Jacoby G.** Extended-spectrum β-lactamases. Antimicrob Agents Chemother 1989;33:1131–1136.

14 **Jacoby GA, Medeiros AA.** More extended-spectrum β-lactamases. Antimicrob Agents Chemother 1991;35:1697–1704.

15 **DuBois SK, Marriott MS, Amyes SGB.** TEM- and SHV-derived extended-spectrum β-lactamases: relationship between selection, structure and function. J Antimicrob Chemother 1995;35:7–22.

16 **Arlet G, Rouveau M, Bengoufa D, et al.** Novel transferrable extended-spectrum β-lactamase (SHV-6) from *Klebsiella pneumoniae* conferring selective resistance to ceftazidime. FEMS Microbiol Lett 1991; 81:57–62.

17 **Bradford PA, Urban C, Jaiswal A, et al.** SHV-7, a novel cefotaxime-hydrolyzing β-lactamase identified in *Escherichia coli* isolates from hospitalized nursing home patients. Antimicrob Agents Chemother (in press).

18 **Jacoby, GA.** Genetics of extended-spectrum β-lactamases. Eur J Clin Microbiol Infect Dis 1994;(suppl 1):2–11.

19 **Jarlier V, Nicolas MH, Fournier G, Philippon, A.** Extended broad spectrum β-lactamases conferring transferrable resistance to newer β-lactam agents in Enterobacteriaceae: hospital prevalence and susceptibility patterns. Rev Infect Dis 1988;10:867–878.

20 **Medeiros AA.** Nosocomial outbreaks of multiresistant bacteria: extended-spectrum β-lactamases have arrived in North America. Ann Intern Med 1993;119:428–430.

21 **Quinn JP.** Clinical significance of extended-spectrum β-lactamases. Eur J Clin Microbiol Infect Dis 1994;13(suppl 1):39–42.

22 **DeChamps C, Sauvant MP, Chanal C, et al.** Prospective survey of colonization and infections caused by Expanded-Spectrum-β-lactamase-Producing members of the family *Enterobacteriacae.* J Clin Microbiol 1989;27:2887–2890.

23 **Naumovski L, Quinn JP, Miyashiro D, et al.** Outbreak of ceftazidime resistance due to extended spectrum β-lactamase in isolates from cancer patients. Antimicrob Agents Chemother 1992;36:1991–1996.

24 **Meyer KS, Urban C, Egan JA, et al.** Nosocomial outbreak of *Klebsiella* infection resistant to late generation cephalosporins. Ann Intern Med 1993;119:353–358.

25 **Rice LB, Willey SH, Papanicolaou GA, et al.** Outbreak of ceftazidime resistance caused by extended-spectrum β-lactamases at a Massachusetts chronic-care facility. Antimicrob Agents Chemother 1990;34: 2193–2199.

26 **Thomson KS, Cherubin CC, Sanders CC.** Outbreak of extended-spectrum β-lactamase-producing Enterobacteriaceae associated with use of ceftazidime. Presented at the 33rd Interscience Conference on Antimicrobial Agents and Chemotherapy, New Orleans, October 1993.

27 **Thomson KS, Sanders CC, Washington JA II.** High-level resistance to cefotaxime and ceftazidime in *Klebsiella pneumoniae* isolates from Cleveland, Ohio. Antimicrob Agents Chemother 1991;35:1001–1003.

28 **Thomson KS, Sanders CC.** Detection of extended-spectrum β-lactamases in members of the family Enterobacteriaceae: comparison of the double-disk and three-dimensional tests. Antimicrob Agents Chemother 1992;36:1877–1882.

29 **Moland ES, Thomson KS.** Extended spectrum β-lactamases of Enterobacteriaceae. J Antimicrob Chemother 1994;33:666–668.

30 **Ferraro MJ, Jacoby GA, Katsanis G, et al.** Improving the reliability of extended-spectrum β-lactamase detection by the Vitek System. Presented at the 32nd Interscience Conference on Antimicrobial Agents and Chemotherapy, Anaheim, October 1992.

31 **Sanders CC, Washington JA II, Barry AL, Shubert C.** Assessment of the Vitek ESBL

test. Presented at the 34th Interscience Conference on Antimicrobial Agents and Chemotherapy, Orlando, October 1994.

32 **Pangon B, Bizet C, Buré A, et al.** In vivo selection of a cephamycin-resistant, porin-deficient mutant of *Klebsiella pneumoniae* producing a TEM-3 β-lactamase. J Infect Dis 1989;159:1005–1006.

33 **Smith CE, Tillman BS, Howell AW, et al.** Failure of ceftazidime-amikacin therapy for bacteremia and meningitis due to *Klebsiella pneumoniae* producing an extended-spectrum β-lactamase. Antimicrob Agents Chemother 1990;34:1290–1293.

34 **Sirot J, Chanal C, Petit A, et al.** *Klebsiella pneumoniae* and other Enterobacteriaceae producing novel plasmid-mediated β-lactamases markedly active against third-generation cephalosporins: epidemiologic studies. Rev Infect Dis 1988;10:850–859.

35 **Brun-Buisson C, Legrand P, Philippon A, et al.** Transferrable enzymatic resistance to third generation cephalosporins during nosocomial outbreak of multiresistant *Klebsiella pneumoniae*. Lancet 1987;2:302–306.

36 **Papanicolaou GA, Medeiros AA, Jacoby GA.** Novel plasmid-mediated β-lactamase (MIR-1) conferring resistance to oxyimino- and α-methoxy β-lactams in clinical isolates of *Klebsiella pneumoniae*. Antimicrob Agents Chemother 1990;34:2200–2209.

37 **Bauernfeind A, Chong Y, Schweighart S.** Extended broad spectrum β-lactamase in *Klebsiella pneumoniae* including resistance to cephamycins. Infection 1989;17:316–321.

38 **Bauernfeind A, Schweighart S, Dornbusch K, Giamarellou H.** A transferrable cephamycinase (CMY-ase) in *Klebsiella pneumoniae*. Presented at the 30th Interscience Conference on Antimicrobial Agents and Chemotherapy, Atlanta, October 1990.

39 **Payne DJ, Woodford N, Amyes SGB.** Characterization of the plasmid-mediated β-lactamase BIL-1. J Antimicrob Chemother 1992;30:119–127.

40 **Horii T, Arakawa Y, Ohta M, et al.** Plasmid-mediated Amp C-type β-lactamase isolated from *Klebsiella pneumoniae* confers resistance to broad-spectrum β-lactams, including moxalactam. Antimicrob Agents Chemother 1993;37:984–990.

41 **Tzouvelekis LS, Tzelepi E, Mentis AF, Tsakris A.** Identification of novel plasmid-mediated β-lactamase with chromosomal cephalosporinase characteristics from *Klebsiella pneumoniae*. J Antimicrob Chemother 1993;31:645–654.

42 **Leiza MG, Perez-Diaz JC, Ayala J, et al.** Gene sequence and biochemical characterization of FOX-1 from *Klebsiella pneumoniae*, a new Amp C-type plasmid-mediated β-lactamase with two molecular variants. Antimicrob Agents Chemother 1994;38: 2150–2157.

43 **Pörnull KJ, Rodrigo G, Dornbusch K.** Production of a plasmid-mediated AmpC-like β-lactamase by a *Klebsiella pneumoniae* septicemia isolate. J Antimicrob Chemother 1994;34:943–954.

44 **Jenks PJ, Hu YM, Danel F, et al.** Plasmid-mediated production of Class 1 (AmpC) β-lactamase by two *Klebsiella pneumoniae* isolates in the UK. J Antimicrob Chemother 1995;35:235–236.

45 **Fosberry AP, Payne DJ, Lawlor EJ, Hodgson JE.** Cloning and sequence analysis of bla_{BIL-1}, a plasmid-mediated class C β-lactamase gene in *Escherichia* coli BS. Antimicrob Agents Chemother 1994;38: 1182–1185.

46 **Tzouvelekis LS, Tzelepi E, Mentis AF.** Nucleotide sequence of a plasmid-mediated cephalosporinase gene (bla_{LAT-1}) found in *Klebsiella pneumoniae*. Antimicrob Agents Chemother 1994;38:2207–2209.

Human Ehrlichiosis in the United States

JACQUELINE E. DAWSON

There are currently two potentially fatal forms of human ehrlichiosis in the United States. Both of these tickborne pathogens cause an acute febrile illness similar to Rocky Mountain spotted fever (1,2). Many physicians believe that the historical diagnosis of "spotless" Rocky Mountain spotted fever may have been due to one of these ehrlichial species. Indeed, the clinical presentation of both ehrlichial diseases is extremely similiar to Rocky Mountain spotted fever; however, a rash is observed in a minority of ehrlichiosis patients. Both of these diseases, human ehrlichiosis due to *Ehrlichia chaffeensis* and human granulocytic ehrlichiosis (HGE), have only been recently recognized (1,2).

In March 1986, a 51-year-old man was bitten by ticks while visiting his family in Malvern, Arkansas (3). Two weeks later, while back at his home in Detroit, Michigan, he developed an acute syndrome characterized by fever, headache, malaise, and myalgia. A physical examination in a Detroit hospital on April 14 revealed a critically ill man. His oral temperature was 39.7°C, his pulse was 110 beats/min, and his respiratory rate was 28. The white blood cell count was 4600/mm^4, with 47% polymorphonuclear cells, 48% band forms, 4% monocytes, and 1% lymphocytes. The platelet count was 18,000/mm^4. A peripheral blood smear revealed blue-staining inclusions in the cytoplasm of occasional lymphocytes, atypical lymphocytes, band neutrophils, segmented neutrophils, and monocytes. The frequency of parasitemia ranged from 1 to 2 infected cells per 100 white cells. Serum samples obtained during the acute and convalescent phases of the patient's illness were positive for antibodies reactive to *Ehrlichia canis*. At the time of his diagnosis, the leukocytic rickettsiae of the genus ehrlichia included the species *E. canis*, *E. phagocytophila*, *E. equi*, *E. risticii*, and *E. sennetsu*.

E. sennetsu, the etiologic agent of human sennetsu fever and the only human pathogen in this genus, causes lymphadenopathy, fever, and lethargy (4). This disease, however, has only been reported in western Japan and not in North America (5). This led some investigators to believe that *E. canis* was causing infections in humans (3). It was not until 1990, when *E. chaffeensis* was isolated and subsequently sequenced, that sufficient evidence accumulated to prove that a new ehrlichial species was infecting humans in the United States (6,7).

Even more recently, another form of human ehrlichiosis has been reported in the United States. In June 1992, a 78-year-old man from Gordon, Wisconsin, was hospitalized with an acute febrile illness (8). His presentation was similar to the man from Detroit, with fever, myalgias, headache, leukopenia, and thrombocytopenia (8). Once again, inclusions were observed in the patient's peripheral blood smear. However, this time, the organisms were exclusively observed in neutrophils. All attempts to culture the etiologic agent have been unsuccessful. However, sequencing of the 16S rRNA gene revealed a 99.9% similarity with *E. phagocytophila* (8), a pathogen of sheep and cattle in Europe, India, and South Africa (9), and a 99.8% similarity with *E. equi*, an equine pathogen in the United States (10).

Because neither of these diseases are reportable, an accurate number of cases is not available. However, prospective studies of human ehrlichiosis due to *E. chaffeensis* have shown rates equal to or in excess of the number of cases of Rocky Mountain spotted fever (11).

CLASSIFICATION OF THE EHRLICHIEAE

The genus *Ehrlichia* was established in 1945 in honor of the German bacteriologist Paul Ehrlich (12). This genus of obligate intracellar leukocytic parasites was created to distinguish it from other medically significant genera (*Rickettsia, Coxiella*, and *Chlamydia*). *Ehrlichia* are members of the order Rickettsiales, in the family Rickettsiaceae, which includes the tribes Ehrlichieae, Rickettsieae, and Wolbachieae. Three species are pathogenic for humans, *E. sennetsu, E. chaffeensis*, and the newly recognized human granulocytic ehrlichiosis agent. The latter agents are the only two recognized in the United States. *E. chaffeensis* is apparently most closely related to the canine pathogens, *E. canis* and *E. ewingii* (7). Similarly, the human granulocytic ehrlichial agent appears to be very closely related, if not identical, to *E. phagocytophila* and *E. equi*, both parasites in domestic herbivores (8).

EPIDEMIOLOGY OF *E. CHAFFEENSIS*

Human ehrlichiosis due to *E. chaffeensis* has been diagnosed in more than 400 patients. Ehrlichiosis is particularly common in individuals 60 years and older, although the median age is 44 years (1). Fatalities have occurred in individuals ranging from age 8 to 68 years. Similar to other tickborne diseases, over 70% of patients are men (1).

Since its discovery in 1986, cases have been reported from 30 states in the

United States. In addition, one case has been reported from Portugal (13) and one from Africa (14). Most cases occur between May and October, suggestive of arthropod transmission. Indeed, Fishbein et al (11) stated that tick exposure is a common part of the history for human ehrlichiosis patients, and Petersen et al (15) found that soldiers who tucked their pants into their boots to deter ticks were only half as likely as their cohorts to develop ehrlichiosis. In addition, Everett et al (16) found a few *Amblyomma americanum* and *Dermacentor variabilis* positive for *E. chaffeensis* by the indirect fluorescent antibody technique, and Anderson et al. (17) used the polymerase chain reaction (PCR) technique to amplify the *E. chaffeensis* 16S gene from a pool of *A. americanum*.

EPIDEMIOLOGY OF HUMAN GRANULOCYTIC EHRLICHIOSIS

Human granulocytic ehrlichiosis is so recently discovered that little is known about geographic distribution or reservoir host(s). All 15 cases reported to date (including two fatalities) were seen in Minnesota and Wisconsin (2,8). The patients ranged in age from 29 to 91 years. Bakken et al (2) reported that 92% of the patients examined had a history of arthropod bite within 10 days of onset of illness. Ticks had been attached to 67% of the patients and were identified as either *Ixodes scapularis* or *D. variabilis*.

More recently, Reed et al (18) reported the removal of an adult female *I. scapularis* from a clinically ill patient. The tick was analyzed, along with blood from the patient, by PCR. *Ehrlichia* DNA was detected in both samples. Although this is not definitive evidence that *I. scapularis* transmits the human granulocytic agent, it does support epidemiologic observations Reed et al (18) also reported two additional patients that were seropositive and PCR positive, thereby bringing the total number of HGE cases to 15.

The possibility that *I. scapularis* may be the vector of HGE is highly significant considering the role this tick already plays in transmission of *Borrelia burgdorferi*, the etiologic agent of Lyme disease. It is certainly possible that some of the unconfirmed Lyme disease cases are due to infection with HGE, considering the similarity of the initial presentation, discussed below.

EHRLICHIAL CLINICAL SYNDROME

Ehrlichial diseases are characterized by sudden onset of fever, headache, and malaise. Other commonly encountered symptoms include confusion, myalgia, rigor, sweats, and nausea/vomiting (1,2). Despite the nonspecific signs and symptoms of human ehrlichiosis, laboratory findings are more constant and frequently include thrombocytopenia, leukopenia, elevated liver enzymes, and, occasionally, anemia (1,2). Most patients present between May and October, often with a history of arthropod exposure. Fatalities have been reported with both agents.

One early case report of human ehrlichiosis ascribed to *E. chaffeensis* documented bone marrow hypoplasia and suggested diminished production of leukocytes, erythrocytes, and platelets (19). Other bone marrow findings have included myeloid hyperplasia, megakaryocytosis, granulomas, marrow histiocytosis, myeloid hypoplasia, pancellular hypoplasia, and normocellular marrow (20).

Postmortem examinations performed in three cases revealed gastrointestinal hemorrhage; mild interstitial pneumonitis; perivascular lymphohistiocytic infiltrates in lung, liver, kidneys, and heart; and bone marrow hyperplasia. Focal hepatocyte necrosis, hepatocyte dropout, Kupffer cell hyperplasia, and erythrophagocytosis were also observed (21).

Immunostaining with biotinylated globulin from a patient convalescing from ehrlichiosis demonstrated the presence of clusters of ehrlichial organisms (morulae) in splenic cords and sinuses, splenic periarteriolar lymphoid sheaths, hepatic sinusoids, lymph nodes, lung microvasculature, bone marrow, kidney, and epicardium (22).

Less is known about the two fatalities that have been attributed to infection with the human granulocytic agent. Both patients died of multiorgan failure after presenting with cough and pulmonary infiltrates that were obvious upon radiography (2). Diagnosis of the first patient was based on autopsy findings a week after death. The second patient's illness was compounded by several factors, including chronic lymphocytic leukemia with Richter's syndrome, high-dose steriod treatment, and previous splenectomy (2).

DIAGNOSIS

Ehrlichia spp. appear as round dark purple-stained dots or clusters of dots (morulae) in the cytoplasm of leukocytes upon direct microscopic examination of peripheral blood smears or buffy coat preparations stained by Romanowsky-type techniques (e.g., Giemsa, Wright, or Diff-Quik) as shown in Figure 8.1. Direct examination of such smears is probably useful only during the acute febrile phase of the infection when organisms are most prevalent. *E. chaffeensis* has been reported occasionally in lymphocytes, atypical lymphocytes, band neutrophils, and segmented neutrophils, but most organisms are observed in monocytes or macrophages (3,23).

The search for *E. chaffeensis* using immunohistologic techniques has been performed not only on peripheral blood smears but on formalin-fixed paraffin-embedded bone marrow biopsy specimens or aspirated marrow. Dumler et al (20) described use of the biotinylated human anti-*E. chaffeensis*, avidin-alkaline phosphatase, or avidin-horseradish peroxidase system. Organisms were detected primarily within histiocytes, but morulae were occasionally present within lymphocytes (20).

The human granulocytic agent has been found in neutrophils and rarely eosinophils (Figure 8.2). Direct examination of buffy coats and peripheral blood

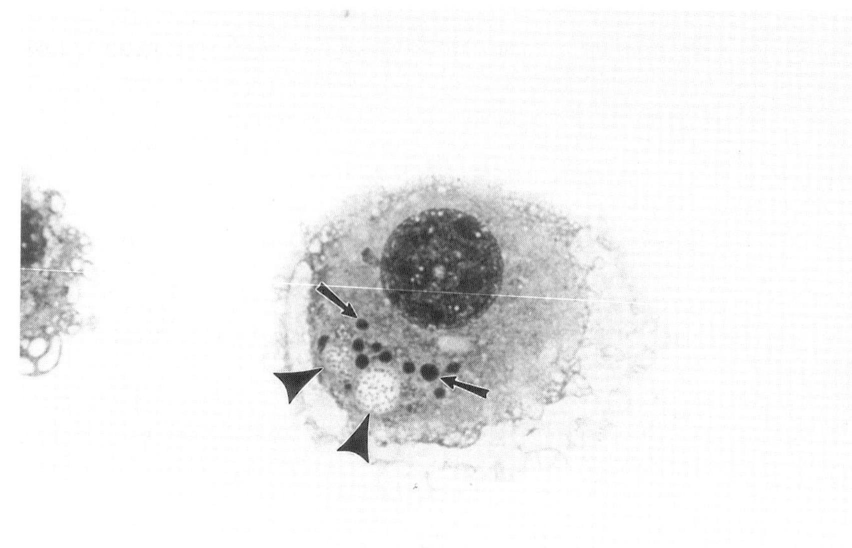

Figure 8.1. Photomicrograph of DH82 cells containing *Ehrlichia chaffeensis* morulae (magnification ×1000). *Arrowheads* indicate loosely packed morulae with individual organisms visible. *Long arrows* indicate densely packed morulae.

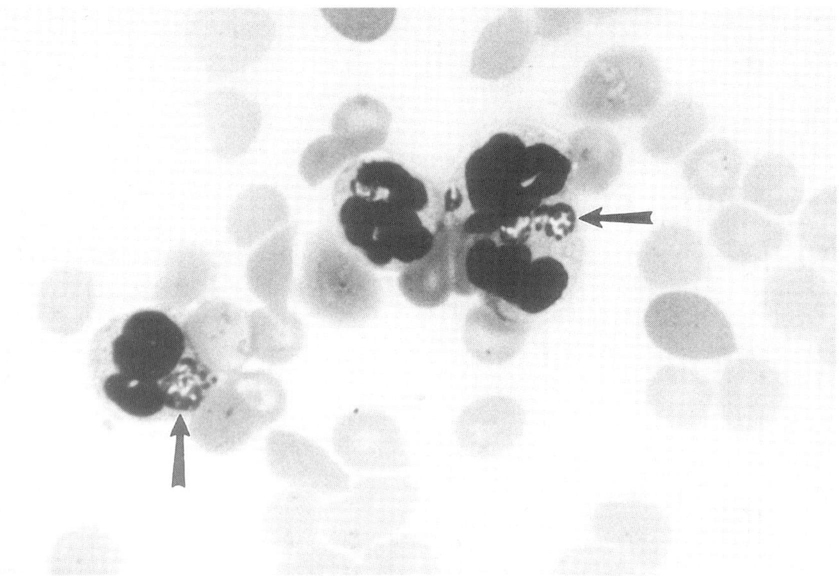

Figure 8.2. Photomicrograph of human neutrophils containing the newly described human granulocytic agent (magnification ×1000). *Long arrows* indicate morulae.

smears is a lengthy process as evidenced by Bakken et al 's (2) need to inspect at least 800 polymorphonuclear granulocytes per smear for evidence of infection with the human granulocytic agent. Immunohistology has also been performed on paraffin-embedded tissue sections from a patient infected with the human granulocytic agent. To locate the etiologic agent in the postmortem specimens, equine anti-*E. equi* and bovine anti-*E. phagocytophila* sera were used in a modified immunohistologic method (2). Numerous small (1 to 3 μm diameter) intracytoplasmic morulae were observed in postmortem spleen and peripheral blood neutrophils that were not present in control tissues (2).

The PCR technique has been used to detect both human ehrlichiosis agents known to occur in the United States. PCR primers derived from variable regions of the 16S rRNA gene sequence have been used to amplify DNA from *E. chaffeensis* (7) and the human granulocytic agent (8). In both instances, sensitivity has been increased by using a nested PCR reaction (8,24). The outside amplification is performed using either primers derived from a highly conserved region of the 16S rRNA gene sequence or universal primers. The specificity of the assay is dependent on the inside primers that bind to the 16S gene of the species in question. Because the granulocytic agent has only been amplified from a few patients, the inside primers were designed to amplify a wider group that includes *E. phagocytophila*, *E. equi*, and the human granulocytic agent. As in the case of successful culture, EDTA blood samples for the PCR technique are optimally drawn during the febrile phase of the disease before antibiotic treatment.

Serologic diagnosis of ehrlichial infections is accomplished by the indirect fluorescent antibody (IFA) test (25). Continuously infected macrophage cultures (DH82 cells) are used as the antigen for *E. chaffeensis IFA* (26). At the Centers for Disease Control and Prevention (CDC), human ehrlichiosis due to *E. chaffeensis* is defined by a fourfold change in immunoglobulin G antibody levels. Until 1990, when *E. chaffeensis* was first isolated, *E. canis* was used as the diagnostic antigen. Comparative tests have shown that *E. chaffeensis* antigen is more sensitive in detecting the homologous antibody during the early stages of the disease (CDC, unpublished data 1994).

Serologically, HGE is detected by testing patients' sera on *E. phagocytophila*-infected neutrophils or *E. equi*-infected leukocytes (8). The majority of patients had a higher antibody titer when *E. equi*-infected cells were used as antigen. However, two patients had a 1:80 titer with *E. phagocytophila* antigen and were less than 1:80 on *E. equi* (2).

PREVENTION AND TREATMENT

Epidemiologic evidence suggests that both forms of human ehrlichiosis are transmitted by ticks. Therefore, precautions against tick exposure must be taken. A study of military personnel documented that permethrin-impregnated clothing is an effective prevention measure (27). However, the availability of

Emergence of *Vibrio Cholerae* O139

R. BRADLEY SACK
M. JOHN ALBERT
A. KASEM SIDDIQUE

Ever since *Vibrio cholerae* was first identified more than 100 years ago by Koch, it has been axiomatic that only the serogroup designated as O1 was capable of causing epidemic cholera. Thus, the observation in late 1992 of an epidemic of cholera caused by a newly identified non-O1 serogroup (later designated as *V. cholerae* O139, the next consecutive number in the typing scheme) came as an unexpected unprecedented event (1–3). Not only had a "new" bacterial pathogen taken its place in the notorious list of pathogens lethal for humans, but this new pathogen belonged to a particularly virulent bacterial species, the only one capable of causing worldwide pandemic disease. Now, more than 2 years after its appearance, there continues to be considerable speculation as to its ultimate behavior: will this organism continue to spread out of its birthplace in the Bay of Bengal to involve the world in the eighth pandemic of cholera?

Fortunately, this organism appeared in a region of the world in which it could be quickly recognized. Within a few months of its discovery, diagnostic sera had been produced to follow the spread of the epidemic, the organism was being characterized in many laboratories around the world, and strategies for vaccine production were being formulated. This rapid response by the global scientific community was exemplary and must be among the most successful ever mounted.

BACKGROUND

Cholera has been known since earliest recorded history in the region of the Ganges River delta, which is now primarily Bangladesh and a small part of India (4,5). Beginning in the early 19th century, however, it spread out of its asiatic "home" to involve the entire world in the form of seven pandemics, causing considerable mortality wherever it struck. Because there was no adequate treatment of any kind until the early 1900s, mortality rates of 50% to 70% were recorded during the early pandemics (4,5).

The causative agent was not identified until 1884 during the fifth pandemic; therefore, the serogroups causing the first four pandemics will probably never be known for certain. The subsequent three pandemics were known to be caused by serogroup O1. The last one, the seventh, which is still in progress, however, was caused by a biotype variant of the O1 serogroup, designated El Tor to differentiate it from the known "classical" O1 vibrios. The behavior of the El Tor vibrios may be instructive in our understanding of the new O139 vibrio (5).

The El Tor vibrio was first discovered in 1905 at the El Tor quarantine station in Egypt in the intestinal contents of deceased pilgrims returning from Mecca (4). It was thought to be a curiosity at the time. In 1936 it was found in the Celebes in Indonesia, where it caused cholera-like disease, but remained in a relatively small geographic area. Because the organism was not a classic vibrio, the clinical disease it caused was initially (and temporarily) designated "paracholera," even though it was identical to true cholera in all respects (5). Not until 1960 did El Tor vibrios begin to move from Indonesia to gradually cover nearly the entire world. Thirty-five years after the pandemic began, it is still causing severe disease on a global scale. Still unknown are the reasons how or why this El Tor vibrio, localized for many years, suddenly developed pandemic potential. Being able to survive and multiply in an aquatic environment (including zooplankton and phytoplankton) (6) seems like the most important feature of its "success," but the characteristics of the vibrio that facilitated this survival advantage are not known.

V. cholerae El Tor, being a biotype of classical vibrios, shares most of the known virulence properties of classical *V. cholerae* (i.e., cell wall antigens, enterotoxin). Thus, persons living in an area endemic for classical cholera are at least partially immune to El Tor cholera. Despite this, El Tor caused large epidemics of cholera in these partially immune populations, and over a period of only a few years, displaced nearly all classic strains, thereby becoming the endemic strain (5). Bangladesh is the only place in the world where classic *V. cholerae* are still isolated (7), but these isolations are now sporadic and rare. In a like manner, in nonimmune populations, which make up most of the rest of the world, El Tor has first caused large epidemics and then has usually persisted as an endemic disease in those same geographic areas.

Because *V. cholerae* O139 has cell wall antigens that are different from the O1 serogroup, it was thought that populations living in areas endemic for O1 cholera would not have significant immunity to infection with the O139 vibrio. Indeed, this has proven to be the case (see later sections). Therefore, all the world is essentially nonimmune to this new cholera vibrio.

Because, unlike El Tor, the O139 vibrio made its first appearance as both a clinically virulent and a potent epidemic-causing organism, it may already harbor all the necessary characteristics that allow it to survive well in the environment and thus be potentially a pandemic strain.

EPIDEMIOLOGY

Although there is some controversy about the exact time and place, it is clear that *V. cholerae* O139 was first isolated sometime in mid-1962 in the south of India (Vellore and Madras). The isolates were sent to the National Institute of Cholera and Enteric Diseases (NICED), Calcutta, for identification (8). The first outbreak of cholera in which these organisms were recognized as being etiologic occurred in Madras in October 1992 (1). Within a month, similar isolates were being identified from other parts of south India (Madurai and Vellore) and Calcutta. Within several months of its isolation in Calcutta, a large epi-

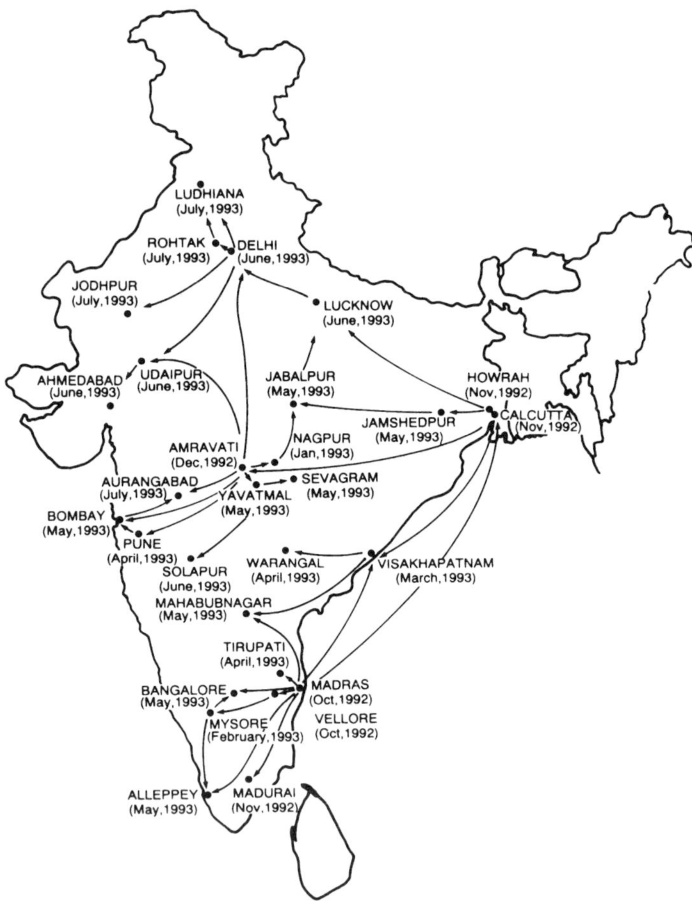

Figure 9.1. Spread of *V. cholerae* O139 in India. Sites marked had serogroup O139 confirmed by the NICED, Calcutta, using specific anti-O139 antiserum. Arrows indicating probable direction of spread are speculative and based on first isolation of O139 in a given area. (Reproduced with permission from Nair et al, J Infect Dis 1994;169:1033.)

demic occurred there. During 1993, the O139 vibrio spread throughout India, causing major outbreaks in a number of cities and largely displacing the endemic El Tor vibrio (9) In all of these outbreaks, those primarily affected by the disease were adults. Figure 9.1 illustrates the rapid spread of the disease in India.

In Bangladesh (2,3,10) the recognition of *V. cholerae* O139 came as the result of an outbreak of cholera in the latter part of 1992 in the small islands off the coast of the Sunderban areas of the southwestern coast. This outbreak was first recognized when it reached the mainland in December 1992, and a team of physicians and epidemiologists from the International Center for Diarrheal Disease Research, Bangladesh (ICDDR,B), were sent to provide diagnostic and clinical support. An unusual clinical pattern in the outbreak was noted: most of the patients were adults, in contrast to the usual outbreaks in Bangladesh in which the majority of patients are children, reflecting the endemic nature of the disease. Initially, these stool samples all grew non-O1 vibrios, which at that time could not be further identified.

In the third week of January 1993, the large Muslim gathering of "Bishwa Istama" (an annual event) was held on the banks of the Turag river about 20 km north of Dhaka. About 2 million pilgrims from all over Bangladesh and the Indian subcontinent gathered, dwelling in crowded generally unhygienic provisions. An outbreak of cholera-like illness occurred during this time, and several persons (locals and foreigners) were treated at the diarrhea hospital of the ICDDR,B in Dhaka; only *V. cholerae* non-O1 were isolated from these patients. Because the possibility of a new vibrio was not yet recognized (the isolates from the outbreak in the south had not yet been characterized or recognized as a single serotype), these strains were not saved (11). It is possible (and can only be surmised) that the O139 vibrios were brought to Dhaka from the south of Bangladesh or India by the pilgrims and perhaps thereafter carried back to their homelands.

In February 1993, large numbers of patients with cholera associated with non-O1 vibrios were being seen at the same hospital, and about 1 month later a similar outbreak was seen in the rural diarrhea hospital of the ICDDR,B in Matlab, about 45 km south of Dhaka (3). As in the outbreaks in the south coastal areas of the country, disproportionate numbers of patients were adults.

By this time it was recognized that the strains from India and those from Bangladesh were of the same O139 serogroup as typed in the laboratory of Dr. T. Shimada (12), and the synonym "Bengal" was suggested for these isolates, because the strains had first appeared in several coastal regions of the Bay of Bengal. Polyclonal diagnostic antisera were quickly prepared in India, Bangladesh, and Japan and made available to laboratories involved in cholera diagnosis.

During 1993, *V. cholerae* spread to most parts of Bangladesh (10), as illustrated in Figure 9.2, except for the northern part of the country. An estimated 170,000 cases and 2000 deaths were reported by the government of Bangladesh in the

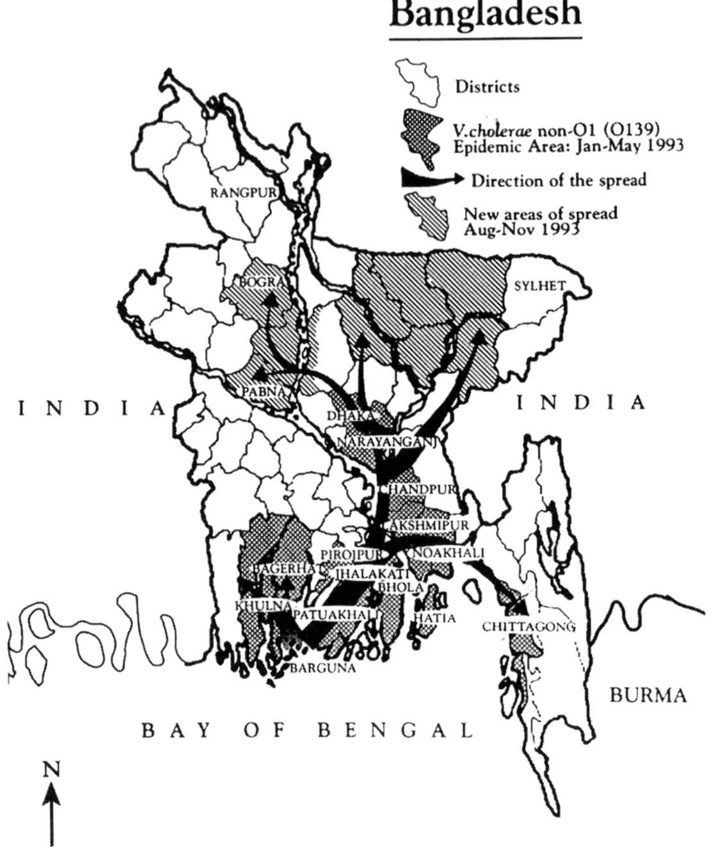

Figure 9.2. Spread of *V. cholerae* O139 in Bangladesh in 1993; isolates were confirmed at the ICDDR,B using specific anti-O139 antiserum. Arrows indicating direction of spread are based on investigation of outbreaks. (Reproduced with permission from Siddique, AK, Epidemic Control Preparedness Plogram, Annual Report, 1993, ICDDR,B, p. 36.)

southern part of the country in a 6-month period (13,14). In many areas, the O139 seemed to replace the O1 vibrios; very few infections with O1 vibrios were being seen during cholera outbreaks. This seemed to be only temporary in some areas, however; by the next cholera epidemic at the end of 1993 in Matlab, *V. cholerae* O1 had returned as the predominant isolate in Matlab. This is shown in Figure 9.3.

In 1993, the hospitalization rate for cholera due to *V. cholerae* O139 in a demographic surveillance population of approximately 200,000 persons living

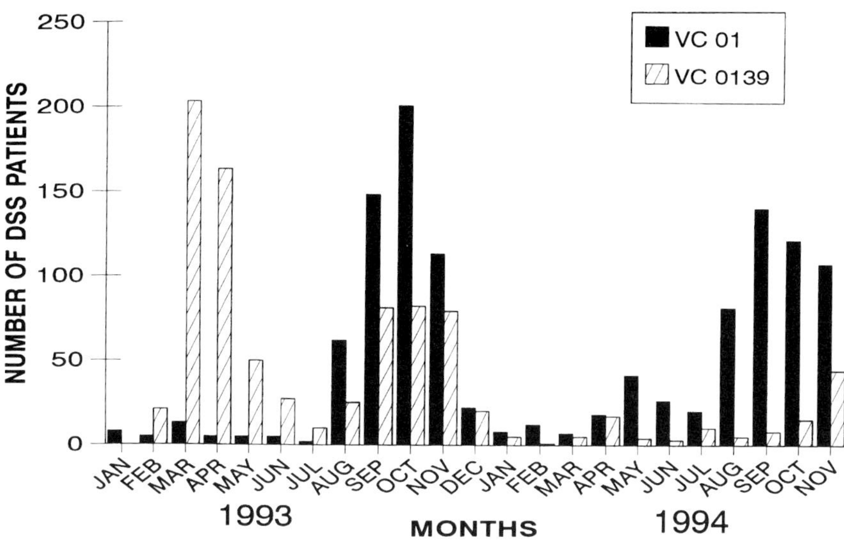

Figure 9.3. Numbers of patients from the Demographic Surveillance System area admitted to the diarrheal hospital in Matlab, Bangladesh, with cholera due to either *V. cholerae* O1 or O139 during 1993 and 1994.

in Matlab was 3.5 per 1000 (13). The attack rates were the same for small children as for adults.

In 1993, *V. cholerae* O139 was also reported from a number of neighboring countries; however, no large outbreaks were reported in these areas. Countries from which these organisms were isolated are Thailand (15), Malaysia, Nepal, Pakistan, and the northwest part of China (16). Several countries also reported imported cases during this time: Japan (17), United States (18), United Kingdom (19), Hong Kong (20), and Singapore (21).

In 1994, the frequency with which O139 vibrios were being isolated decreased. New outbreaks, however, were reported in Vellore, India (22), and in Karachi, Pakistan, but no new countries were invaded. Diagnostic antisera had been supplied to essentially all countries in this region to facilitate recognition of these organisms.

Studies of transmission of *V. cholerae* O139 have been performed in both rural and urban areas in Bangladesh (23,24). In the rural Matlab study, secondary infection rates among family members were 25% within 10 days of the index cases, with 27% of those infected having diarrhea (23). Children under 5 years of age were more frequently infected than adults. Tubewell water, which was free of vibrios at its source, frequently become contaminated with O139 vibrios on storage in the house.

In the Dhaka urban study, 16% of family contacts became infected and 37% of them were symptomatic (24).

ENVIRONMENTAL STUDIES

Relatively few studies have yet been done on the environmental hardiness of these organisms. Cultures of surface waters (ponds, rivers) in Bangladesh were frequently positive for *V. cholerae* O139; of 92 samples cultured, 11 (12%) were positive (25).

Studies done in laboratory microcosms showed that O139 vibrios survive equally as well as El Tor vibrios—up to about 6 weeks in pond water (26,27). *V. cholerae* O139 also can be found in association with plankton in surface waters, as has been shown for O1 vibrios (Huq A, Colwell RR, Chowdhury MAR et al, unpublished data, 1995). Like O1 vibrios, O139 vibrios also become nonculturable and can persist as recognizable vibrios as seen by fluorescent microscopy (27). Recent unpublished studies, as indicated by Huq et al above, demonstrate that they too can remain viable in the nonculturable state.

CLINICAL FEATURES OF THE DISEASE

The syndrome of clinical cholera produced by *V. cholerae* O139 is indistinguishable from that produced by *V. cholerae* O1 in adults and children (3,10,28–30). Patients have a rapid onset of illness; their duration of diarrhea before hospitalization is about 12 hours. Vomiting is almost universal at the onset of their disease. Voluminous quantities of electrolyte-rich rice-watery stool are passed, leading to dehydration and hypovolemic shock. Stool output after correction of dehydration ranges from 4 to 12 ml/kg body weight/hr; total stool output over the course of the illness in adults given appropriate antibiotics may be as high as 10 to 15 liters. The small bowel is heavily colonized with vibrios, as confirmed by small bowel biopsies and by high bacterial counts in jejunal fluid; large amounts of cholera enterotoxin are found in the stool (3). Convalescent antibody responses occur to the cell wall antigens of the vibrio and the cholera enterotoxin (3).

Patients respond to standard therapy for cholera. Intravenous rehydration is usually required initially in hospitalized patients, because most are severely dehydrated. This is followed by oral rehydration therapy when the patient is no longer in shock. Patients with only moderate or mild dehydration at the time of presentation can usually be treated with oral rehydration therapy alone.

Antibiotics are important adjuncts to treatment. All O139 vibrios have been sensitive to tetracyclines, which are the drugs of choice (3,31). Antibiotic treatment diminishes the volume of stool passed and the duration of illness by about 50%. If antibiotics are not given, the disease may last 3 to 4 days, whereas with antibiotics, it is predictably about 36 hours.

Mortality in untreated disease is estimated to be 50% or more, as was seen during the July 1994 Zaire outbreak caused by *V. cholerae* O1 (32). With adequate treatment, mortality should be less than 1%; essentially anyone who arrives at a treatment facility with a heartbeat should not die from cholera.

LABORATORY STUDIES

V. cholerae O139 exhibits striking resemblance to *V. cholerae* O1 in almost all characteristics.

Morphology

It is a gram-negative, facultative, anaerobic, curved bacillus, measures 2 to 3 μm by 0.5 μm, and has a single polar flagellum (Fig. 9.4). As a result of these morphologic features, it shows the typical darting motility of *V. cholerae*.

Culture

The cultural characteristics of *V. cholerae* O139 are identical to those of *V. cholerae* O1. It grows on all nonselective and selective media used for the cultivation and isolation of *V. cholerae* O1. It grows in media containing 0 to 3%, but not 8%, salt. Of note is that it thrives in media with a high alkalinity (as alkaline-peptone-water), which can be used for enrichment of *V. cholerae* O139 from mixed cultures as in the case of *V. cholerae* O1. The same two solid media used for selective cultivation of *V. cholerae* O1 are also used for *V. cholerae* O139.

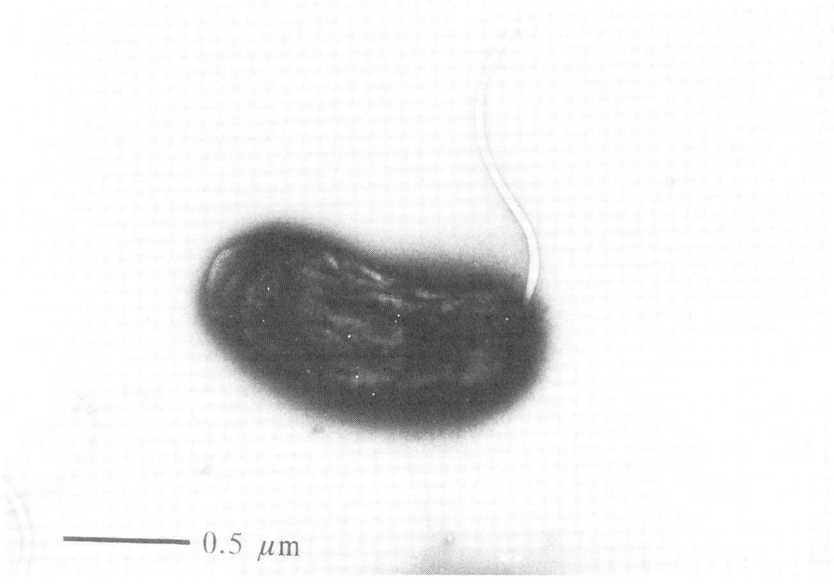

Figure 9.4. Transmission electron microscopy of a negatively stained *V. cholerae* O139 Bengal, which shows a curved organism with an uniform flagellum. (Photo courtesy of Dr. M. Ehara, Institute of Tropical Medicine, University of Nagasaki, Nagasaki, Japan.)

On one such medium, thiosulfate-citrate-bile salt-sucrose (TCBS) agar, *V. cholerae* O139 produces typical yellow colonies as a result of sucrose fermentation (3,25,31). However, we have found that occasional strains of *V. cholerae* O139 can be sucrose nonfermenters or late-fermenters. Such strains will give rise to green colonies after 20 to 24 hours incubation of the plates. Adequate attention should be paid to such strains if they are not to be missed (33). The second selective medium, taurocholate-tellurite-gelatin agar (TTGA) (34), which is routinely used at the clinical microbiology laboratory of the ICDDR,B, produces colonies typical of *V. cholerae* O1. The colonies are grayish with dark centers surrounded most often by a zone of opacity (due to gelatinase activity).

On several media including Luria agar, gelatin agar, and TTGA, like certain *V. cholerae* non-O1 strains, *V. cholerae* O139 produces two types of colonies: opaque and translucent. Some strains produce either form, and others produce a mixture of both. Opaque colonies on gelatin-containing media, such as gelatin agar and TTGA, produce, in addition, a zone of opacity around the colonies as a result of gelatinase activity, whereas this characteristic is absent or minimal with translucent colonies. Upon prolonged incubation (beyond 24 hours), however, this distinction between the colonies becomes blurred as translucent forms become opaque. As in other *V. cholerae* non-O1 strains, this colony variation is correlated with the presence of a capsular layer (35,36). Opaque colonies possess a capsule, whereas this capsular layer is negligible or absent in translucent colonies (see below) (36).

Physiology and Biochemistry

Like all vibrios, *V. cholerae* O139 is positive for indophenol oxidase and ferments a variety of sugars without gas production. Of note is that, like O1 vibrios, it ferments D-(+)-mannose and sucrose but not L-(+)-arabinose and thus belongs to Heiberg group 1 vibrios (37). Like the El Tor biotype of O1 vibrios, it is positive for Vogues-Proskauer reaction, shows variable hemolysis of sheep erythrocytes in conventional tube test but consistent hemolysis in the CAMP test (Lesmana M, Albert MJ, unpublished data 1994), and agglutinates erythrocytes from a variety of species, including chicken. It possesses κ-type phage but is resistant to Mukherjee's phages specific for classical and El Tor vibrios (3,38). It is also resistant to polymyxin B (50 μg disc) and vibriostatic compound O/129 (2,4-diamino-6,7-diisopropylpteridine, 10 μg and 150 μg discs) (25,31).

Antimicrobial Susceptibility

In the early part of the epidemic, *V. cholerae* O139 isolates from Bangladesh were reported to be susceptible to tetracycline, ampicillin, chloramphenicol, erythromycin, and ciprofloxacin but resistant to cotrimoxazole and streptomycin (3). Isolates from Calcutta, India, were also reported to be susceptible to the commonly used antimicrobial agents but resistant to cotrimoxazole, streptomycin, and furazolidone (1). All of these data were obtained by disc diffusion method. More recently, in another study (39), the minimum inhibitory concentrations (MICs) of 39 antimicrobial agents to 173 isolates obtained from India, Bangladesh, and Thailand during 1992 to 1993 were tested. The newer quinolones (norfloxacin, ofloxacin, tosufloxacin, ciprofloxacin, sparfloxacin, BAYy3118, and DU6859a) showed the greatest activity (MICs $\leq$ 0.06 μg/mL). All isolates were susceptible to tetracycline (MICs, 0.25 to 0.5 μg/mL). Approximately 95% of the isolates were resistant to chloramphenicol (MICs, 4 to 8 μg/mL), furazolidone (MICs, 2 to 8 μg/mL), streptomycin (MICs, 64 $\geq$ 256 μg/mL), sulfamethoxazole (MIC, $\geq$256 μg/mL), trimethoprim (MIC, 128 $\geq$ 256 μg/mL), and vibriostatic compound O/129 (MIC, $\geq$256 μg/mL). Six isolates of *V. cholerae* O139 were resistant to ampicillin, tetracycline, chloramphenicol, kanamycin, gentamicin, sulfamethoxazole, trimethoprim, and O/129. This resistance phenotype was encoded by a 200-kb plasmid in all six strains. Azithromycin, an azalide, was more active against *V. cholerae* O139 than erythromycin. Because this agent also has a good safety record in children, it could be an attractive chemotherapeutic agent of choice in the treatment of cholera (39).

Capsule

Like a majority of *V. cholerae* non-O1 strains but unlike *V. cholerae* O1, *V. cholerae* O139 isolates possess a capsule. However, this capsule seems to be relatively thin, at 18 to 25 nm in thickness (Fig. 9.5). Preliminary analysis of the capsular layer suggests that it is distinct from the lipopolysaccharide (LPS) antigen (see below) and has the following sugars: 3,6-dideoxyhexose (colitose), *N*-acetylquinovosamine, *N*-acetyl glucosamine, glucose, galactose, and galacturonic acid and traces of tetradecanoic and hexadecanoic fatty acids (35,40). Another report also confirmed the presence of the above sugars as components of the capsular layer; however, in place of 3,6-dideoxyhexose, a 3,6-dideoxyxylohexose was identified (41). Yet another report suggested that colitose might be part of LPS (42). Using spontaneously occurring translucent mutant colonies and TnphoA mutants defective in LPS and capsular polysaccharide (CPS) synthesis, it was found that LPS and CPS have cross-reactive epitopes. Furthermore, CPS might be a polymerized form of O-antigen side-chain molecules that are not covalently bound to core polysaccharide and lipid A (43). It is hoped that studies with the mutants should clarify the structure and composition of CPS. The biologic significance of this capsule is under investigation.

In comparison with a heavily capsulated organism like *Klebsiella pneumoniae*, there are differences; whereas *K. pneumoniae* is highly hydrophilic and serum resistant, *V. cholerae* O139 isolates was not hydrophilic but intermediate in serum resistance (44). However, serum resistance of *V. cholerae* O139, as a result of capsule, poses problems in the development of a vibriocidal antibody assay for immune response studies of *V. cholerae* O139 infection. A vibriocidal assay patterned after *V. cholerae* O1 does not result in the killing of *V. cholerae* O139 organisms (45). This is thought to be due to the inhibitory effect of CPS that prevents the effective attachment of the terminal complement complex to the surface of the bacterium which should result in bacterial lysis (46). However, our studies revealed that this inhibitory effect of CPS can be overcome by increasing the complement concentration and decreasing the bacterial numbers compared with the standard vibriocidal assay for *V. cholerae* O1 (Qadri F, Mohi MG, Hossain J, et al., unpublished data). The presence of capsule in *V. cholerae* non-O1 in general is associated with increased virulence, especially of bacteremia due to serum resistance (47). A similar phenomenon has also been demonstrated for *V. cholerae* O139. Intradermal inoculation of mice resulted in

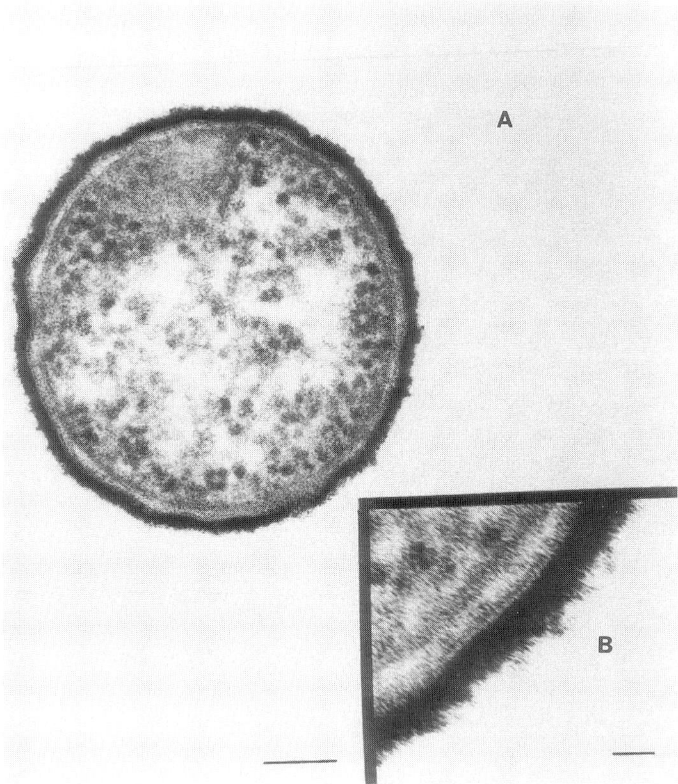

Figure 9.5. (**A**) Transmission electron microscopy of a negatively stained thin section of an isolate of *V. cholerae* O139 Bengal with a distinct electron-dense band (capsule). Bar, 100 nm. (**B**) Higher magnification of the dense band showing fine ultrastructure of the cell wall. Bar, 20 nm. (Photo courtesy of Dr. A. Weintraub, Huddinge Hospital, Karolinska Institute, Stockholm, Sweden.)

bacteremia with *V. cholerae* O139 and not with *V. cholerae* O1 (36). Moreover, there are at least two documented cases of bacteremia due to *V. cholerae* O139—one in an adult patient with chronic liver disorder and another in a malnourished child (48) (Khan AM, Albert MJ, Sarker SA, et al, unpublished data 1994), both of whom presented with *V. cholerae* O139-associated diarrhea.

LPS Antigen

The LPS antigen of *V. cholerae* O139 is distinctly different from that of *V. cholerae* O1. However, the magnitude of biological activities, such as mitogenic activity, lethal toxicity, and Shwartzman reaction in laboratory models for LPSs from *V. cholerae* O1 and O139, are similar (49). The polyclonal antiserum to *V. cholerae* O1 does not agglutinate *V. cholerae* O139 and vice versa. The monoclonal antibodies directed against the A, B, and C antigenic epitopes of *V. cholerae* O1 also do not react with *V. cholerae* O139 (50). Smooth bacterial forms, including *V. cholerae* O1, have three components in their LPS structure: lipid A, core oligosaccharide, and O-antigenic side chain. However, studies on LPS antigen of *V. cholerae* O139 suggested that the LPS is that of a semirough type bacterium in that it contains lipid A, a highly substituted core-oligosaccharide, and no long O-antigenic side chain (51). By sugar analysis, one group of workers identified a 3,6-dideoxyhexose (colitose) as a dominant part of LPS for the first time in any member of the family Vibrionaceae (42). However, another group identified this sugar as a constituent of CPS (35) (vide supra).

Other constituents of LPS are glucose, galactose, glucosamine, heptose, and keto-3-deoxy-D-mannose-octulosonic acid (KDO). Tetradecanoic acid, hexadecanoic acid, 3-hydroxy-dodecanoic acid, and 3-hydroxy-tetradecanoic acids were identified in the lipid A (34,41). *V. cholerae* O139 shares the R antigen with all vibrios. Therefore, the diagnostic antiserum to *V. cholerae* O139 should be cross-absorbed with a rough strain of *V. cholerae* to remove R agglutinins. Furthermore, of the 155 serogroups of *V. cholerae* described so far, only two serogroups, O22 and O155, cross-react with *V. cholerae* O139 in an a,b-a,c type of relationship, where a is the common antigenic epitope and b and c are distinct epitopes (52). This has also made it necessary to absorb the *V. cholerae* O139 diagnostic antiserum with reference *V. cholerae* strains representing serogroups O22 and O155 (52).

Fimbrial Antigens

Fimbrial appendages help in the adherence of vibrios to the intestinal mucosal surface. A variety of fimbrial antigens has been demonstrated in *V. cholerae* O1. These include the toxin-coregulated pilus with a subunit molecular weight of 20 kDa (TcpA) (53), mannose-sensitive hemagglutinin (MSHA) (54), a 16-kDa subunit structure pilus (55), and a hydrophobic pilus of 18 kDa (56). All of these fimbrial antigens of *V. cholerae* O1 have been demonstrated in *V. cholerae* O139 as well (13,31,57,58). In addition, *V. cholerae* O139 produces a curved (wavy) pilus with a subunit molecular weight of 2.8 kDa (minipilus), which is shared by many species of gram-negative bacteria (59). Also, *V. cholerae* O139 produces a pilus with a 20-kDa subunit structure that is present in some non-O1 *V. cholerae* but not *V. cholerae* O1 (60). The finding of a variety of pili in O139 vibrios as in O1 vibrios suggests that *V. cholerae* O139 should be a good colonizer. Accordingly, *V. cholerae* O139 organisms have been recovered from the upper small intestinal fluids (3) and demonstrated to be adherent to the small intestinal mucosal tissue in patients with cholera in the acute stage of the disease (61). Like O1 vibrios, they show a predilection for aggregative adherence to the microfolds of the Peyer's patches where M cells are located. Obviously, the bacteria are effectively presented to the immune system via the M cells (61).

Toxins and Other Soluble Factors

V. cholerae O139 produces a cholera toxin (CT) that is identical to that produced by El Tor vibrios (62). As in the case of El Tor vibrios, optimal production of CT occurs under AKI-SW cultural conditions (57), and the amount of toxin produced sometimes exceeds that produced by El Tor vibrios (50). Patients infected with *V. cholerae* O139 also excrete CT in the stool, sometimes in amounts exceeding those excreted by patients infected with El Tor vibrios (50). It has been observed that the type of toxin produced depends on the medium used. For example, when grown in Casamino acids-yeast extract broth, *V. cholerae* O139 produces a cytotonic enterotoxin, but in brain-heart infusion broth, it produces a toxin that is cytotoxic for Y1 adrenal tumor cells (31). Hemagglutinin/protease is an enzyme that nicks the A subunit of CT. *V. cholerae* O139 produces a hemagglutinin/protease that is identical to that produced by *V. cholerae* O1 and non-O1 vibrios (Naka A, Yamamoto K, Albert MJ, Honda T, unpublished data). The organism also produces a soluble hemolysin that is lethal for sheep erythrocytes. Because it possesses gene sequences for minor toxins of *V. cholerae* O1, such as zonula occludens toxin (Zot) and accessory cholera enterotoxin (Ace), it is presumed that the organism is capable of elaborating these toxins. However, it does not possess the gene sequence for heat-stable enterotoxin of some non-O1 vibrios (NAG-ST) (50).

Invasive Properties

Non-O1 vibrios not infrequently produce extraintestinal infections, especially septicemia, in individuals with chronic underlying disease entities. This capacity is mostly attributed to the possession of capsules by non-O1 vibrios (47). Although *V. cholerae* O1 organisms are prototype organisms of secretory diarrhea, there are reports of bloodstream infections by them (63,64). As alluded to in a preceding section, there are at least two documented cases of bloodstream infection with *V. cholerae* O139. When the ability of O1 and O139 vibrios to invade HEp-2 cells on culture was studied, several bacteria belonging to both serogroups were located intracellularly (31). However, the invasive property of these vibrios needs to be studied in detail. The invasive property may be yet another aspect of the pathogenesis of cholera. It is possible that a mild degree of invasion of intestinal mucosa may not manifest as invasive diarrhea but rather may be an effective mechanism to present CT to the internal milieu of enterocytes.

Molecular Characterization

In *V. cholerae* O1 strains, most of the genes that encode virulence factors are located on a 4.5-kb virulence cassette or core region of the chromosome. The genes that have been identified in the core region are ctxAB (that encodes CT), zot (that encodes zonula occludens toxin), ace (that encodes accessory cholera enterotoxin), and cep (that encodes a pilin antigen for intestinal colonization). This core region is flanked by two or more copies of RS1 elements (repetitive sequence 1, an insertion sequence 2.7-kb long normally found at the junction of tandem duplication of ctxAB responsible for amplification of ctxAB). The RS1 sequence encodes a site-specific recombination system that mediates recombination between CTX genetic element and an 18-bp target sequence on the *V. cholerae* chromosome termed attRS1. The core region and the RS1 element constitute the CTX element, and this element is indeed a site-specific transposon (65). Normally, *V. cholerae* O1 isolates carry multiple copies of the CTX element. Similarly, *V. cholerae* O139 also carries two or more copies of the CTX element. The finding of multiple copies of the CTX element in *V. cholerae* O139 suggests that duplication and amplification of the element may play a role in the virulence of *V. cholerae* O139 strains as in the case of *V. cholerae* O1 strains (66,67). The classical and El Tor biotypes of *V. cholerae* O1 differ in the distribution of the CTX element within the chromosome. In the classic strains, the CTX element is located at two loci, whereas in El Tor strains, it is located at only one locus that is identical to one of the two loci associated with the CTX integration in classic strains (68). Studies by one group of investigators (69) suggested that the CTX elements in *V. cholerae* O139 were located at two loci that are homologous to those identified in classic rather than El Tor biotype of *V. cholerae* O1, although these loci in *V. cholerae* O139 could reside on restriction fragments of variable size. However, studies by another group (65) suggested that chromosomal organization of CTX element in *V. cholerae* O139 resembled that of El Tor and not classical *V. cholerae*. The reason for the discrepancy of findings is not known. Moreover, *V. cholerae* O139 isolates carry the tcpA gene (which encodes the structural subunit of TCP, TcpA) that has structural identity with that of El Tor vibrios (70) and three iron-regulated genes, irgA (a virulence gene), viuA (the gene for the receptor for the siderophore vibriobactin), and fur (an iron-regulating gene) previously described in O1 vibrios in the same chromosomal location as in El Tor vibrios (71). Further relatedness with El Tor vibrios was

REFERENCES

1 **Ramamurthy T, Garg S, Sharma R, et al.** Emergence of novel strain of *Vibrio cholerae* with epidemic potential in southern and eastern India. Lancet 1993;341:703–704.

2 **Albert MJ, Siddique AK, Islam MS, et al.** Large outbreak of clinical cholera due to *Vibrio cholerae* non-O1 in Bangladesh. Lancet 1993;341:704.

3 Cholera Working Group, International Centre for Diarrhoeal Disease Research, Bangladesh. Large epidemic of cholera like disease in Bangladesh caused by *Vibrio cholerae* O139 synonym Bengal. Lancet 1993; 342:387–390.

4 **Pollitzer R.** Cholera. Geneva: World Health Organization, 1959:11–50.

5 **Barua D.** History of cholera. In: Barua D, Greenough WB, eds. Cholera. New York, London: Plenium Medical Book company, 1992:1–36.

6 **Islam MS, Drasar BS, Sack RB.** The aquatic flora and fauna as reservoirs of *Vibrio cholerae*: a review, J Diarrhoeal Dis Res 1994;12:87–96.

7 **Siddique AK, Baqui AK, Eusof A, et al.** Survival of classic cholera in Bangladesh. Lancet 1991;337:1125–1127.

8 **Nair GB, Bhattacharya SK, Shimada T, Takeda Y,** The spread of *Vibrio cholerae* O139 in India. Letter J Infect Dis 1995;171:759.

9 **Nair GB, Ramamurthy T, Bhattacharya SK, et al.** Spread of *Vibrio cholerae* O139 Bengal in India. J Infect Dis 1994;169:1029–1034.

10 **Siddique AK, Zaman K, Akram K, et al.** Emergence of a new epidemic strain of *Vibrio Cholerae* in Bangladesh. Trop Geograph Med 1994;46:147–150.

11 **Albert MJ.** Personal reflections on the discovery of *Vibrio cholerae* O139 synonym Bengal: a tribute to team work and international collaboration. J Diarrhoeal Dis Res 1993;11: 207–210.

12 **Shimada T, Nair GB, Deb BC, et al.** Outbreak of *Vibrio cholerae* non-O1 in India and Bangladesh. Lancet 1993;341:1346–1347.

13 **Sack RB, Albert MJ.** Summary of cholera vaccine workshop. J Diarrhoeal Dis Res 1994;12:138–143.

14 **Rabbani GH, Mahalanabis D.** New strains of *Vibrio cholerae* O139 in India and Bangladesh: lessons from the recent epidemic. J Diarrhoeal Dis Res 1993;11:63–66.

15 **Manas C, Wanpen C, Pikul M, et al.** *Vibrio cholerae* O130 Bengal in Bangkok. Lancet 1993;342:430–431.

16 World Health Organization. Cholerae caused by *Vibrio cholerae* O139 Weekly epidemiological record. 1994;69:214–216.

17 **Kurazono T, Yamada F, Yamaguchi M, et al.** The first report of traveller's diarrhoea associated with a newly discribed toxigenic *Vibrio cholera* O139 strain in Japan. J Jpn Assoc Infect Dis 1994;68:8–12.

18 Centers for Disease Control and Prevention. Imported cholerae associated with a newly described toxigenic *Vibrio cholerae* O139 strain—California, 1993. JAMA 1993;270: 428–429.

19 **Cheasty T, Rowe B, Said B, Frost J.** *Vibrio cholerae* serogroup O139 in England and Wales. Lancet 1993;307:1007.

20 **Yuen K-Y, Yam W-C, Wong SS-Y, et al.** *Vibrio cholerae* O139 synonym Bengal in Hong Kong. Clin Infect Dis 1994;19:553.

21 **Tay L, Goh KT, Lim YS.** *Vibrio cholerae* O139 "Bengal" in Singapore. J Trop Med Hyg 1994;97:317–320.

22 **Jesudason MV, John TJ.** Major shift in prevalence of non-O1 and El Tor *Vibrio cholerae*. Lancet 1993;341:1090–1091.

23 **Yunus M, Sack RB, Zaman K, et al.** Transmission of *Vibrio cholerae* O139 Bengal among family contacts of index cases in a rural area in Bangladesh. Third commonwealth conference on diarrhoea and malnutriton, Shatin, Hongkong, November 1994.

24 **Faruque ASG, Mahalanabis D, Albert MJ, Hoque SS.** Studies of infection with *Vibrio cholerae* O139 synonym Bengal in family contacts of index cases. Trans R Soc Trop Med Hyg 1994;88:439.

25 **Islam MS, Hasan MK, Miah MA, et al.** Isolation of *Vibrio cholerae* O139 synonym Bengal from the aquatic environment in Bangladesh: implications for disease transmission. Appl Environ Microbiol 1994;60: 1684–1686.

26 **Okitsu T, Morozumi H, Murase T, et al.** Survival of *Vibrio cholerae* O139 in water from a river. J Jpn Assoc Infect Dis 1994;68: 744–750.

27 **Islam MS, Hasan MK, Miah MA, et al.** Non-culturable *Vibrio cholerae* O139. Presented at the 94th General Meeting of the American Society for Microbiology, Las Vegas, Nevada, May 1994.

28 **Bhattacharya SK, Bhattcharya MK, Dutta D, et al.** *Vibrio cholerae* O139 in Calcutta. Arch Dis Child 1994;71:161–162.

29 **Bhattacharya SK, Bhattacharya MK, Nair**

GB, et al. Clinical profile of acute diarrhoea cases infected with the new epidemic strain of *Vibrio cholerae* O139: designation of the disease as cholera. J Infect 1993;27:11–15.

30 **Mahalanabis D, Faruque ASG, Albert MJ, et al.** An epidemic of cholera due to *Vibrio cholerae* O139 In Dhaka, Bangladesh: clinical and epidemiological features. Epidemiol Infect 1994;112:463–471.

31 **Albert MJ.** *Vibrio cholerae* O139 Bengal. J Clin Microbiol 1994;32:2345–2349.

32 **Siddique AK, Salam A, Islam MS, et al.** Why treatment centres failed to prevent cholera deaths among Rwandan refugees in Goma, Zaire. Lancet 1995;345:359–361.

33 **Ansaruzzaman M, Rahman M, Kibriya AKMG, et al.** Isolation of sucrose late-fermenting and nonfermenting variants of *Vibrio cholerae* O139 Bengal: implications for diagnosis of cholera. J Clin Microbiol 1995; 33:1339–1340.

34 **Monsur KA.** A highly selective gelatin-taurocholate-tellurite medium for the isolation of *Vibrio cholerae*. Trans R Soc Trop Med Hyg 1961;55:440–442.

35 **Weintraub A, Widmalm G, Jansson P-E, et al.** *Vibrio cholerae* O139 Bengal possesses a capsular polysaccharide which may confer increased virulence. Microb Pathog 1994;16: 235–241.

36 **Johnson JA, Salles CA, Panigrahi P, et al.** *Vibrio cholerae* O139 synonym Bengal is closely related to *Vibrio cholerae* O1 El Tor, but has important differences. Infect Immun 1994;62:2108–2110.

37 **Heiberg B.** The biochemical reactions of vibrios. J Hyg 1936;36:114–117.

38 **Higa N, Honma Y, Albert MJ, Iwanaga M.** Characterization of *Vibrio cholerae* O139 synonym Bengal isolated from patients with cholera-like disease in Bangladesh. Microbiol Immunol 1993;37:971–974.

39 **Yamamoto T, Nair GB, Albert MJ, et al.** Survey of in vitro susceptibilities of *Vibrio cholerae* O1 and O139 to antimicrobial agents. Antimicrob Agents Chemother 1995; 39:241–244.

40 **Weintraub A, Matheson L, Jansson P-E, et al.** Characterization of the carbohydrate antigens present in the cell wall of *Vibrio cholerae* O139 Bengal. In: Proceedings of the 30th Joint Conference on Cholera and Related Diarrhoeal Diseases. Fukuoka, Japan: US-Japan Cooperative Medical Science Program, 1994:58–61.

41 **Preston LM, Xu QW, Johnson JA, et al.** Preliminary structure determination of the capsular polysaccharide of *Vibrio cholerae* O139 Bengal AI1837. J Bacteriol 1995;177:835–838.

42 **Hisatsune K, Kondo S, Isshiki Y, et al.** O-antigenic polysaccharide of *Vibrio cholerae* O139 Bengal, a new epidemic strain for recent cholera in the Indian subcontinent. Biochem Biophys Res Commun 1993;196: 1309–1315.

43 **Waldor MK, Colwell R, Mekalanos JJ.** The *Vibrio cholerae* O139 serogroup antigen includes an O-antigen capsule and lipopolysaccharide virulence determinants. Proc Natl Acad Sci USA 1994;91:11388–11392.

44 **Meno Y, Amako K.** Biological meaning of the capsule-like layer of *Vibrio cholerae* O139. In: Proceedings of the 30th Joint Conference on Cholera and Related Diarrhoeal Diseases. Fukuoka, Japan: US-Japan Cooperative Medical Science Program, 1994:67–71.

45 **Tacket CO, Morris JG, Losonsky GA, et al.** Volunteer studies investigating the pathogenicity of *Vibrio cholerae* O139 and the protective efficacy conferred by both primary infection and by vaccine strain CVD 112. In: Proceedings of the 30th Joint Conference, on Cholera and Related Diarrheal Diseases. Fukuoka, Japan: U.S.-Japan Cooperative Medical Science Program, 1994:142–147.

46 **Goldman RL, Joiner K, Leive L.** Serum-resistant mutants of *Escherichia coli* O111 contain increased lipopolysaccharide, lack an O antigen-containing capsule, and cover more of their lipid A core with O-antigen. J Bacteriol 1984;159:877–882.

47 **Johnson JA, Panigrahi P, Morris JG Jr.** Non-O1 *Vibrio cholerae* NRT36S produces a polysaccharide capsule that determines colony morphology, serum resistance, and virulence in mice. Infect Immun 1992;60: 864–869.

48 **Jesudason MV, Cherion AM, John TJ.** Blood stream invasion by *Vibrio cholerae* O139. Lancet 1993;342:431.

49 **Shimizu T, Yanagihara Y, Isshiki Y, et al.** Biological activities of lipopolysaccharide isolated from *Vibrio cholerae* O139, a new epidemic strain for recent cholera in Indian subcontinent. Microbiol Immunol 1994;38: 471–474.

50 **Nair GB, Shimada T, Kurazono H, et al.** Characterization of phenotypic, serological and toxigenic traits of *Vibrio cholerae* O139 Bengal. J Clin Microbiol 1994;32:2775–2779.

51 **Manning PA, Stroeher UH, Morona R.** Molecular basis for O-antigenic biosynthesis in *Vibrio cholerae* O1: Ogawa-Inaba switching.

In: Wachsmuth IK, Blake PA, Olsvik O, eds. *Vibrio cholerae* and cholera: molecular to global perspectives. Washington, D.C.: American Society for Microbiology, 1994:77–94.

52 **Shimada T, Arakawa F, Itoh K, et al.** Two strains of *Vibrio cholerae* non-O1 possessing somatic (O) antigen factors in common with *V. cholerae* serogroup O139 synonym "Bengal." Curr Microbiol 1994;29:331–333.

53 **Hall RH, Losonsky G, Silveira APD, et al.** Immogenicity of *Vibrio cholerae* O1 toxin-coregulated pili in experimental and clinical cholera. Infect Immun 1991;59:2508–2512.

54 **Johnson G, Holmgren J, Svennerholm A-M.** Identification of a mannose-binding pilus of *Vibrio cholerae* El Tor. Microb Pathog 1991;11:433–441.

55 **Iwanaga M, Nakasone N, Yamashiro T, Higa N.** Pili of *Vibrio cholerae* widely distributed in serogroup O1 strains. Microbiol Immunol 1993;37:23–28.

56 **Ehara M, Iwami M, Ichinose Y, et al.** Purification and characterization of fimbriae from fimbriate *Vibrio cholerae* O1 strain Bgd 17. Trop Med 1991;33:109–125.

57 **Waldor MK, Mekalanos JJ.** ToxR regulates virulence gene expression in non-O1 strains of *Vibrio cholerae* that cause epidemic cholera. Infect Immun 1994;62:72–78.

58 **Nakasone N, Yamahiro T, Albert MJ, Iwanaga M.** Pili of a *Vibrio cholerae* O139. Microbiol Immunol 1994;38:225–227.

59 **Yamashiro T, Nakasone N, Honma Y, et al.** Purification and characterization of *Vibrio cholerae* O139 pili. FEMS Microbiol Lett 1994;115:247–252.

60 **Sengupta TK, Sengupta DK, Nair GB, Ghose AC.** Epidemic isolates of *Vibrio cholerae* O139 express antigenically distinct types of colonization pili. FEMS Microbiol Lett 1994;118:265–272.

61 **Yamamoto T, Albert MJ, Sack RB.** Adherence to the human small intestines of capsulated *Vibrio cholerae* O139. FEMS Microbiol Lett 1994;119:229–236.

62 **Hall RH, Khambaty FM, Kothary MH, et al.** *Vibrio cholerae* non-O1 serogroup associated with cholera gravis genetically and physiologically resembles O1 El Tor cholera strains. Infect Immun 1994;62:3859–3863.

63 **Jamil B, Ahmed A, Sturm AW.** *Vibrio cholerae* O1 septicemia. Lancet 1992;340:910–911.

64 **Rao A, Stockwell BA.** The Queensland cholera incidence of 1977. I. The index case. Bull World Health Organ 1980;58:663–664.

65 **Waldor MK, Mekalanos JJ.** Emergence of new cholera pandemic: molecular analysis of virulence determinants in *Vibrio cholerae* O139 and development of a live vaccine prototype. J Infect Dis 1994;170:278–283.

66 **Iida T, Shrestha J, Yamamoto K, et al.** Cholera isolates in relation to the "eighth pandemic." Lancet 1993;342:926.

67 **Das B, Ghosh RK, Sharma L, et al.** Tandem repeats of cholera toxin gene in *Vibro cholerae* O139. Lancet 1993;342:1173–1174.

68 **Goldberg I, Mekalanos JJ.** Effect of a recA mutation on cholera toxin gene amplification and deletion events. J Bacteriol 1986; 165:723–731.

69 **Lebens M, Holmgren J.** Structure and arrangement of the cholera toxin genes in *Vibrio cholerae* O139. FEMS Microbiol Lett 1994;117:197–202.

70 **Rhine JA, Taylor RK.** TcpA pilin sequences and colonization requirements for O1 and O139 *Vibrio cholerae*. Mol Microbiol 1994;13: 1013–1020.

71 **Calia KE, Murtagh M, Ferraro MJ, Calderwood SB.** Comparison of *Vibrio cholerae* O139 and *V. cholerae* classical and El Tor biotypes. Infect Immun 1994;62:1504–1506.

72 **Popovic T, Fields PI, Olsvik O, et al.** Molecular subtyping of toxigenic *Vibrio cholerae* O139 causing epidemic cholera in India and Bangladesh, 1992–1993. J Infect Dis 1995;171: 122–127.

73 **Comstock LE, Maneval D Jr, Panigrahi P, et al.** The capsule and O antigen in Vibrio cholerae O139 Bengal are associated with a genetic region not present in *Vibrio cholerae* O1. Infect Immun 1995;63:317–323.

74 **Waldor MK, Mekalanos JJ.** *Vibrio cholerae* O139 specific gene sequences. Lancet 1994; 343:1366.

75 **Faruque SM, Alim ARMA, Roy SK, et al.** Molecular analysis or rRNA and cholera toxin genes carried by the new epidemic strain of toxigenic *Vibrio cholerae* O139 Bengal. J Clin Microbiol 1994;32:1050–1053.

76 **Kurazono H, Okuda J, Takeda Y, et al.** *Vibrio cholerae* O139 Bengal isolated from India, Bangladesh and Thailand are clonal as determined by pulsed-field gel electrophoresis. J Infect 1994;29:109–110.

77 **Bhadra RK, Choudhury SR, Das J.** *Vibrio cholerae* O139 El Tor biotype. Lancet 1994; 343:728.

78 **Cravioto A, Beltran P, Delgado G, et al.** Non-O1 *Vibrio cholerae* O139 Bengal is ge-

netically related to *V. cholerae* O1 El Tor Ogawa isolated in Mexico. J Infect Dis 1994;169:1412–1413.

79 **Berche P, Poyart C, Abachin E, et al.** The novel epidemic strain O139 is closely related to the pandemic strain O1 of *Vibrio cholerae*. J Infect Dis 1994;170:701–704.

80 **Olsvik O, Wahlberg J, Petterson B, et al.** Use of automated sequencing of PCR-generated amplicons to identify three types of cholera toxin subunit B in *Vibrio cholerae* O1 strains. J Clin Microbiol 1993;31:22–25.

81 **Yam W-C, Yuen K-Y, Wong S-S-Y, Que T-L.** *Vibrio cholerae* O139 susceptible to vibriostatic agent O/129 and co-trimoxazole. Lancet 1994;344:404–405.

82 **Qadri F, Azim T, Chowdhury A, et al.** Production, characterization and application of monoclonal antibodies to *Vibrio cholerae* O139 synonym Bengal. Clin Diagn Lab Immunol 1994;1:51–54.

83 **Garg S, Ramamurthy T, Mukhopadhyay AK, et al.** Production and cross-reactivity patterns of a panel of high affinity monoclonal antibodies to *Vibrio cholerae* O139 Bengal. FEMS Immunol Med Microbiol 1994;8: 293–298.

84 **Qadri F, Chowdhury A, Hossain J, et al.** Development and evaluation of rapid monoclonal antibody-based coagglutination test for direct detection of *Vibrio cholerae* O139 synonym Bengal in stool samples. J Clin Microbiol 1994;32:1589–1590.

85 **Qadri F, Hasan JAK, Hossain J, et al.** Evaluation of the monclonal antibody-based kit Bengal SMART for rapid detection of *Vibrio cholerae* O139 synonym Bengal in stool samples. J Clin Microbiol 1995;33:732–734.

86 **Albert JM, Alam K, Ansaruzzaman M, et al.** Lack of cross-protection against diarrhea due to *Vibrio cholerae* (Bengal Strain) after oral immunization of rabbits with *V. cholerae* O1 vaccine strain CVD103-HgR. J Infect Dis 1994;169:230–231.

87 **Albert MJ, Alam K, Rahman AS, et al.** Lack of cross-protection against diarrhea due to *Vibrio cholerae* O1 after oral immunization of rabbits with *V. Cholerae* O139 Bengal. J Infect Dis 1994;169:709–10.

88 **Kaper JB, Morris JG, Levine MM.** Cholera. Clin Microbiol Rev 1995;8:48–86.

89 **Waldor MK, Coster TS, Killeen KP, et al.** *Vibrio cholerae* O139: genetic analysis, immunobiology, and volunteer studies of live attenuated vaccines. In: Proceedings of the 30th Joint Conference on Cholera and Related Diarrheal Diseases. Fukuoka, Japan: U.S.-Japan Cooperative Medica. Science Program, 1994:148–152.

90 **Rivas M, Toma C, Millwebsky E, et al.** Cholera isolates in relation to the "eighth" pandemic. Lancet 1993;342:925–926.

underdiagnosis in others who have adult respiratory distress syndrome (ARDS) (42). Noninfectious infiltrates may appear because of atelectasis, pulmonary edema, or postoperative changes (43). On chest x-ray, only air-bronchograms correlate significantly with pneumonia in intubated patients. No radiologic signs distinguish pneumonia if ARDS is present (44). Purulent respiratory secretions often occur because of chronic endotracheal intubation and can be misinterpreted as lower respiratory tract inflammation (45).

Because of the deficiencies of traditional diagnostic methods, members of a consensus conference of critical care physicians called for improved criteria for pneumonia in mechanically ventilated patients, particularly for research purposes (46). The panel suggested that researchers should make the diagnosis of pneumonia based on histopathology (lung biopsy) or protected quantitative cultures of lower respiratory secretions (46). They touted quantitative cultures as the best method to distinguish colonizing bacteria, present in low numbers, from pathogenic bacteria growing to high concentrations (47). Investigators have used several methods for obtaining samples of lower respiratory secretions uncontaminated by oropharyngeal organisms. These range from relatively noninvasive procedures, such as endotracheal aspiration, to bronchoscopically obtained aspirates, brushings, and lavages (48). Each of these techniques can provide material for culture or for immediate microscopic examination. Culture provides essential information about the bacteria's antibiotic susceptibility pattern. In contrast, immediate microscopic examination provides data quickly for therapeutic decisions (47).

Endotracheal aspiration (EA) is the method clinicians most commonly use to obtain specimens for Gram stain and culture from intubated patients (48). However, because the trachea is proximate to the oropharynx, upper airway bacteria may contaminate endotracheal specimens. Several recent studies (Table 10.4) have examined the diagnostic utility of EA to predict pneumonia in intubated patients. Unfortunately, the studies used different "gold standards"

Table 10.4. Endotracheal Aspiration

Study	*N*	*Method*	*Gold Standard*	*Sensitivity (%)*	*Specificity (%)*
Salata et al (49)	51	EA culture	Sterile fluid culture, histology	86	59
Salata et al (49)	51	Elastin fibers	Sterile fluid culture, histology	52	73
Torres et al (50)	25	EA culture	Autopsy, clinical response	100	29
Jordá et al (54)	40	EA culture	Clinical criteria	44	100
Torres et al (51)	27	EA culture	No clinical infection	Not available	52

to define which patients truly had pneumonia. This lack of standardization is a common problem in nosocomial pneumonia research, making comparisons among studies difficult. In studies that used more stringent criteria for pneumonia, such as cultures from sterile sites or histopathology, EA with growth of 10^5 cfu/mL detected 86% to 100% of infections (49,50). Many noninfected patients also had positive EA cultures, so that the specificity of EA was only 29% to 59% (49–51). Salata et al (49) noted that aspirates containing elastin fibers, produced by tissue destruction, predicted pneumonia. In addition, they reported that higher organism counts on semiquantitative EA Gram stains significantly correlated with pneumonia ($P < 0.05$). However, they did not report the sensitivity and specificity of Gram stains. The mean numbers of organisms on EA Gram stains of colonized and infected patients appeared similar, perhaps obscuring an appropriate break point for infection (49).

The low specificity of EA stimulated investigators to develop other lower respiratory tract sampling methods. One example is the protected catheter aspirate (PCA). In performing this procedure, the investigator inserts a plugged catheter into the bronchial tree, either with bronchoscopic guidance or blindly. The plug is extruded, and a relatively sterile sample of lower respiratory secretions is then aspirated (48). Table 10.5 depicts the results of several studies evaluating the diagnosis of nosocomial pneumonia by PCA in intubated patients. With PCA, cultures growing 10^3 cfu/mL usually indicate true infection. This level corresponds to 10^5 cfu/mL in the lung before the small (0.01 mL) sample is diluted 100-fold (47). In part because the area sampled is also small, the sensitivity of PCA measures only 60% to 70% in most studies (50,52–54). The specificity of PCA improves significantly over EA, ranging from 84% to 100% (50,52–54).

Investigators have more extensively studied a similar technique, the protected specimen brush (PSB). In this approach, a small brush is bronchoscopically inserted into the bronchial tree to collect a sample for culture

Table 10.5. Protected Catheter Aspirate

Study	*N*	*Method*	*Gold Standard*	*Sensitivity (%)*	*Specificity (%)*
Torres et al (50)	25	Blind PCA culture	Histology, clinical response to Abx	61	100
Torres et al (50)	25	PCA culture	Histology, clinical response to Abx	66	100
Torres et al (52)	34	PCA culture	Clinical criteria	72	86
Pham et al (53)	55	PCA culture	Sterile fluid culture cavity, histology	100	84
Jordá et al (54)	40	Blind PCA culture	Clinical criteria	61	100
Jordá et al (54)	40	PCA culture	Clinical criteria	65	100

Table 10.8. Positive Predictive Values (PPV) at Selected Prevalence Values (10%, 50%, 90%)

Technique	*Sensitivity (%)*	*Specificity (%)*	*PPV*		
			10%	*50%*	*90%*
EA	52–100	29–100	8–100	45–100	88–100
PCA	61–100	64–100	16–100	63–100	94–100
PSB	65–100	60–100	15–100	62–100	94–100
BAL	80–100	75–100	26–100	76–100	97–100

one of the few studies that has examined reliability, comparing the results of 32 pairs of successive PSB samples in patients with suspected pneumonia. They found that 24% of paired samples yielded different organisms. In 37% of paired samples, bacterial growth was on opposite sides of the 10^3 cfu/mL threshold level, leading to differing predictions of the probability of pneumonia (62). Reanalyzing these data, the authors showed that successive PSB samples had a κ coefficient of 0.25 for predicting pneumonia, a rather low correlation. If single investigators have difficulty reproducing test results, one can imagine how different centers could come to varying conclusions based on the same diagnostic techniques.

Clearly, more research is necessary to improve the diagnosis of nosocomial pneumonia. Several new techniques hold promise. However, most studies investigating them have had small sample sizes, and several have been poorly standardized. The reliability of these new techniques is largely unproven. Larger better controlled studies should be performed before these diagnostic techniques are widely adopted. Future trials should also incorporate other questions in addition to diagnostic accuracy and reliability. They should measure the effects of the new techniques on clinicians' choices of antibiotic therapy and patient outcome (63).

RISK FACTORS

Clinicians need to understand the epidemiology of nosocomial pneumonia to discover interventions that will help prevent or improve its outcome. In the process, they must define risk factors for pneumonia or death that are dependent on unmodifiable host factors, as well as the modifiable factors. Any study of interventions must account for confounding risks in the population it examines; many of these risks will be unmodifiable.

Several groups of investigators have analyzed risk factors for nosocomial pneumonia in large study populations, often using powerful multivariate regression techniques (Table 10.9) (3,12,14–16,18,20,21,23,35,64–67). Most have used traditional clinical definitions of pneumonia, with the accompanying di-

Table 10.9. Risk Factors for Nosocomial Rneumonia

Factor	*Odds Ratio (Range)*	*References*
Age	2.1–4.6	(23,65)
COPD	1.9–3.7	(16,18,23)
Low albumen	12.4–15.6	(21,65)
Neuromuscular disease	3.9–18	(12,65)
Decreased consciousness	1.9–5.8	(15,23)
Impaired reflexes	2.9–3.5	(12,15)
Trauma	2.6–3.0	(15,20)
Severity of illness	2.9–6.4	(15,21,64)
Aspiration	5–10.6	(18,23)
ICP monitor	4.2	(14)
Endotracheal intubation	3.0–12.9	(1,15,18,23,65)
Emergent intubation	2.7	(20)
Prolonged mechanical Ventilation	1.2–3.1	(12,18)
Thoracic/upper abdominal Surgery	4.3–6.0	(21,23,67)
Nasogastric intubation	6.5	(67)

Risk factors for nosocomial pneumonia identified by multivariate analysis. Most studies used clinical definitions to identify pneumonia. (COPD: Chronic Obstructive Pulmonary Disease; ICP: Intracranial Pressure Monitor.)

agnostic inaccuracies. Only a handful of recent reports have relied on quantitative culture procedures (PSB or BAL) to diagnose pneumonia in their study patients (16,25,35,64). As more studies use new techniques to diagnose pneumonia, it will be important to compare their results with epidemiologic studies using older definitions of pneumonia.

A patient's underlying disease state may predispose him or her to nosocomial pneumonia. Some aspects of risk relate to older age (23,64,65) and to chronic conditions such as chronic obstructive pulmonary disease (16,18,23), poor nutrition manifested as low albumen (21,65), and the presence of neuromuscular disease (12,65). Other aspects of risk involve acute events such as decreased level of consciousness (15,23), impaired airway reflexes (12,15), and trauma, particularly to the head or chest (15,20), all of which may lead to pneumonia. Several measures of severity of illness, including the Acute Physiology and Chronic Health Evaluation II (APACHE II), the American Society of Anesthesiologists (ASA), the McCabe-Jackson, and the Injury Severity Score, have independently correlated with the development of pneumonia (15,20,21,64). These studies clearly depict the injured, severely ill, older patient as one whose impaired mental status prevents him or her from protecting the airway. Not surprisingly, aspiration is also strongly associated with nosocomial pneumonia (18,23).

Therapeutic measures have also proved to be important risk factors. Some procedures, such as intracranial pressure monitoring (14), reflect the patient's underlying disease. The most commonly correlated procedure, endotracheal intubation, occurs frequently in patients with underlying lung disease. However, intubation also bypasses airway defenses to allow bacteria into the lower respiratory tract (1,15,18,23,65). The risk of intubation increases if physicians perform the procedure emergently (20) or if the duration of mechanical ventilation is prolonged (12,16,18). Other procedures that compromise the integrity of the respiratory system are risk factors for pneumonia as well. These include surgery to the thorax or upper abdomen (21,23,67) and nasogastric intubation (67).

One can similarly divide risks for death from hospital-acquired pneumonia into patient factors and treatment factors (Table 10.10). Patient-related risks arise from either underlying disease or from the pneumonia itself. Several epidemiologic analyses have found that both older age (3,23) and the presence of an ultimately or rapidly fatal underlying disease (18,23) were associated with a fatal outcome. Underlying neoplasia also worsened prognosis (3). Several gauges of pneumonia severity point to increased mortality. Bilateral lung involvement (23), a high alveolar-arterial oxygen gradient (66), worsening respiratory failure, and septic shock (18) predictably lead to death more often. In addition, if the nosocomial pneumonia is caused by a broadly antibiotic-resistant or more virulent organism, such as *Acinetobacter*, *Pseudomonas*, or *S. aureus*, infected patients are more likely to die (23,35,39,64,66).

Most investigators studying how treatment affects the outcome of nosocomial pneumonia have focused on the influence of antibiotics. Some

Table 10.10. Risk Factors for Death with Nosocomial Pneumonia

Risk Factor	*Odds Ratio (Range)*	*References*
Age (gr)	1.1–4.6	(3,23)
Neoplasia	1.6	(3)
Fatal underlying disease	4.8–8.8	(18,23)
Bilateral pneumonia	6.3	(23)
High A-a gradient	4.0	(66)
Worsening respiratory Failure	11.9	(18)
Septic shock	2.8	(18)
Resistant/virulent organism	2.5–8.7	(23,25,35)
Inappropriate antibiotics	5.8–32.5	(18,23)
Prior antibiotic treatment	9.2	(35)

Risk factors for mortality from nosocomial pneumonia identified by multivariate analysis.

series have reported that more patients died if they were treated with antibiotics to which the infecting organism was resistant (18,23). Interestingly, Rello et al (35) found that any antibiotic treatment before the development of pneumonia heralded a poor outcome. Their analysis showed that prior antibiotic use also correlated with pseudomonal nosocomial pneumonia (35). If antibiotic exposure leads to infection with more resistant and/or more virulent organisms, this could in part explain the higher mortality.

INTERVENTIONS

The ultimate goal of understanding the epidemiology of hospital-acquired pneumonia is to design interventions to prevent it or to improve its outcome. Because the pathogenesis of nosocomial pneumonia is complex (Figure 10.1), several points lie open to attack. Some interventions rely on simple measures, such as altering the patient's position, decreasing endobronchial secretions, and maintaining gastric acidity. Others are both more complicated and more controversial. The use of selective digestive decontamination falls into the latter

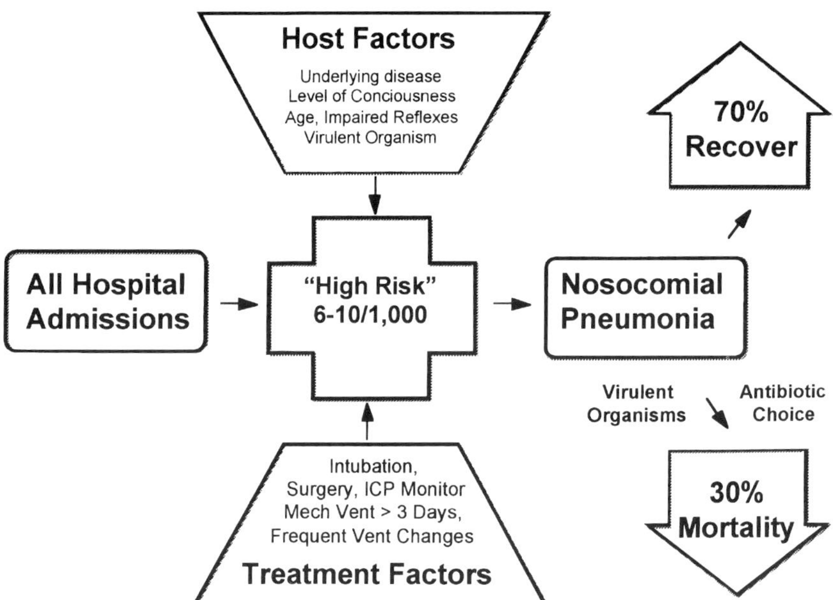

Figure 10.1. The pathogenesis of nosocomial involves the intersection of complex risk factors, arising from both host and medical treatment. Many of these factors, along with characteristics of the pneumonia, determine outcome as well.

category (68). The individual clinician must decide which strategies are most likely to reduce the incidence of nosocomial pneumonia and then pursue their implementation.

Body Position

There is good evidence that placing patients in a semirecumbent position reduces their aspiration of oropharyngeal secretions. Torres et al (30) compared aspiration of radiolabeled tracer in intubated patients, both while supine and while elevated to a 45° angle. Patients aspirated 10-fold less tracer while semirecumbent. Differences in the volume of aspiration became more pronounced the longer patients remained supine (30). Placing patients in a semirecumbent position is a good example of a low-cost intervention with potentially far reaching beneficial effects.

Subglottic Secretion Drainage

Another strategy designed to prevent the aspiration of oropharyngeal secretions is to continuously remove them by suction before they accumulate below the glottis. Specially designed endotracheal tubes allow the removal of subglottic secretions through a dorsal lumen opening above the cuff (69). Two studies of the efficacy of subglottic drainage have demonstrated that the special endotracheal tube reduced the incidence of nosocomial pneumonia by 50% (69,70). The rate of oropharyngeal colonization with *H. influenzae* and gram-positive cocci decreased by nearly 50% over 6 to 10 days, accompanied by a corresponding fall in rates of pneumonia caused by these organisms (69). Colonization with *Pseudomonas* and pseudomonal pneumonia, however, did not change. If further investigators confirm the value of subglottic drainage, it will add another simple yet effective barrier to infection.

Stress Ulcer Prophylaxis

In critically ill patients, gastric secretions are often heavily colonized with bacteria, forming a reservoir for infection. Bacterial concentration climbs with the decreased acidity brought about by stress ulcer prophylaxis with histamine receptor antagonists or antacids (29,71,72). A number of prospective randomized trials have compared stress ulcer prophylaxis with these agents to sucralfate, an agent that maintains a low gastric pH (29,71–78) (Figure 10.2). The investigators examined rates of clinically diagnosed pneumonia in the different treatment groups. Several investigators found no significant difference in nosocomial pneumonia incidence (72,73,75,77). However, others reported lower rates of pneumonia in the sucralfate group. This difference either achieved or closely approached statistical significance (29,71,74,76,78). In addition, two recent meta-analyses have supported these findings (79,80). The Hospital Infection Control Advisory Committee of the Centers for Disease Control

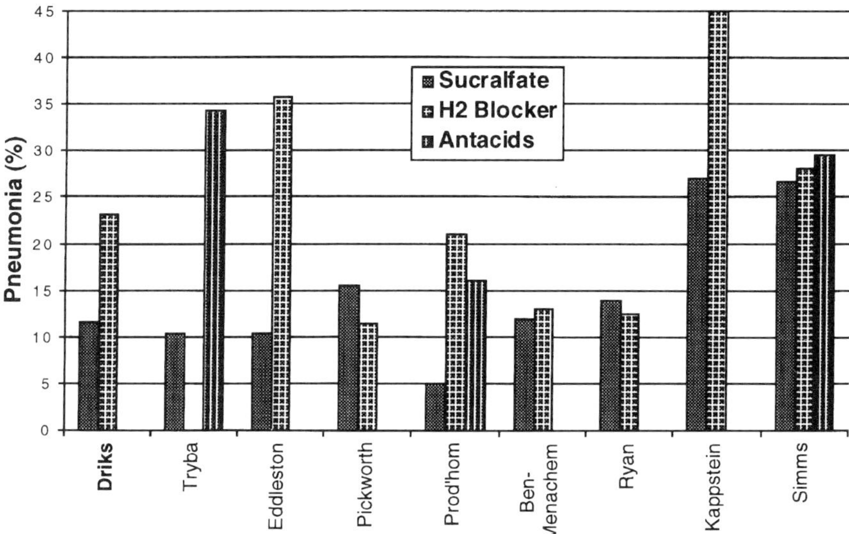

Figure 10.2. Summary of the results of prospective controlled trials investigating the use of stress ulcer prophylaxis and the development of nosocomial pneumonia. Rates of pneumonia were generally lower with sucralfate, which maintains gastric acidity, than with antacids or histamine receptor antagonists.

and Prevention currently recommends using agents for stress ulcer prophylaxis that do not raise gastric pH (68).

Selective Digestive Decontamination

Another strategy designed to reduce oropharyngeal and gastric bacterial colonization is selective digestive decontamination (SDD). Investigators have applied nonabsorbable antibiotics to patients' mouths and gastrointestinal tracts to lower the bacterial burden. In most studies, they have used polymyxin, an aminoglycoside, and amphotericin B, sometimes in combination with a fluoroquinalone or a third-generation cephalosporin given systemically (81). Trials of SDD have almost universally shown a decrease in oropharyngeal and gastric bacterial colonization (82–88). Gram-negative bacilli were particularly reduced in number. Many investigators have also demonstrated significant reductions in rates of nosocomial pneumonia in mechanically ventilated patients (87–90). However, several other groups have not found reduced rates of pneumonia with SDD (82–84,91). If one limits consideration to the few SDD trials that were randomized, double-blind, and placebo controlled, the conclusions about its efficacy remain uncertain (Figure 10.3) (82,89–91). Most importantly, none of these better controlled studies have shown any improvement in overall mortality with SDD prophylaxis (82,89–91). Such an improvement in

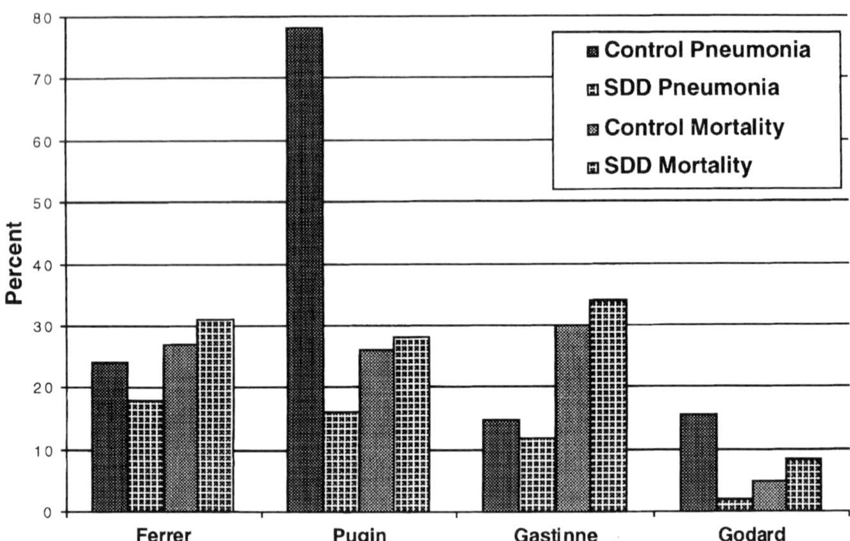

Figure 10.3. Summary of double-blind controlled trials of the use of SDD to prevent pneumonia. Rates of pneumonia were somewhat lower with SDD than in controls, but overall mortality was not significantly different.

outcome was rare even in unblinded trials (87). An additional concern is the possible induction of antibiotic resistance in colonizing organisms. Some centers that have used SDD have reported an increase in highly antibiotic resistant gram-negative bacilli in the ICU (92). Others have noted greater patient colonization with gram-positive cocci (84). The latter is particularly worrisome given the current proliferation of vancomycin resistant enterococci. SDD clearly remains a controversial intervention with unproven long-term benefit, and it cannot be recommended.

Antibiotic Therapy

Ideally, antibiotic therapy for nosocomial pneumonia should be determined by the susceptibility of the causative organism. All too frequently, however, clinicians fail to find the etiology of nosocomial pneumonia, particularly early in the course when treatment is most crucial. This leaves them with empiric antibiotic therapy. As Fagon et al (39) discovered in their prospective study of pneumonia treatment, when physicians must decide about antibiotic regimens based on clinical information, they often choose incorrectly. Despite the uncertainty, there is growing consensus about empiric antibiotic choices for hospital acquired pneumonia (93,94).

Traditionally, physicians have used a combination of a β-lactam (penicillin or cephalosporin) and an aminoglycoside to treat nosocomial pneumonia (94–96). Together, these agents frequently can be shown to act synergistically against gram-negative bacilli. Because neither β-lactams nor aminoglycosides achieve high concentrations in bronchial secretions compared with serum levels, clinicians believed synergism was important for effective treatment (94,97). Studies have shown that synergism is crucial for the treatment of pseudomonal pneumonia (98). Synergism also helps prevent the development of antibiotic resistance in other bacteria, such as *Enterobacter cloacae* (94,95). There is growing evidence, however, that monotherapy with a newer broad-spectrum agent may be equally effective as combination therapy for some groups of patients. Several studies have described equal cure rates in less critically ill patients who were treated with third-generation cephalosporins or combination therapy (33,96).

Clinicians are currently faced with a choice of regimens with apparent equivalent efficacy. Monotherapy may reduce cost and patient antibiotic exposure. Combination therapy has an added margin of safety for more virulent organisms (94,97). Recent guidelines drafted by the Canadian Hospital Acquired Pneumonia Consensus Conference provide a useful framework for making such choices (93). They recommend monotherapy for patients who are not critically ill, unless *Pseudomonas* or another antibiotic resistant organism is isolated. Clinicians may add other antibiotics for patients with specific risk factors. For instance, patients who have grossly aspirated should be treated for anaerobes; those on high-dose corticosteroids should receive a macrolide for *Legionella*. They also recommend that all critically ill patients be treated with combination therapy for presumed *Pseudomonas* pneumonia (93). If a less-virulent microorganism is subsequently isolated, antibiotic therapy can be narrowed appropriately (94). These guidelines present a reasonable distillation of the current literature regarding antibiotic therapy for nosocomial pneumonia. Optimally, investigators should evaluate their efficacy in practice to see whether they meet their goals of successful treatment with reduced cost and antibiotic exposure.

CONCLUSIONS

Hospital-acquired pneumonia remains a common nosocomial infection associated with a high mortality. It has stimulated numerous investigators to examine all aspects of its epidemiology, diagnosis, and treatment. Despite volumes of research, much remains unclear. The traditional clinical definition of nosocomial pneumonia has been challenged, but no alternative has been widely accepted in its place. The epidemiology of nosocomial pneumonia, which was based on the traditional definition, must be re-examined. Finally, antibiotic therapy and other preventive interventions must be prospectively evaluated in light of new definitions and insights.

REFERENCES

1 **Cross AS, Roup B.** Role of respiratory assistance devices in endemic nosocomial pneumonia. Am J Med 1981;70:681–685.

2 **Horan TC, White JW, Jarvis WR, et al.** Nosocomial infection surveillance, 1984. MMWR 1986;35:17SS–29SS.

3 **Leu H-S, Kaiser DL, Mori M, et al.** Hospital-acquired pneumonia: attributable mortality and morbidity. Am J Epidemiol 1989; 129:1258–1267.

4 **Broderick A, Mori M, Nettleman MD, et al.** Nosocomial infections: validation of surveillance and computer modeling to identify patients at risk. Am J Epidemiol 1990;131:734–742.

5 **Boyce JM, Potter-Bynoe G, Dziobek L, Solomon SL.** Nosocomial pneumonia in Medicare patients. Hospital costs and reimbursement patterns under the prospective payment system. Arch Intern Med 1991; 151:1109–1114.

6 **Emori TG, Gaynes RP.** An overview of nosocomial infections, including the role of the microbiology laboratory. Clin Microbiol Rev 1993;6:428–442.

7 **Haley RW, Culver DH, White JW, et al.** The efficacy of infection surveillance and control programs in preventing nosocomial infections in US hospitals. Am J Epidemiol 1985; 121:182–205.

8 **Wenzel RP.** Hospital-acquired pneumonia: overview of the current state of the art for prevention and control. Eur J Clin Microbiol Infect Dis 1989;8:56–60.

9 National Center for Health Statistics. National hospital discharge survey; annual summary, 1991. Vital Health Stat [13] 1993; 15:7–8.

10 **Craven DE, Steger KA, Duncan RA.** Prevention and control of nosocomial pneumonia. In: Wenzel RP, ed. Prevention and control of nosocomial infections. 2nd ed. Baltimore: Williams & Wilkins, 1993;580–599.

11 **Craven DE, Kunches LM, Lichtenberg DA, et al.** Nosocomial infection and fatality in medical and surgical intensive care unit patients. Arch Intern Med 1988;148:1161–1168.

12 **Mosconi P, Langer M, Cigada M, Mandelli M.** Intensive Care Unit Group for Infection Control. Epidemiology and risk factors of pneumonia in critically ill patients. Eur J Epidemiol 1991;7:320–327.

13 **Jarvis WR, Edwards JR, Culver DH, et al.** Nosomial infection rates in adult and pediatric intensive care units in the United States. Am J Med 1991;91(suppl 3B):185S–191S.

14 **Craven DE, Kunches LM, Kilinsky V, et al.** Risk factors for pneumonia and fatality in patients receiving continuous mechanical ventilation. Am Rev Respir Dis 1986;133: 792–796.

15 **Chevret S, Hemmer M, Carlet J, Langer M.** Incidence and risk factors of pneumonia acquired in intensive care units. Results from a multicenter prospective study on 996 patients. European Cooperative Group on Nosocomial Pneumonia. Intensive Care Med 1993;19:256–264.

16 **Jiménez P, Torres A, Rodríguez-Roisín R, et al.** Incidence and etiology of pneumonia acquired during mechanical ventilation. Crit Care Med 1989;17:882–885.

17 **Rello J, Quintana E, Ausina V, et al.** Incidence, etiology, and outcome of nosocomial pneumonia in mechanically ventilated patients. Chest 1991;100:439–444.

18 **Torres A, Azner R, Gatell JM, et al.** Incidence, risk, and prognosis factors of nosocomial pneumonia in mechanically ventilated patients. Am Rev Respir Dis 1990;142:523–528.

19 **Wenzel RP, Osterman CA, Donowitz LG, et al.** Identification of procedure-related nosocomial infections in high-risk patients. Rev Infect Dis 1981;3:701–707.

20 **Rodriguez JL, Gibbons KJ, Bitzer LG, et al.** Pneumonia: incidence, risk factors, and outcome in injured patients. J Trauma 1991;31:907–912. Discussion 912–914.

21 **Garibaldi RA, Britt MR, Coleman ML, et al.** Risk factors for postoperative pneumonia. Am J Med 1981;70:677–680.

22 **Pannuti CS, Gingrich R, Pfaller MA, Wenzel RP.** Nosocomial pneumonia in adult patients undergoing bone marrow transplantation: a 9-year study. J Clin Oncol 1991;9:77–84.

23 **Celis R, Torres A, Gatell JM, et al.** Nosocomial pneumonia: a multivariate analysis of risk and prognosis. Chest 1988; 93:318–324.

24 **Bartlett JG, O'Keefe P, Tally FP, et al.** Bacteriology of hospital-acquired pneumonia. Arch Intern Med 1986;146:868–871.

25 **Fagon JY, Chastre J, Hance AJ, et al.** Nosocomial pneumonia in ventilated patients: a cohort study evaluating attributable

mortality and hospital stay. Am J Med 1993;94:281–288.

26 **Pannuti C, Gingrich R, Pfaller MA, et al.** Nosocomial pneumonia in patients having bone marrow transplant: attributable mortality and risk factors. Cancer 1992;69:2653–2662.

27 **Kappstein I, Schulgen G, Beyer U, et al.** Prolongation of hospital stay and extra costs due to ventilator-associated pneumonia in an intensive care unit. Eur J Clin Microbiol Infect Dis 1992;11:504–508.

28 **Torres A, el-Ebiary M, González J, et al.** Gastric and pharyngeal flora in nosocomial pneumonia acquired during mechanical ventilation. Am Rev Respir Dis 1993;148: 352–357.

29 **Prod'hom G, Leuenberger P, Koerfer J, et al.** Nosocomial pneumonia in mechanically ventilated patients receiving antacid, ranitidine, or sucralfate as prophylaxis for stress ulcer. A randomized controlled trial. Ann Intern Med 1994;120:653–662.

30 **Torres A, Serra-Batlles J, Ros E, et al.** Pulmonary aspiration of gastric contents in patients receiving mechanical ventilation: the effect of body position. Ann Intern Med 1992;116:540–543.

31 **Levine SA, Niederman MS.** The impact of tracheal intubation on host defenses and risks for nosocomial pneumonia. Clin Chest Med 1991;12:523–543.

32 **Rodriguez JL.** Hospital-acquired gram-negative pneumonia in critically ill, injured patients. Am J Surg 1993;165(2A suppl):34S–42S.

33 **Schleupner CJ, Cobb DK.** A study of the etiologies and treatment of nosocomial pneumonia in a community-based teaching hospital. Infect Control Hosp Epidemiol 1992;13:515–525.

34 **Schaberg DR, Culver DH, Gaynes RP.** Major trends in the microbial etiology of nosocomial infection. Am J Med 1991; 91(suppl 3B):72S–75S.

35 **Rello J, Ausina V, Ricart M, et al.** Impact of previous antimicrobial therapy on the etiology and outcome of ventilator-associated pneumonia. Chest 1993;104:1230–1235.

36 **Doebbeling BN, Wenzel RP.** The epidemiology of *Legionella pneumophila* infections. Semin Respir Infect 1987;2:206–221.

37 **Valenti WM, Hall CB, Douglas RG Jr, et al.** Nosocomial viral infections. I. Epidemiology and significance. Infect Control 1979;1: 33–37.

38 **Hall CB.** Nosocomial viral respiratory infections: perennial weeds on pediatric wards. Am J Med 1981;70:670–676.

39 **Fagon JY, Chastre J, Hance AJ, et al.** Evaluation of clinical judgment in the identification and treatment of nosocomial pneumonia in ventilated patients. Chest 1993;103:547–553.

40 **Johanson WG Jr, Peirce AK, Sanford JP, Thomas GD.** Nosocomial respiratory infections with gram-negative bacilli: the significance of colonization of the respiratory tract. Ann Intern Med 1972;77:710–716.

41 **Wollschlager CM, Khan FA, Khan A.** Utility of radiography and clinical features in the diagnosis of community-acquired pneumonia. Clin Chest Med 1987;8:393–404.

42 **Meduri GU.** Diagnosis of ventilator-associated pneumonia. Infect Dis Clin North Am 1993;7:295–329.

43 **Bryant LR, Mobin-Uddin K, Dillon ML, Griffen WO.** Misdiagnosis of pneumonia in patients needing mechanical respiration. Arch Surg 1973;106:286–288.

44 **Wunderink RG, Woldenberg LS, Zeiss J, et al.** The radiologic diagnosis of autopsy-proven ventilator-associated pneumonia. Chest 1992;101:458–463.

45 **Bartlett JG, Faling LJ, Willey S.** Quantitative tracheal bacteriologic and cytologic studies in patients with long-term tracheostomies. Chest 1978;74:635–639.

46 **Pingleton SK, Fagon J-Y, Leeper KV.** Patient selection for the clinical investigation of ventilator-associated pneumonia: criteria for evaluating diagnostic techniques. Chest 1992;102(5 suppl):553S–556S.

47 **Baselski VS, el-Torky M, Coalson JJ, Griffin JP.** The standardization of criteria for processing and interpreting laboratory specimens in patients with suspected ventilator-associated pneumonia. Chest 1992; 102(5 suppl 1):571S–579S.

48 **Griffin JJ, Meduri GU.** New approaches in the diagnosis of nosocomial pneumonia. Medi Clin North Am 1994;78:1091–1122.

49 **Salata RS, Lederman MM, Shlaes DM, et al.** Diagnosis of nosocomial pneumonia in intubated, intensive care unit patients. Am Rev Respir Dis 1987;135:426–432.

50 **Torres A, de la Bellacasa JP, Rodriguez-Roisin R, et al.** Diagnostic value of telescoping plugged catheters in mechanically ventilated patients with bacterial pneumonia using the Metras catheter. Am Rev Respir Dis 1988;138:117–120.

51 **Torres A, Martos A, de la Bellacasa JP, et al.** Specificity of endotracheal aspiration, pro-

tected specimen brush, and bronchoalveolar lavage in mechanically ventilated patients. Am Rev Respir Dis 1993;147:952–957.

52 **Torres A, de la Bellacasa JP, Xaubet A, et al.** Diagnostic value of quantitative cultures of bronchoalveolar lavage and telescoping plugged catheters in mechanically ventilated patients with bacterial pneumonia. Am Rev Respir Dis 1989;140:306–310.

53 **Pham LH, Brun-Buisson C, Legrand P, et al.** Diagnosis of nosocomial pneumonia in mechanically ventilated patients: comparison of a plugged telescoping catheter with the protected specimen brush. Am Rev Respir Dis 1991;143:1055–1061.

54 **Jordá R, Parras F, Ibañez J, et al.** Diagnosis of nosocomial pneumonia in mechanically ventilated patients by the blind protected telescoping catheter. Intensive Care Med 1993;19:377–382.

55 **Chastre J, Viau F, Brun P, et al.** Prospective evaluation of the protected brush for the diagnosis of pulmonary infections in ventilated patients. Am Rev Respir Dis 1984;130: 924–929.

56 **Chastre J, Fagon J-Y, Soler P, et al.** Diagnosis of nosocomial bacterial pneumonia in intubated patients undergoing ventilation: comparison of the usefulness of bronchoalveolar lavage and the protected specimen brush. Am J Med 1988;85:499–506.

57 **Fagon J-Y, Chastre J, Hance AJ, et al.** Detection of nosocomial lung infection in ventilated patients: use of a protected specimen brush and quantitative culture techniques in 147 patients. Am Rev Respir Dis 1988; 138:110–116.

58 **Solé-Violán J, Rodríguez de Castro F, Rey A, et al.** Usefulness of microscopic examination of intracellular organisms in lavage fluid in ventilator-associated pneumonia. Chest 1994;106:889–894.

59 **Meduri GU, Beals DH, Maijub AG, Baselski V.** Protected bronchoalveoloar lavage: a new bronchoscopic technique to retrieve uncontaminated distal airway secretions. Am Rev Respir Dis 1991;143:855–864.

60 **Marquette CH, Wallet F, Nevière R, et al.** Diagnostic value of direct examination of the protected specimen brush in ventilator-associated pneumonia. Eur Respir J 1994;7: 105–113.

61 **Gaussorgues P, Piperno D, Bachmann P, et al.** Comparison of nonbronchoalveolar lavage to open lung biopsy for the bacteriologic diagnosis of pulmonary infections in mechanically ventilated patients. Intensive Care Med 1989;15:94–98.

62 **Timsit JF, Misset B, Francoual S, et al.** Is protected specimen brush an reproducible method to diagnose ICU-acquired pneumonia? Chest 1993;104:104–108.

63 **Cook DJ, Brun-Buisson C, Guyatt GH, Sibbald WJ.** Evaluation of new diagnostic technologies: bronchoalveolar lavage and the diagnosis of ventilator-associated pneumonia. Crit Care Med 1994;22:1314–1322.

64 **Fagon J-Y, Chastre J, Domart Y, et al.** Nosocomial pneumonia in patients receiving continuous mechanical ventilation: prospective analysis of 52 episodes with use of a protected specimen brush and quantitative culture techniques. Am Rev Respir Dis 1989;139:877–884.

65 **Hanson LC, Weber DJ, Rutala WA, Samsa GP.** Risk factors for nosocomial pneumonia in the elderly. Am J Med 1992;92:161–166.

66 **Malangoni MA, Crafton R, Mocek FC.** Pneumonia in the surgical intensive care unit: factors determining successful outcome. Am J Surg 1994;167:250–255.

67 **Joshi N, Localio AR, Hamory BH.** A predictive risk index for nosocomial pneumonia in the intensive care unit. Am J Med 1992; 93:135–142.

68 **Tablan OC, Anderson LJ, Arden NH, et al.** Guideline for prevention of nosocomial pneumonia. Infect Control Hosp Epidemiol 1994;15:587–590.

69 **Vallés J, Artigas A, Rello J, et al.** Continuous aspiration of subglottic secretions in preventing ventilator-associated pneumonia. Ann Intern Med 1995;122:179–186.

70 **Mahul P, Auboyer, C, Jospe R, et al.** Prevention of nosocomial pneumonia in intubated patients: respective role of mechanical subglottic secretions drainage and stress ulcer prophylaxis. Intensive Care Med 1992;18:20–25.

71 **Eddleston JM, Vohra A, Scott P, et al.** A comparison of the frequency of stress ulceration and secondary pneumonia in sucralfate- or ranitidine-treated intensive care unit patients. Crit Care Med 1991;19: 1491–1496.

72 **Simms HH, DeMaria E, McDonald L, et al.** Role of gastric colonization in the development of pneumonia in critically ill trauma patients: results of a prospective randomized trial. J Trauma 1991;31:531–536. Discussion 536–537.

73 **Ben-Menachem T, Fogel R, Patel RV, et al.** Prophylaxis for stress-related gastric hemorrhage in the medical intensive care unit. A randomized, controlled, single-blind study. Ann Intern Med 1994;121:568–575.

74 **Tryba M.** Risk of acute stress bleeding and nosocomial pneumonia in ventilated intensive care unit patients: sucralfate versus antacids. Am J Med 1987;83(suppl 3B):117–124.

75 **Pickworth KK, Falcone RE, Hoogeboom JE, Santanello SA.** Occurrence of nosocomial pneumonia in mechanically ventilated trauma patients: a comparison of sucralfate and ranitidine. Crit Care Med 1993;21:1856–1862.

76 **Driks MR, Craven DE, Celli BR, et al.** Nosocomial pneumonia in intubated patients given sucralfate as compared with antacids or histamine type 2 blockers: the role of gastric colonization. N Engl J Med 1987;317:1376–1382.

77 **Ryan P, Dawson J, Teres D, et al.** Nosocomial pneumonia during stress ulcer prophylaxis with cimentidine and sucralfate. Arch Surg 1993;128:1353–1357.

78 **Kappstein I, Schulgen G, Friedrich T, et al.** Incidence of pneumonia in mechanically ventilated patients treated with sucralfate or cimetidine as prophylaxis for stress bleeding: bacterial colonization of the stomach. Am J Med 1991;91(suppl 2A):125S–131S.

79 **Cook DJ, Reeve BK, Scholes LC.** Histamine-2-receptor antagonists and antacids in the critically ill population: stress ulceration versus nosocomial pneumonia. Infect Control Hosp Epidemiol 1994;15:437–442.

80 **Tryba M.** Sucralfate versus antacids or H_2-antagonists for stress ulcer prophylaxis: a meta-analysis on efficacy and pneumonia rate. Crit Care Med 1991;19:942–949.

81 **Duncan RA, Steger KA, Craven DE.** Selective decontamination of the digestive tract: risks outweigh benefits for intensive care unit patients. Semin Respir Infect 1993;8: 308–324.

82 **Ferrer M, Torres A, González J, et al.** Utility of selective digestive decontamination in mechanically ventilated patients. Ann Intern Med 1994;120:389–395.

83 **Aerdts SJA, van Dalen R, Clasener HAL, et al.** Antibiotic prophylaxis of respiratory tract infection in mechanically ventilated patients: a prospective, blinded, randomized trial of the effect of a novel regimen. Chest 1991;100:783–791.

84 **Brun-Buisson C, Legrand P, Rauss A, et al.** Intestinal decontamination for control of nosocomial multiresistant gram-negative bacilli: study of an outbreak in an intensive care unit. Ann Intern Med 1989;110:873–881.

85 **Flaherty J, Nathan C, Kabins SA, Weinstein RA.** Pilot trial of selective decontamination for prevention of bacterial infection in an intensive care unit. J Infect Dis 1990;162:1393–1397.

86 **Kerver AJH, Rommes JH, Mevissen-Verhage EAE, et al.** Prevention of colonization and infection in critically ill patients: a prospective randomized study. Crit Care Med 1988;16:1087–1093.

87 **Ulrich C, Harinck-de Weerd JE, Bakker NC, et al.** Selective decontamination of the digestive tract with norfloxacin in the prevention of ICU-acquired infections: a prospective randomized study. Intensive Care Med 1989;15:424–431.

88 **Unertl K, Ruckdeschel G, Selbmann HK, et al.** Prevention of colonization and respiratory infections in long-term ventilated patients by local antimicrobial prophylaxis. Intensive Care Med 1987;13:106–113.

89 **Godard J, Guillaume C, Reverdy M-E, et al.** Intestinal decontamination in a polyvalent ICU: a double-blind study. Intensive Care Med 1990;16:307–311.

90 **Pugin J, Auckenthaler R, Lew DP, Suter PM.** Oropharyngeal decontamination decreases incidence of ventilator-associated pneumonia. A randomized, placebo-controlled double-blind clinical trial. JAMA 1991;265:2704–2710.

91 **Gastinne H, Wolff M, Delatour F, et al.** A controlled trial in intensive care units of selective decontamination of the digestive tract with nonabsorbable antibiotics. The French Study Group on Selective Decontamination of the Digestive Tract. N Engl J Med 1992;326:594–599.

92 **Nardi G, Valentinis U, Proietti A, et al.** Epidemiological impact of prolonged systematic use of topical SDD on bacterial colonization of the tracheobronchial tree and antibiotic resistance. A three year study. Intensive Care Med 1993;19:273–278.

93 **Mandell LA, Marrie TJ, Niederman MS.** The Canadian Hospital Acquired Pneumonia Consensus Conference Group. Initial antimicrobial treatment of hospital acquired pneumonia in adults: a conference report. Can J Infect Dis 1993;4:317–321.

94 **Niederman MS.** An approach to empiric

therapy of nosocomial pneumonia. Med Clin North Am 1994;78:1123–1141.

95 **Aoun M, Klastersky J.** Drug treatment of pneumonia in the hospital. What are the choices? Drugs 1991;42:962–973.

96 **LaForce FM.** Systemic antimicrobial therapy of nosocomial pneumonia: monotherapy versus combination therapy. Eur J Clin Microbiol Infect Dis 1989;8:61–68.

97 **Unertl KE, Lenhart FP, Forst H, Peter K.** Systemic antibiotic treatment of nosocomial pneumonia. Intensive Care Med 1992;18: S28–S34.

98 **Hilf M, Yu VL, Sharp J, et al.** Antibiotic therapy for *Pseudomonas aeruginosa* bacteremia: outcome correlations in a prospective study of 200 patients. Am J Med 1989;87:540–546.

Acute Bacterial Meningitis in Adults

ALLAN R. TUNKEL
W. MICHAEL SCHELD

Bacterial meningitis remains a significant problem worldwide, despite the availability of effective bactericidal antimicrobial agents. This review focuses on the epidemiology, etiology, clinical presentation, diagnosis, and management of bacterial meningitis in adult patients, with special emphasis on recommendations for antimicrobial therapy based on changing susceptibility patterns of meningeal pathogens and the data for use of adjunctive dexamethasone therapy in adults.

EPIDEMIOLOGY AND ETIOLOGY

The overall annual attack rate for bacterial meningitis in the United States was approximately 3.0 cases per 100,000 population as described in a surveillance study of 27 states from 1978 through 1981 (1). *Haemophilus influenzae* type b, *Neisseria meningitidis*, and *Streptococcus pneumoniae* were the most common pathogens isolated during this study, accounting for 81% of cases; in a subsequent surveillance study of five states and Los Angeles county, these three pathogens accounted for 77% of cases (2). Bacterial meningitis is also a significant problem in hospitalized patients. In one review of 493 episodes of bacterial meningitis in adults (≥16 years of age) at the Massachusetts General Hospital from 1962 through 1988 (3), 40% of episodes were nosocomial in origin with a mortality rate of 35% for single episodes. Of interest, the overall mortality rate for patients in the study (both community-acquired and nosocomial meningitis) was 25%, which did not significantly change over the 27-year study period. In patients with community-acquired meningitis, risk factors for death included age at least 60 years, obtundation on admission, and onset of seizures within the first 24 hours.

Bacterial meningitis is also a significant problem in other areas of the world. A large retrospective review of approximately 4100 cases of bacterial meningitis at the Hospital Couta Maia in Salvador, Brazil, from 1973 through 1982 revealed an attack rate of 45.8 cases per 100,000 population and an overall case fatality rate of 33% (4); 50% of the deaths occurred within the first 48 hours of hospitalization. Most cases (62%) were caused by *H. influenzae* type b, *N. meningitidis*, and *S. pneumoniae*.

Although *H. influenzae* type b was the most common etiologic agent of bacterial meningitis in the United States (~45% to 48% of cases) (1,2), the vast majority of cases occurred in infants and children under the age of 6 years. However, the incidence of *H. influenzae* type b disease has fallen dramatically since the introduction of *H. influenzae* type b conjugate vaccines (5). In adult patients the incidence of likely meningeal pathogens is much different (Table 11.1) (6). The following sections review the epidemiology and etiology for specific meningeal pathogens in adults with bacterial meningitis.

Streptococcus pneumoniae

S. pneumoniae is the most frequently isolated meningeal pathogen in adults. Overall, pneumococci account for 13% to 17% of cases of meningitis in the United States, with a mortality rate ranging from 19% to 26% (1,2). Patients with pneumococcal meningitis often have contiguous or distant foci of infection (e.g., pneumonia, otitis media, mastoiditis, sinusitis, or endocarditis). In addition, serious infection may be observed in patients with underlying conditions such as previous splenectomy, asplenic states (i.e., sickle cell anemia), multiple myeloma, hypogammaglobulinemia, alcoholism, malnutrition, chronic liver or renal disease, malignancy, and diabetes mellitus (7,8). Pneumococci are also the most common etiologic agents in bacterial meningitis associated with basilar skull fracture and cerebrospinal fluid (CSF) leak (9).

Table 11.1. Bacterial Etiology of Meningitis in Patients over 15 Years of Age

Organism	***Incidence (%)***
Streptococcus pneumoniae	30–50
Neisseria meningitidis	10–35
Haemophilus influenzae	1–3
Gram-negative bacilli	1–10
Group B streptococci	5
Staphylococci	5–15
Listeria monocytogenes	5

SOURCE: Roos KL, Tunkel AR, Scheld WM. Acute bacterial meningitis in children and adults. In: Scheld WM, Whitley RJ, Durack DT, eds. Infections of the central nervous system. New York: Raven Press, 1991:335–409.

Neisseria meningitidis

N. meningitidis most commonly causes bacterial meningitis in children and young adults. In the United States, serogroup B strains account for approximately 51% of isolates (1), usually as part of sporadic outbreaks, although the incidence of serogroup C disease has recently equaled that of serogroup B in the United States (10). Serogroups A and C may cause disease as part of epidemics in patient populations living in closed communities, such as military barracks, households, college dormitories, boarding schools, and day care centers (6). There have been recent outbreaks of serogroup C meningococcal disease in North America (11,12). The increased incidence in some areas of Canada was largely because of the emergence of a single clone of serogroup C *N. meningitidis* (12); the predominant strain, multilocus enzyme electrophoretic type 15, was associated with a higher case fatality rate than other serogroup C strains. The incidence of meningococcal infection is increased in patients with deficiencies in the terminal complement components (C5, C6, C7, C8, and perhaps C9) (13) and dysfunctional properdin (14), suggesting an important role for the complement pathway in resistance against meningococcal infection.

Haemophilus influenzae Type b

H. influenzae type b was the most frequent cause of bacterial meningitis in the United States before the introduction of conjugate vaccines, although most episodes occur in infants and children under the age of 6 years; the peak incidence in the United States is between 6 and 12 months of age (15). If this organism is isolated in adult patients with bacterial meningitis, this should suggest the presence of certain underlying conditions (e.g., sinusitis, otitis media, epiglottitis, pneumonia, diabetes mellitus, alcoholism, previous splenectomy, asplenic states, basilar skull fracture with CSF leak, or hypogammaglobulinemia) (16,17).

Listeria monocytogenes

In adults, listerial infection is most common in the elderly, alcoholics, and in those patients with cancer or who are immunosuppressed (e.g., renal transplant recipients) (18,19). Other conditions that may increase risk of *Listeria* infection include diabetes mellitus, liver disease, chronic renal disease, collagen-vascular disorders, and conditions associated with iron overload. Despite the increased incidence of *Listeria* infection in patients with deficiencies in cell-mediated immunity, meningitis is found infrequently in patients with human immunodeficiency virus infection (20,21). Meningitis can also occur in previously healthy adults (20). Outbreaks of *Listeria* infection have been associated with the consumption of contaminated cole slaw, raw vegetables, milk, and cheese (18), suggesting that the gastrointestinal tract is the usual portal of entry for this infection.

DIAGNOSIS

The typical CSF findings in patients with bacterial meningitis are shown in Table 11.2 (29). Despite these typical findings, it is sometimes difficult to make a distinction between bacterial and other causes of meningitis based on the CSF formula when the CSF Gram stain and culture are negative. A recent analysis found that a CSF glucose concentration less than 34 mg/dL, a CSF-blood glucose ratio less than 0.23, a CSF protein concentration greater than 220 mg/dL, greater than 2000/μL CSF leukocytes, or greater than 1180/μL CSF neutrophils were individual predictors of bacterial, rather than viral, meningitis with 99% certainty or better (34). This analysis was validated in a retrospective chart review when applied to a geographically distinct and exclusively adult population comprised of primary care and referral patients (35), although proof of this prediction model's utility in clinical practice will require prospective application.

In patients with a CSF formula consistent with bacterial meningitis, but in whom the CSF Gram stain is negative, several rapid diagnostic tests have been developed to aid in the diagnosis (36); these include latex agglutination and staphylococcal coagglutination which detect the antigens of various meningeal pathogens. Currently available latex agglutination tests detect the antigens of *S. pneumoniae*, some *N. meningitidis*, *H. influenzae* type b, *E. coli* K1, and *Streptococcus agalactiae*. However, many of the test kits do not include tests for group B meningococci, and other kits are poor for this organism, probably because of

Table 11.2. Typical CSF Findings in Patients with Bacterial Meningitis

CSF Parameter	*Typical Findings*
Opening pressure	>180 mm H_2O[a]
White blood cell count	1000–5000/μL (range <100 to >10,000)[b]
Percentage of neutrophils	≥80%[c]
Protein	100–500 mg/dL
Glucose	≤40 mg/dL[d]
Lactate	≥35 mg/dL
Gram stain	Positive in 60–90%[e]
Culture	Positive in 70–85%[f]
Bacterial antigen detection	Positive in 50–100%

[a] Values over 600 mm H_2O suggest the presence of cerebral edema, intracranial suppurative foci, or communicating hydrocephalus.
[b] Patients with very low CSF white blood cell counts (0 to 20/μL) tend to have a poor prognosis.
[c] About 30% of patients with *Listeria monocytogenes* meningitis have an initial lymphocyte predominance in CSF.
[d] The CSF-serum glucose ratio is <0.31 in ~70% of patients.
[e] The likelihood of detecting the organism by Gram stain correlates with the concentration of bacteria in CSF; concentrations of ≤10^3 cfu/mL is associated with positive Gram stain ~25% of the time and concentrations ≥10^5 cfu/mL leads to positive microscopy in up to 97% of cases.
[f] Yield of CSF cultures may decrease in patients who have received prior antimicrobial therapy.

the poor immunogenicity of group B meningococcal polysaccharide. One of these tests should be performed on all CSF specimens from patients with presumed bacterial meningitis, especially in cases in which the Gram stain is negative or in patients who have received prior antimicrobial therapy. In one report, 15 (25%) of 61 patients with bacterial meningitis who had received prior antimicrobial therapy had negative CSF cultures but positive CSF bacterial antigen tests (37). It must be emphasized, however, that a negative bacterial antigen test does not rule out the diagnosis of meningitis caused by a specific pathogen.

More recently, polymerase chain reaction (PCR) on CSF specimens has been used to amplify DNA in patients with meningitis caused by *N. meningitidis* and *L. monocytogenes* (38–40). In one study of patients with meningococcal meningitis, PCR had a sensitivity and specificity of 91%. However, there may be problems with false-positive results when using PCR, although further refinements in this technique may lead to its usefulness in patients with bacterial meningitis in whom the CSF Gram stain, bacterial antigen tests, and cultures are negative.

TREATMENT

In a patient who presents clinically with a suspected diagnosis of bacterial meningitis, the initial diagnostic approach is to perform a lumbar puncture. If the CSF formula is consistent with a diagnosis of bacterial meningitis, antimicrobial therapy should be initiated rapidly (within 30 minutes of presentation) based on results of Gram stain or rapid bacterial antigen tests. However, if no etiologic agent can be identified by these means or if there is a delay (i.e., greater than 30 minutes from time of presentation) in the performance of a lumbar puncture, empiric antimicrobial therapy should be initiated based on the patient's age and underlying disease status (Table 11.3) (29). One reason for a delay in performance of a lumbar puncture is the patient with focal signs on neurologic exam or evidence of papilledema on funduscopic examination. These patients should have a computed tomography (CT) scan before lumbar puncture because of the potential risk of herniation if an intracranial mass lesion is present (41). Although antimicrobial therapy administered before CSF examination may decrease the positive yield from CSF cultures, pretreatment blood cultures, the CSF formula, and/or bacterial antigen tests will likely provide evidence for or against a diagnosis of bacterial meningitis.

Although precise data on the time to administration of antimicrobial agents in patients who present with bacterial meningitis are lacking (42), we believe the standard should be rapid administration (i.e., within 30 minutes of presentation). Two recent retrospective studies examining early antimicrobial administration in patients with meningococcal disease give relevance to this recommendation. One study was a retrospective analysis of 46 consecutive patients with meningococcal disease admitted to a hospital in England during

Table 11.3. Empiric therapy of purulent meningitis in adults based on predisposing factor[a]

Predisposing Factor	*Common Bacterial Pathogens*	*Antimicrobial Therapy*
Age 18–50 years	*Streptococcus pneumoniae*, *Neisseria meningitidis*	Third-generation cephalosporin[b,c]
Age >50 years	*Streptococcus pneumoniae*, *Neisseria meningitidis*, *Listeria monocytogenes*, aerobic gram-negative bacilli	Third-generation cephalosporin[b] plus ampicillin
Immunocompromised host	*Streptococcus pneumoniae*, *Neisseria meningitidis*, *Listeria monocytogenes*, aerobic gram-negative bacilli (including *Pseudomonas aeruginosa*)	Vancomycin plus ampicillin plus a ceftazidime
Basilar skull fracture	*Streptococcus pneumoniae*, *Haemophilus influenzae*, group A β-hemolytic streptococci	Third-generation cephalosporin[b]
Head trauma; postneurosurgery	*Staphylococcus aureus*, *Staphylococcus epidermidis*, aerobic gram-negative bacilli (including *Pseudomonas aeruginosa*)	Vancomycin plus ceftazidime
CSF shunt	*Staphylococcus epidermidis*, *Staphylococcus aureus*, aerobic gram-negative bacilli (including *Pseudomonas aeruginosa*), *Propionibacterium acnes*	Vancomycin plus ceftazidime

[a] Vancomycin should be added to empiric therapeutic regimens when highly penicillin- or cephalosporin-resistant strains of *Streptococcus pneumoniae* are suspected; see text for details.
[b] Cefotaxime or ceftriaxone
[c] Add ampicillin if meningitis caused by *Listeria monocytogenes* is suspected.

which time a campaign was instituted for administration of antimicrobial therapy before presentation to the hospital (43); none of the 13 patients given parenteral penicillin by the referring physician died versus eight deaths in 33 patients admitted without such treatment. In another retrospective review of hospital notes and laboratory and public health medical department records of patients in Southwest England with presumed meningococcal meningitis, parenteral benzylpenicillin given by general practitioners before hospital admission was associated with a reduced mortality rate (from 9% to 5%) (44); the mortality rate was further reduced in patients who presented with a hemorrhagic rash (from 12% to 5%). Although retrospective in nature and not specifically reviewing patients with meningitis, these data suggest that early administration of antimicrobial therapy to patients with meningococcal disease improves outcome.

Furthermore, some patients with bacterial meningitis should receive adjunctive dexamethasone therapy immediately upon presentation. The available clinical data in infants and children support the routine use of adjunctive dexamethasone (0.15 mg/kg every 6 hours for 4 days), administered concomitant with or just before the first dose of the antimicrobial agent, in patients with suspected or proven *H. influenzae* type b meningitis (29,45,46). *We do not routinely recommend the use of adjunctive dexamethasone in adult patients with bacterial meningitis except in those with severely impaired mental status, cerebral edema, or markedly elevated intracranial pressure.* The rationale for use of this agent is discussed in greater detail below.

Antimicrobial Therapy

Once a bacterial pathogen is isolated, antimicrobial therapy can be modified for optimal treatment (Table 11.4) (29); recommended dosages for adults are shown in Table 11.5. The following sections review our recommendations for specific antimicrobial agents in adult patients with bacterial meningitis. Specific attention is paid to recent changes in antimicrobial susceptibility patterns of meningeal pathogens.

S. pneumoniae The therapy of pneumococcal meningitis has undergone major evolution in recent years as a result of changes in susceptibility of this organism to penicillin (47–49). In the past, pneumococci were uniformly susceptible to penicillin G with minimal inhibitory concentrations (MICs) of no more than 0.06 μg/mL. There have now been numerous reports throughout the world, including the United States, documenting strains that are relatively (MIC 0.1–1.0 μg/mL) and highly penicillin-resistant (MIC $\geqslant$ 2.0 μg/mL); the mechanism of this resistance is a result of alterations in the structure and molecular size of penicillin-binding proteins. The majority of resistant pneumococcal strains isolated from CSF is serotypes 6, 14, 19, and 23; most of those isolated in the United States disseminated from a multiresistant serotype 23F clone isolated from Spain as early as 1978 (50). The first relatively penicillin-resistant strain of *S. pneumoniae* (MIC 0.6 μg/mL) was isolated in 1967 in Australia, and the first highly resistant strain (MIC 4–8 μg/mL) from South Africa in 1978. Since these initial reports, the incidence of penicillin-resistant pneumococci has been increasing. In the United States from 1979 through 1987, 4.5% of pneumococcal strains (most isolated from Alaska, New Mexico, and Oklahoma) were either relatively or highly resistant to penicillin (51). More recently, in a surveillance study of 13 hospitals in 12 states from October 1, 1991 to September 30, 1992, 16.4% of pneumococcal isolates were resistant to at least

Table 11.4. Specific Antimicrobial Therapy for Bacterial Meningitis

Microorganism	*Standard Therapy*	*Alternative Therapies*
Streptococcus pneumoniae		
Penicillin MIC < 0.1 μg/mL	Penicillin G or ampicillin	Third-generation cephalosporin[a]; chloramphenicol; vancomycin
Penicillin MIC 0.1–1.0 μg/mL	Third-generation cephalosporin[a]	Vancomycin
Penicillin MIC ≥ 2.0 μg/mL	Vancomycin[b]	Imipenem[c]; meropenem[d,e]
Neisseria meningitidis	Penicillin G or ampicillin	Third-generation cephalosporin[a]; chloramphenicol
Haemophilus influenzae		
β-Lactamase negative	Ampicillin	Third-generation cephalosporin[a]; chloramphenicol; aztreonam
β-Lactamase positive	Third-generation cephalosporin[a]	Chloramphenicol; aztreonam; fluoroquinolone
Enterobacteriaceae	Third-generation cephalosporin[a]	Aztreonam; fluoroquinolone; trimethoprim-sulfamethoxazole
Pseudomonas aeruginosa	Ceftazidime[f]	Aztreonam[f]; fluoroquinolone[f]; meropenem[e,f]
Listeria monocytogenes	Ampicillin or penicillin G[f]	Trimethoprim-sulfamethoxazole
Streptococcus agalactiae	Ampicillin or penicillin G[f]	Third-generation cephalosporin[a]; vancomycin
Staphylococcus aureus		
Methicillin sensitive	Nafcillin or oxacillin	Vancomycin
Methicillin resistant	Vancomycin	
Staphylococcus epidermidis	Vancomycin ± rifampin	

[a] Cefotaxime or ceftriaxone.
[b] Addition of rifampin or a third-generation cephalosporin should be considered.
[c] Use is associated with an increased risk of seizures.
[d] Currently under study in patients with pneumococcal meningitis.
[e] Not yet licensed for clinical use in the United States.
[f] Addition of an aminoglycoside should be considered.

Table 11.5. Recommended Dosages of Antimicrobial Agents for Meningitis in Adults with Normal Renal and Hepatic Function

Antimicrobial Agent	*Total Daily Dose*	*Dosing Interval (hr)*
Amikacin[a]	15 mg/kg	8
Ampicillin	12 gm	4
Aztreonam	6–8 gm	6–8
Cefotaxime	6–12 gm	4–8
Ceftazidime	6 gm	8
Ceftriaxone	2–4 gm	12–24
Chloramphenicol[b]	4–6 gm	6
Ciprofloxacin	800–1200 mg	8–12
Gentamicin[a]	3–5 mg/kg	8
Imipenem	2 gm	6
Nafcillin	9–12 gm	4
Oxacillin	9–12 gm	4
Penicillin G	24 million units	4
Rifampin[c]	600 mg	24
Tobramycin[a]	3–5 mg/kg	8
Trimethoprim-sulfamethoxazole[d]	10 mg/kg	12
Vancomycin[a,e]	2–3 g	8–12

[a] Need to monitor peak and trough serum concentrations.
[b] Higher dose recommended for pneumococcal meningitis.
[c] Oral administration.
[d] Dosage based on trimethoprim component.
[e] May need to monitor CSF concentrations in severely ill patients.

one of the following antimicrobial agents: penicillins, cephalosporins, macrolides, trimethoprim-sulfamethoxazole, and chloramphenicol (52). A subsequent surveillance study of 40 medical centers in the United States documented that about 20% of pneumococci were penicillin resistant (53). Despite these impressive epidemiologic data, it pales in comparison with data obtained from other areas of the world. In Spain, the incidence of penicillin resistance rose from 6% in 1979 to 44% in 1989 (54). The highest incidence of resistance has been documented in Hungary with a rate of 58% in a surveillance study from 1988 to 1989 (55). The development of penicillin resistance has been associated with a number of factors, including age less than 10 or greater than 50 years, immunosuppression, prolonged hospitalization, children in day care settings, infection by pneumococcal serotypes 14 and 23, and frequent use of prophylactic antimicrobial therapy (e.g., to prevent otitis media) (47,56).

These changes in pneumococcal susceptibility have important implications in the therapy of pneumococcal meningitis (57). Because sufficient CSF concentrations of penicillin are difficult to achieve with standard parenteral regimens (initial CSF concentrations ~1 μg/mL), penicillin alone can never be recommended as empiric therapy when *S. pneumoniae* is considered a likely pathogen or even when *S. pneumoniae* is isolated, pending results of susceptibility testing.

Several alternative antimicrobial regimens have been examined in clinical studies in the therapy of pneumococcal meningitis caused by penicillin-resistant strains (Table 11.6). Chloramphenicol has been used, although chloramphenicol resistance in pneumococci has been reported. In addition, clinical failure has occurred even when the organism was susceptible to chloramphenicol by disc diffusion and MIC testing. In a South African study in which disc diffusion demonstrated chloramphenicol susceptibility, 20 of 25 children with pneumococcal meningitis treated with chloramphenicol had unsatisfactory outcomes defined as poor clinical response, serious neurologic sequelae, and death (58). It appeared that despite chloramphenicol susceptibility on disc testing, the chloramphenicol minimal bactericidal concentrations (MBCs) for the penicillin-resistant isolates were significantly higher than the penicillin-sensitive isolates, likely resulting in subtherapeutic CSF bactericidal activity. Another study from northwest England found that 83% of their penicillin-resistant pneumococci had an MBC to chloramphenicol of greater than 4 μg/mL (59), *supporting the concept that chloramphenicol should not be used in patients with suspected or proven penicillin-resistant pneumococcal meningitis.*

In patients with meningitis caused by relatively penicillin-resistant pneumococci, the third-generation cephalosporins (cefotaxime or ceftriaxone) are considered the treatment of choice (57,60). Although previous reports documented that ceftizoxime had essentially the identical in vitro spectrum as the other third-generation cephalosporins against pneumococci, a recent study demonstrated that pneumococcal strains relatively or highly resistant to penicillin were less susceptible to ceftizoxime than cefotaxime and ceftriaxone (61), indi-

Table 11.6. Potential Antimicrobial Regimens for Therapy of Meningitis Caused by Penicillin-Resistant *Streptococcus pneumoniae*

Chloramphenicol
Third-generation cephalosporin[a]
Third-generation cephalosporin[a] plus ampicillin
Third-generation cephalosporin[a] plus vancomycin
Third-generation cephalosporin[a] plus rifampin
Vancomycin
Vancomycin plus rifampin
Vancomycin plus rifampin plus third-generation cephalosporin[a]
Imipenem[b]
Meropenem[c]

[a] Cefotaxime or ceftriaxone.
[b] Proconvulsant activity may preclude its use in meningitis.
[c] Not currently licensed for clinical use in the United States.

cating that *ceftizoxime should not be used to treat suspected or proven pneumococcal infections in areas where resistance to penicillin is prevalent*. Unfortunately, pneumococcal strains have also emerged that are resistant to the third-generation cephalosporins. In one report of three pediatric patients who had recently received oral antibiotics, therapy for pneumococcal meningitis consisted of either cefuroxime or cefotaxime (62). Susceptibility testing of the isolates revealed relative or high-level penicillin resistance as well as resistance to the third-generation cephalosporins (MIC ranging from 4 to >32 μg/mL, which may be higher than achievable CSF concentrations with these agents). After initial clinical deterioration in all three patients, a subsequent change in antimicrobial therapy to vancomycin plus chloramphenicol resulted in CSF sterilization. Another report decribed a patient with pneumococcal meningitis (MIC to penicillin and cefotaxime of 1.0 μg/mL) who failed therapy with cefotaxime (63). However, a study of five children with penicillin- and cephalosporin-resistant pneumococcal meningitis revealed that chidren with strains that had MICs to cefotaxime or ceftriaxone of no more than 1.0 μg/mL may be adequately treated with these antimicrobial agents (64). The National Committee for Clinical Laboratory Standards has established guidelines stating that pneumococcal isolates associated with meningitis for which the MICs are at least 0.5 μg/mL should be considered resistant to the third-generation cephalosporins. However, investigators at the Centers for Disease Control and Prevention have recommended that a 30-μg ceftizoxime disc be used for screening (65); ceftizoxime produces a sufficiently large separation between cephalosporin-sensitive and cephalosporin-resistant pneumococcal isolates. A zone of inhibition of less than 15 mm correlates with a cefotaxime or ceftriaxone MIC greater than 2 μg/mL. This discrepancy indicates the need for further clinical data before definitive recommendations can be made regarding the cephalosporin breakpoint for *S. pneumoniae*.

Vancomycin is considered the treatment agent of choice for pneumococcal meningitis caused by highly penicillin- or cephalosporin-resistant strains (57,60); some authorities also recommend the addition of rifampin, although there are no clinical data to support this recommendation. Rifampin can never be used as monotherapy because of the rapid development of resistance. Vancomycin has been evaluated in the therapy of confirmed pneumococcal meningitis caused by relatively penicillin-resistant strains (66). Unfortunately, clinical failure occurred in 4 of 11 patients treated with vancomycin; in two of the failures, CSF vancomycin concentrations were undetectable at 48 hours and a third patient had recurrence of clinical symptoms on day 8, possibly secondary to decreasing meningeal inflammation and deficient blood-brain barrier penetration of vancomycin. This concept has been supported by data in an experimental rabbit model of pneumococcal meningitis, in which the CSF penetration of vancomycin was consistently and substantially reduced, and CSF sterilization delayed, in animals receiving dexamethasone therapy (67). These data indicate that vancomycin may not be optimal therapy for treatment of pneumococcal meningitis, and we do not favor vancomycin monotherapy for this disease. Patients receiving vancomycin therapy need to be carefully monitored clinically for therapeutic failure; measurement of CSF vancomycin concentrations may also be beneficial. Due to concerns regarding erratic CSF penetration of vancomycin, consideration should be given to the intrathecal route of administration in patients with a poor clinical response, although there are no data that this approach improves outcome.

Several other antimicrobial agents have also been used clinically in patients with pneumococcal meningitis. There are reports from Spain of successful treatment of patients with penicillin-resistant pneumococcal meningitis with imipenem (68), although the proconvulsant activity of imipenem may limit its usefulness. Meropenem, a new carbapenem with less seizure proclivity than imipenem, may be an effective alternative. Meropenem had poor efficacy in an experimental rabbit model of meningitis, possibly related to its rapid metabolism in rabbits resulting in only short periods of supra-MICs in CSF (69); clinical studies with meropenem, however, are promising (70). Other antimicrobial agents have been evaluated in in vitro systems and in experimental animal models of pneumococcal meningitis (48); these include the fluoroquinolones (e.g., CP-99,219, clinafloxacin, sparfloxacin), streptogramins (e.g., RP 59500), macrolides, and clindamycin. However, these agents cannot be recommended for therapy of pneumococcal meningitis pending their evaluation in well-designed clinical trials.

Based on the above data, it is recommended that the third-generation cephalosporins (cefotaxime or ceftriaxone) be used in patients when relatively penicillin-resistant pneumococcal strains are suspected or isolated and vancomycin (in combination) be used for highly penicillin- or cephalosporin-resistant isolates. As an empiric regimen, the combination of vancomycin plus a third-generation cephalosporin is recommended based on data in an experimental rabbit model of pneumococcal meningitis in which the combination of vancomycin plus ceftriaxone was synergistic (69). Clearly, patients with pneumococcal meningitis need to be followed very carefully for evidence of clinical failure.

N. meningitidis Penicillin G and ampicillin remain the drugs of choice for therapy of meningococcal meningitis. These recommendations may change in the future, however, with the emergence of strains of *N. meningitidis* that are relatively resistant to penicillin (MIC 0.1 to 1.0 μg/ml). The prevalence of penicillin-resistant meningococci has remained low and has not changed significantly in the United States over the last decade; only 3 of 100 meningococcal isolates submitted to the Centers for Disease Control and Prevention for the year 1991 were relatively penicillin-resistant versus none of the more than 900 isolates tested from 1980 through 1990 (71). In other areas of the world, however, the prevalence of resistant isolates has been increasing. Of 3264 strains of *N. meningitidis* isolated from blood and CSF in Spain during 1978 to 1985, only one resistant isolate was observed, whereas 9 (5%) of 168 invasive isolates relatively resistant to penicillin were found in the first 6 months of 1986; this reached 20% in 1989 (72). This resistance has been reported to be mediated by a reduced affinity of the antibiotic for penicillin-binding proteins 2 and 3 (72,73). Fortunately, patients with meningitis caused by these isolates have recovered with standard penicillin therapy so their clinical significance is unclear. However, if there are concerns about penicillin therapy for patients with resistant meningococcal isolates, therapy with ceftriaxone is recommended based on in vitro susceptibility data (74).

***H. influenzae* Type b** Although meningitis caused by *H. influenzae* type b is uncommon in adult patients, it may cause meningitis in certain clinical circumstances (see above). Because of the emergence of β-lactamase–producing strains of *H. influenzae* type b (1) and because chloramphenicol has been shown in one prospective study to be bacteriologically and clinically inferior to cefotaxime and ceftriaxone (75), the third-generation cephalosporins are the recommended agents of choice for empiric therapy when *H. influenzae* type b meningitis is suspected. Although the second-generation cephalosporin, cefuroxime, was initially thought to be efficacious, several randomized studies that compared cefuroxime to ceftriaxone for therapy of childhood bacterial meningitis have documented a more rapid rate of CSF sterilization and a lower incidence of hearing impairment in the patients receiving ceftriaxone (76,77). Although all studies evaluating the efficacy of antimicrobial agents for *H. influenzae* type b meningitis have been performed in infants and children, we believe this data should be extrapolated to the adult patient with meningitis caused by this organism.

Enteric Gram-Negative Bacilli The third-generation cephalosporins have revolutionized the therapy of meningitis caused by enteric gram-negative bacilli (78–80). Previous mortality rates with standard regimens (usually an aminoglycoside with or without chloramphenicol) ranged from about 40% to 90%. Cure rates with the third-generation cephalosporins have ranged from 78% to 94%. Ceftazidime, a third-generation agent with enhanced in vitro activity against *P. aeruginosa*, resulted in cure of 19 of 24 patients with *P. aeruginosa* meningitis when used alone or in combination with an aminoglycoside (81); in this situation, we believe that combination therapy should be used for a 3-week treatment course. Concomitant intraventricular or intrathecal aminoglycoside therapy may be needed in patients not responding to parenteral antimicrobial agents (82).

Several other antimicrobial agents have also been evaluated in patients with meningitis caused by enteric gram-negative bacilli. Imipenem was efficacious in one case of *Acinetobacter* meningitis (83), although a high rate of seizure activity (33%) in patients with meningitis treated with imipenem may limit its usefulness (84). High-dose meropenem (2 gm every 8 hours) given for 18 weeks was successful in a lymphoma patient with *P. aeruginosa* meningitis who failed ceftazidime plus gentamicin therapy (85) and when given for 20 days in a trauma patient with nosocomial multiresistant *P. aeruginosa* (86). The fluoroquinolones (e.g., ciprofloxacin, pefloxacin) have been used successfully in some patients with enteric gram-negative bacillary meningitis (87), although the limited published literature available on the fluoroquinolones suggests that their primary area of usefulness is for therapy of multidrug-resistant gram-negative organisms (e.g., *P. aeruginosa*) or when the response to conventional β-lactam therapy is slow. These agents should never be used as empiric therapy for purulent meningitis of unknown etiology because of their poor in vitro activity against *S. pneumoniae*. Newer cephalosporins (e.g., cefepime, cefpirome) are currently under clinical investigation in patients with meningitis. A recent prospective randomized trial found cefepime to be safe and therapeutically equivalent to cefotaxime for management of bacterial meningitis in infants and children (88); most cases were caused by *H. influenzae* type b.

L. monocytogenes For patients with *L. monocytogenes* meningitis, therapy should consist of ampicillin or penicillin G (18,19), with the addition of an aminoglycoside considered in proven infection due to documented in vitro synergy and enhanced killing in vivo in experimental animal models of infection. However, therapy with ampicillin compared with ampicillin plus gentamicin has never been evaluated in a controlled clinical trial. In the penicillin-allergic patient, trimethoprim-sulfamethoxazole, which is bactericidal against *Listeria* in vitro, should be used. Despite favorable in vitro susceptibility results, chloramphenicol and vancomycin have been associated with unacceptably high failure rates in patients with *Listeria* meningitis, although intraventricular vancomycin was successful in one case of recurrent *L. monocytogenes* meningitis (89). Although rifampin in bacteriostatic against *L. monocytogenes* in vitro, it was no better than penicillin alone in an experimental rabbit model of meningitis (90). Meropenem, which is active in vitro and in experimental animal models of *L. monocytogenes* meningitis, may be a useful alternative in the future (29). The third-generation cephalosporins and fluoroquinolones are inactive in meningitis caused by *L. monocytogenes*.

Corticosteroid Therapy

Rationale Despite the availability of effective bactericidal antimicrobial agents, the morbidity and mortality from bacterial meningitis remains unacceptably high. A major cause of mortality and sequelae are intracranial complications arising during the acute phase of the disease. In a recent prospective clinical study of 86 consecutive patients with bacterial meningitis between the ages of 15 and 87 years, complications occurred in 43 patients (91). The major central nervous system complications were angiographically documented cerebrovascular involvement, brain swelling, hydrocephalus, and intracranial hemorrhage; seven patients had cerebral herniation, three with a lethal course.

These data indicate the need to develop adjunctive strategies for the therapy of bacterial meningitis in the hopes of improving outcome.

To develop a rationale for the use of adjunctive therapy in patients with bacterial meningitis, the pathogenesis and pathophysiology of bacterial meningitis must be understood (92–94). Bacterial meningitis begins by host acquisition of a new organism by nasopharyngeal colonization, followed by local invasion. Once gaining access to the bloodstream, meningeal pathogens overcome host defense mechanisms as a result of the presence of a polysaccharide capsule that inhibits neutrophil phagocytosis and resists classic complement-mediated bactericidal activity. Subsequently, there is meningeal invasion, although the precise location and mechanism of central nervous system invasion are poorly understood. Once meningeal pathogens gain access to the subarachnoid space, local host defense mechanisms are inadequate to control the infection. With continued bacterial replication, an intense subarachnoid space inflammatory response is generated, which leads to many of the pathophysiologic consequences of bacterial meningitis. These include further increases in blood-brain barrier permeability with development of vasogenic edema, increased CSF outflow resistance that may produce hydrocephalus and interstitial edema and cytotoxic edema that is a result of swelling of cellular elements of the brain. All of these factors contribute to increased intracranial pressure in bacterial meningitis. The subarachnoid space inflammatory response can also lead to cerebral vasculitis and resultant infarction; when combined with the increased intracranial pressure, there may be regional alterations in cerebral blood flow.

Investigations over the last two decades have determined that administration of antimicrobial agents to experimental animals with bacterial meningitis may enhance the subarachoid space inflammatory response, perhaps contributing to the excess morbidity and mortality in patients with bacterial meningitis. In the experimental rabbit model of pneumococcal meningitis, it has been shown that the generation of pneumococcal cell wall components after treatment with bacteriolytic antibiotics may contribute to increased subarachnoid space inflammation (95,96). For gram-negative bacteria, such as *H. influenzae* type b, lipopolysaccharide appears to be the important virulence factor, and several experimental studies have demonstrated that the intracisternal inoculation of purified *H. influenzae* type b lipopolysaccharide induces subarachnoid space inflammation in a time- and dose-dependent manner (97,98). In addition, recent evidence supports the hypothesis that pneumococcal cell wall components or lipopolysaccharide induces subarachnoid space inflammation through local central nervous system release of various inflammatory cytokines, such as tumor necrosis factor-α (TNF-α) and interleukin-1β (IL-1β) (99,100). Other inflammatory mediators (including IL-6, IL-8, platelet-activating factor, and macrophage inflammatory proteins 1 and 2) may also be important (101–104). It appears that these cytokines have multiple complex and interrelated activities in the central nervous system, contributing to tissue damage during bacterial meningitis. As a result of these studies, various experimental and clinical trials were undertaken to determine whether attenuation of the subarachnoid space inflammatory response might be beneficial in patients with bacterial meningitis.

Experimental Studies

As stated above, the generation of pneumococcal cell wall components during antibiotic-induced autolysis in the experimental rabbit model of pneumococcal meningitis may contribute to a marked subarachnoid space inflammatory response. This inflammatory response was reduced by agents, such as methylprednisolone and oxindanac, which inhibit the cyclooxygenase pathway of arachidonic acid metabolism (105). Methylprednisolone has also been shown to produce a significant reduction in the mass of leukocytes within the meninges of rabbits with pneumococcal meningitis (106) and to reduce the CSF outflow resistance (defined as factors that inhibit the flow of CSF from the subarachnoid space to the major dural sinuses) to a greater extent than in untreated or penicillin-treated rabbits with pneumococcal meningitis (107). The effects of methylprednisolone and another corticosteroid agent, dexamethasone, on brain water content (which reflects cerebral edema), CSF pressure, and CSF lactate were determined in rabbits with pneumococcal meningitis (108). Each agent completely reversed the development of brain edema, but only dexamethasone reduced the increases in CSF pressure and lactate; only methylprednisolone was associated with increased CSF concentrations of bacteria. However, neither agent was superior to ampicillin alone in reduction of cerebral edema or increased intracranial pressure, and no comparison was made between ampicillin alone and ampicillin plus corticosteroid, a comparison that would have been relevant to the potential clinical utility of adjunctive corticosteroid in bacterial meningitis.

This question was subsequently examined in a rabbit model of *H. influenzae* type b meningitis, in which therapy with ceftriaxone was compared with the combination of ceftriaxone plus dexamethasone (109). Combination therapy consistently reduced brain water content, CSF pressure, and CSF lactate to a greater extent than ceftriaxone alone, although the differences were not statistically significant, and, by 29 hours, the values were comparable whether the animals received antibiotic alone, dexamethasone alone, or the combination. The authors of this study suggested that dexamethasone might be more beneficial if administered early, or even before, antibiotic-induced autolysis and release of microbial products. Using the same animal model, it was determined that a significant increase in CSF lipopolysaccharide concentrations occurred 2 hours after ceftriaxone administration, which was followed by a rise in CSF TNF concentrations (110). Simultaneous administration of ceftriaxone and dexamethasone did not affect the appearance of lipopolysaccharide in CSF but led to a marked attenuation in CSF TNF concentrations 8 hours later and a reduction in the resultant CSF leukocytosis, with a trend toward earlier improvement in various CSF parameters (glucose, lactate, and protein). These data indicated that dexamethasone, in conjunction with antimicrobial agents, appears to improve a number of parameters of subarachnoid space inflammation. One essential effect of dexamethasone was blockade of release of cytokines from mononuclear cells and astrocytes, the probable sources of cytokines during bacterial meningitis.

Clinical Studies Based on these studies from experimental animal models of meningitis, several clinical trials were undertaken to examine the utility of adjunctive dexamethasone in patients with bacterial meningitis. Within the last decade, there have been several well-designed, randomized, placebo-controlled trials on the use of adjunctive dexamethsone in infants and children with bacterial meningitis caused predominantly by *H. influenzae* type b (111–114). These trials demonstrated significant improvements in neurologic and/or audiologic sequelae in the patients receiving adjunctive dexamethasone and led to the recommendation for use of this agent, administered concomitant with or 15 to 20 minutes before the first dose of an antimicrobial agent, in all infants and children with suspected *H. influenzae* type b meningitis.

Unfortunately, there is only one recent trial that has examined the utility of adjunctive dexamethasone therapy in adults with bacterial meningitis. In this trial, conducted in Egypt, 429 children and adults with bacterial meningitis were randomized to receive antimicrobial therapy (ampicillin plus chloramphenicol) with or without adjunctive dexamethasone (115); this study was not placebo controlled. The results demonstrated a significant reduction in the mortality rate and overall neurologic sequelae in the subset of patients with pneumococcal meningitis who received adjunctive dexamethasone therapy (Table 11.7). However, no significant differences were observed in time to afebrility or improvement in CSF parameters, the antimicrobial agents were administered intramuscularly, there was no documentation of possible adverse effects, more than 60% of the patients presented in a comatose state, and most patients (370 of 429) had inadequate therapy for 3 to 5 days before hospitalization. Furthermore, no benefits in terms of mortality or hearing impairment were

Table 11.7. Mortality Rate and Audiologic Sequelae After Adjunctive Dexamethasone Therapy for Pneumococcal Meningitis

	No. Deaths/Total (%)	*No. Hearing Loss/Total (%)*
With dexamethasone	7/52 (13.5)	0/45 (0)
Without dexamethasone	22/54 (40.7)	4/32 (12.5)
P	<0.01	<0.05

SOURCE: Girgis NI, Farid Z, Mikhail IA, et al. Dexamethasone treatment for bacterial meningitis in children and adults. Pediatr Infect Dis J 1989;8:848–851.

observed in the patients with meningitis caused by *N. meningitidis* or *H. influenzae* type b who received adjunctive dexamethasone.

These data indicate the need for additional studies before the routine use of adjunctive dexamethasone can be recommended for adult patients with bacterial meningitis. Although some authors have recommended the use of adjunctive dexamethasone in all cases of meningitis with a likely bacterial etiology (i.e., demonstrable bacteria on Gram stain, which may predict the patients at greatest risk of bacteriolysis-induced exacerbation of subarachnoid space inflammation) (94), there are no clinical data to support this recommendation. Adult patients most likely to benefit from adjunctive dexamethasone are those with severely impaired mental status (stupor or coma), documented cerebral edema (e.g., by CT scan), and/or evidence of markely elevated intracranial pressure (29); we recommend the use of dexamethasone in these clinical situations. However, the use of adjunctive dexamethasone is of particular concern in patients with meningitis caused by highly penicillin- or cephalosporin-resistant *S. pneumoniae*, in which the diminished CSF inflammatory response might significantly reduce vancomycin penetration into CSF with a delay in CSF sterilization.

REFERENCES

1 **Schlech WF III, Ward JI, Band JD, et al.** Bacterial meningitis in the United States, 1978 through 1981. The national bacterial meningitis surveillance study. JAMA 1985; 253:1749–1754.

2 **Wenger JD, Hightower AW, Facklam RR, et al.** Bacterial meningitis in the United States, 1986: report of a multistate surveillance study. J Infect Dis 1990;162:1316–1323.

3 **Durand ML, Calderwood SB, Weber DJ, et al.** Acute bacterial meningitis in adults. A review of 493 episodes. N Engl J Med 1993;328:21–28.

4 **Bryan JP, de Silva HR, Tavares A, et al.** Etiology and mortality of bacterial meningitis in northeastern Brazil. Rev Infect Dis 1990;12:128–135.

5 **Vadheim CM, Greenberg DP, Eriksen E, et al.** Eradication of *Haemophilus influenzae* type b disease in Southern California. Arch Pediatr Adolesc Med 1994:148:51–56.

6 **Roos KL, Tunkel AR, Scheld WM.** Acute bacterial meningitis in children and adults. In: Scheld WM, Whitley RJ, Durack DT, eds. Infections of the central nervous system. New York: Raven Press, 1991:335–409.

7 **Geiseler PJ, Nelson KE, Levin S, et al.** Community-acquired purulent meningitis: a review of 1,316 cases during the antibiotic era, 1954–1976. Rev Infect Dis 1980;2:725–745.

8 **Musher DM.** Infections caused by *Streptococcus pneumoniae*: clinical spectrum, pathogenesis, immunity, and treatment. Clin Infect Dis 1992;14:801–809.

9 **Kaufman BA, Tunkel AR, Pryor JC, Dacey RG Jr.** Meningitis in the neurosurgical patient. Infect Dis Clin North Am 1990;4:677–701.

10 **Pinner RW, Gellin BG, Bibb WF, et al.** Meningococcal disease in the United States—1986. J Infect Dis 1991;164:368–374.

11 **Jackson LA, Schuchat A, Reeves MW, Wenger JD.** Serogroup C meningococcal outbreaks in the United States. An emerging threat. JAMA 1995;273:383–389.

12 **Whalen CM, Hockin JC, Ryan A, Ashton F.** The changing epidemiology of invasive meningococcal disease in Canada, 1985 through 1992. Emergence of a virulent clone of *Neisseria meningitidis*. JAMA 1995;273:390–394.

13 **Ross SC, Densen P.** Complement deficiency states and infection: epidemiology, pathogenesis and consequences of neisserial and other infections in an im-

mune deficiency. Medicine (Baltimore) 1984;64:243–273.

14 **Sjöholm AG, Kuijpre EF, Tijssen CC, et al.** Dysfunctional properdin in a Dutch family with meningococcal disease. N Engl J Med 1988;319:33–37.

15 **Broome CV.** Epidemiology of *Haemophilus influenzae* type b infections in the United States. Pediatr Infect Dis J 1987;6:779–782.

16 **Spagnuolo PJ, Ellner JJ, Lerner PI, et al.** *Haemophilus influenzae* meningitis: the spectrum of disease in adults. Medicine (Baltimore) 1982;61:74–85.

17 **Farley MM, Stephens DS, Brachman PS, et al.** Invasive *Haemophilus influenzae* disease in adults. A prospective, population-based surveillance. N Engl J Med 1992;116: 806–812.

18 **Gellin BG, Broome CV.** Listeriosis. JAMA 1989;261:1313–1320.

19 **Cherubin CE, Appleman MD, Heseltine PNR, et al.** Epidemiologic spectrum and current treatment of listerosis. Rev Infect Dis 1991;13:1108–1114.

20 **Decker CF, Simon GL, DiGioia RA, Tuazon CU.** *Listeria monocytogenes* infections in patients with AIDS: report of five cases and review. Rev Infect Dis 1991; 13:413–417.

21 **Berenguer J, Solera J, Diaz MD, et al.** Listeriosis in patients infected with human immunodeficiency virus. Rev Infect Dis 1991;13:115–119.

22 **Zuniga M, Aguado JM, Vada J.** *Listeria monocytogenes* meningitis in previously healthy adults: long-term follow-up. Q J Med 1992;85:911–915.

23 **Schlesinger LS, Ross SC, Schaberg DR.** *Staphylococcus aureus* meningitis. A broad-based epidemiologic study. Medicine (Baltimore) 1987;66:148–156.

24 **Jensen AG, Espersen F, Skinhoj P, et al.** *Staphylococcus aureus* meningitis. A review of 104 nationwide, consecutive cases. Arch Intern Med 1993;153:1902–1908.

25 **Cherubin CE, Marr JS, Sierra MF, Becker S.** *Listeria* and gram-negative bacillary meningitis in New York City, 1972–1979. Am J Med 1981;71:199–209.

26 **Cameron ML, Durack DT.** Helminthic infections of the central nervous system. In: Scheld WM, Whitley RJ, Durack DT, eds. Infections of the central nervous system. New York: Raven Press, 1991:825–858.

27 **Farley MM, Harvey RC, Stull T, et al.** A population-based assessment of invasive disease due to group B streptococci in non-pregnant adults. N Engl J Med 1993;328: 1807–1811.

28 **Dunne DW, Quagliarello V.** Group B streptococcal meningitis in adults. Medicine (Baltimore) 1993;72:1–10.

29 **Tunkel AR, Scheld WM.** Acute meningitis. In: Mandell GL, Bennett JE, Dolin R, eds. Principles and practice of infectious diseases, 4th ed. New York: Churchill Livingstone, 1994:831–865.

30 **Gorse GJ, Thrupp LD, Nudleman KL, et al.** Bacterial meningitis in the elderly. Arch Intern Med 1989;149:1603–1606.

31 **Tunkel AR, Scheld WM.** Central nervous system infection in the compromised host. In: Rubin RH, Young LS, eds. Clinical approach to infection in the compromised host. 3rd ed. New York: Plenum Publishing Corp, 1994:163–210.

32 **Schoenbaum SC, Gardner P, Shillito J.** Infections of cerebrospinal fluid shunts: epidemiology, clinical manifestations, and therapy. J Infect Dis 1975;131:543–552.

33 **Kaufman BA, McLone DG.** Infections of cerebrospinal fluid shunts. In: Scheld WM, Whitley RJ, Durack DT, eds. Infections of the central nervous system. New York: Raven Press, 1991:561–585.

34 **Spanos A, Harrell FE Jr, Durack DT.** Differential diagnosis of acute meningitis. An analysis of the predictive value of initial observation. JAMA 1989;262:2700–2707.

35 **McKinney WP, Heudebert GR, Harper SA, et al.** Validation of a clinical prediction rule for the differential diagnosis of acute meningitis. J Gen Intern Med 1994;9:8–12.

36 **Gray LD, Fedorko DP.** Laboratory diagnosis of bacterial meningitis. Clin Microbiol Rev 1992;5:130–145.

37 **Bhisitkul DM, Hogan AE, Tanz RR.** The role of bacterial antigen detection tests in the diagnosis of bacterial meningitis. Pediatr Emerg Care 1994;10:67–71.

38 **Jaton K, Sahili R, Bille J.** Development of polymerase chain reaction assays for detection of *Listeria monocytogenes* in clinical cerebrospinal fluid samples. J Clin Microbiol 1992;30:1931–1936.

39 **Kristiansen BE, Ask E, Jenkins A, et al.** Rapid diagnosis of meningococcal meningitis by polymerase chain reaction. Lancet 1991;337:1568–1569.

40 **Ni H, Knight AI, Cartwright K, et al.** Polymerase chain reaction for diagnosis of meningococcal meningitis. Lancet 1992;340: 1432–1434.

41 **Marton KI, Gean AD.** The spinal tap: a

new look at an old test. Ann Intern Med 1986;104:840–848.

42 **Meadow WL, Lantos J, Tanz RR, et al.** Ought "standard care" be the "standard of care"? A study of the time to administration of antibiotics in children with meningitis. Am J Dis Child 1993;147:40–44.

43 **Strang JR, Pugh EJ.** Meningococcal infections: reducing the case fatality rate by giving penicillin before admission to hospital. Br Med J 1992;305:141–143.

44 **Cartwright K, Reilly S, White D, Stuart J.** Early treatment with parenteral penicillin in meningococcal disease. Br Med J 1992;305:143–147.

45 **McGowan JE Jr, Chesney PJ, Crossley KB, LaForce FM.** Guidelines for the use of systemic corticosteroids in the management of selected infections. J Infect Dis 1992;165:1–13.

46 **Tunkel AR.** Bacterial meningitis: non-antibiotic modes of therapy. Curr Opin Infect Dis 1993;6:638–643.

47 **Appelbaum PC.** Antimicrobial resistance in *Streptococcus pneumoniae*: an overview. Clin Infect Dis 1992;15:77–83.

48 **Friedland IR, McCracken GH JR.** Management of infections caused by antibiotic-resistant *Streptococcus pneumoniae.* N Engl J Med 1994;331:377–382.

49 **Austrian R.** Confronting drug-resistant pneumococci. Ann Intern Med 1994;121: 807–809.

50 **McDougal LK, Facklam R, Reeves M, et al.** Analysis of multiply antimicrobial-resistant isolates of *Streptococcus pneumoniae* from the United States. Antimicrob Agents Chemother 1992;36:2176–2184.

51 **Spika JS, Facklam RR, Plikaytis BD, Oxtoby MJ.** Antimicrobial resistance to *Streptococcus pneumoniae* in the United States, 1979–1987: the pneumococcal surveillance working group. J Infect Dis 1991;163:1273–1278.

52 **Breiman RF, Butler JC, Tenover FC, et al.** Emergence of drug-resistant pneumococcal infections in the United States. JAMA 1994;271:1831–1835.

53 **Jones RN, Kehrberg E, Erwin ME, Sader H.** Epidemiologic studies of emerging antimicrobial resistance in USA hospitals: report from a forty medical center surveillance of parenteral drug susceptibility. In: Program and Abstracts of the 34th Interscience Conference on Antimicrobial Agents and Chemotherapy. Washington, DC: American Society for Microbiology, 1994:87.

54 **Fenoll A, Bourgnon CM, Munoz R, et al.** Serotype distribution and antimicrobial resistance of *Streptococcus pneumoniae* isolates causing systemic infections in Spain, 1979–1989. Rev Infect Dis 1991;13:56–60.

55 **Marton A, Gulyas M, Munoz R, Tomasz A.** Extremely high incidence of antibiotic resistance in clinical isolates of *Streptococcus pneumoniae* in Hungary. J Infect Dis 1991;163:542–548.

56 **Garcia-Leoni ME, Cercenado E, Rodeno P, et al.** Susceptibility of *Streptococcus pneumoniae* to penicillin: a prospective microbiologic and clinical study. Clin Infect Dis 1992;14:427–435.

57 **Schwartz MT, Tunkel AR.** Therapy of penicillin-resistant pneumococcal meningitis. Zentralbl Bakteriol 1995;282:7–12.

58 **Friedland IR, Klugman KP.** Failure of chloramphenicol therapy in penicillin-resistant pneumococcal meningitis. Lancet 1992;339:405–408.

59 **Ridgway EJ, Allen KD, Neal TJ, et al.** Penicillin-resistant pneumococcal meningitis. Lancet 1992;339:931.

60 **Friedland IR, Istre GR.** Management of penicillin-resistant pneumococcal infections. Pediatr Infect Dis J 1992;11:433–435.

61 **Haas DW, Stratton CW, Griffin JP, et al.** Diminished activity of ceftizoxime in comparison to cefotaxime and ceftriaxone against *Streptococcus pneumoniae.* Clin Infect Dis 1995;20:671–676.

62 **Sloas MM, Barrett FF, Chesney PJ, et al.** Cephalosporin treatment failure in penicillin- and cephalosporin-resistant *Streptococcus pneumoniae* meningitis. Pediatr Infect Dis J 1992;11:622–626.

63 **Catalan MJ, Fernandez JM, Vazquez A, et al.** Failure of cefotaxime in the treatment of meningitis due to relatively resistant *Streptococcus pneumoniae.* Clin Infect Dis 1994;18:766–769.

64 **Tan TQ, Schutze GE, Mason EO Jr, Kaplan SL.** Antibiotic therapy and acute outcome of meningitis due to *Streptococcus pneumoniae* considered intermediately susceptible to broad-spectrum cephalosporins. Antimicrob Agents Chemother 1994;38: 918–923.

65 **John CC.** Treatment failure with use of a third-generation cephalosporin for penicillin-resistant pneumococcal meningitis. Case report and review. Clin Infect Dis 1994;18:188–193.

66 **Viladrich PF, Gudiol F, Linares J, et al.** Evaluation of vancomycin for therapy of adult pneumococcal meningitis. Antimicrob Agents Chemother 1991;35:2467–2472.

67 **Paris MM, Hickey SM, Uscher MI, et al.** Effect of dexamethasone on therapy of experimental penicillin- and cephalosporinresistant pneumococcal meningitis. Antimicrob Agents Chemother 1994;38: 1320–1324.

68 **Asensi F, Otero MC, Perez-Tamarit D.** Risk/benefit in the treatment of children with imipenem-cilastatin for meningitis caused by penicillin-resistant pneumococcus. J Chemother 1991;5:133–134.

69 **Friedland IR, Paris M, Ehrett S, et al.** Evaluation of antimicrobial regimens for treatment of experimental penicillin- and cephalosporin-resistant pneumococcal meningitis. Antimicrob Agents Chemother 1993;37:1630–1636.

70 **Lopez E, The Meropenem Study Group.** Meropenem versus cefotaxime or ceftriaxone for bacterial meningitis. In: Program and Abstracts of the 33rd Interscience Conference on Antimicrobial Agents and Chemotherapy. Washington, DC: American Society for Microbiology, 1993:236.

71 **Jackson LA, Tenover FC, Baker C, et al.** Prevalence of *Neisseria meningitidis* relatively resistant to penicillin in the United States, 1991. J Infect Dis 1994;169:438–441.

72 **Saez-Nieto JA, Lujan R, Berron S, et al.** Epidemiology and molecular basis of penicillin-resistant *Neisseria meningitidis* in Spain: a 5-year history (1985–1989). Clin Infect Dis 1992;14:394–402.

73 **Mendelman PM, Campos J, Chaffin DO, et al.** Relatively penicillin G resistance in *Neisseria meningitidis* and reduced affinity of penicillin-binding protein 3. Antimicrob Agents Chemother 1988;32:706–709.

74 **Trallero EP, Arenzana JM, Ayestaran I, Baroja IM.** Comparative activity in vitro of 16 antimicrobial agents against penicillin-susceptible meningococci and meningococci with diminished susceptibility to penicillin. Antimicrob Agents Chemother 1989;33:1622–1623.

75 **Peltola J, Anttila M, Renkonen OV, The Finnish Study Group.** Randomised comparison of chloramphenicol, ampicillin, cefotaxime, and ceftriaxone for childhood bacterial meningitis. Lancet 1989;1:1281–1287.

76 **Lebel MH, Hoyt MJ, McCracken GH Jr.** Comparative efficacy of ceftriaxone and cefuroxime for treatment of bacterial meningitis. J Pediatr 1989;114:1049–1054.

77 **Schaad UB, Suter S, Gianella-Borradori A, et al.** A comparison of ceftriaxone and cefuroxime for the treatment of bacterial meningitis in children. N Engl J Med 1990;322:141–147.

78 **Cherubin CE, Corrado ML, Nair SR et al.** Treatment of gram-negative bacillary meningitis: role of the new cephalosporin antibiotics. Rev Infect Dis 1982;4:S453–S464.

79 **Landesman SH, Corrado ML, Chah PM, et al.** Past and current roles of cephalosporin antibiotics in treatment of meningitis. Emphasis on use in gram-negative bacillary meningitis. Am J Med 1981;71:693–703.

80 **Cherubin CE, Eng RHK, Norrby R, et al.** Penetration of newer cephalosporins into cerebrospinal fluid. Rev Infect Dis 1989; 11:526–548.

81 **Fong IW, Tomkins KB.** Review of *Pseudomonas aeruginosa* meningitis with special emphasis on treatment with ceftazidime. Rev Infect Dis 1985;7:604–612.

82 **Saha V, Stansfield R, Masterton R, Edem T.** The treatment of *Pseudomonas aeruginosa* meningitis—old regime or newer drugs? Scand J Infect Dis 1993;25:81–83.

83 **Rodriguez K, Dickinson GM, Greenman RL.** Successful treatment of gram-negative bacillary meningitis with imipenem/cilastatin. South Med J 1985;78:732–733.

84 **Wong VK, Wright HT Jr, Ross LA, et al.** Imipenem/cilastatin treatment of bacterial meningitis in children. Pediatr Infect Dis J 1991;10:122–125.

85 **Donnelly JP, Horrevorts AM, Sauerwein RW, De Pauw BE.** High-dose meropenem in meningitis due to *Pseudomonas aeruginosa*. Lancet 1992;339:1117.

86 **Chmelik V, Gutvirth J.** Meropenem treatment of post-traumatic meningitis due to *Pseudomonas aeruginosa*. J Antimicrob Chemother 1993;32:922–923.

87 **Tunkel AR, Scheld WM.** Treatment of bacterial meningitis. In: Wolfson JS, Hooper DC, eds. Quinolone antimicrobial agents. Washington, DC: American Society for Microbiology, 1993:481–495.

88 **Saez-Llorens X, Castano E, Garcia R, et al.** Prospective randomized comparison of cefepime and cefotaxime for treatment of bacterial meningitis in infants and children. Antimicrob Agents Chemother 1995;39:937–940.

89 **Richards SJ, Lambert CM, Scott AC.** Recurrent *Listeria monocytogenes* meningitis

treated with intraventricular vancomycin. J Antimicrob Chemother 1992;29:351–353.

90 **Scheld WM.** Evaluation of rifampin and other antibiotics against *Listeria monocytogenes* in vitro and in vivo. Rev Infect Dis 1983;5:S593–S599.

91 **Pfister HW, Feiden W, Einhäupl KM.** Spectrum of complications during bacterial meningitis in adults. Results of a prospective clinical study. Arch Neurol 1993;50: 575–581.

92 **Tunkel AR, Wispelwey B, Scheld WM.** Bacterial meningitis: recent advances in pathophysiology and treatment. Ann Intern Med 1990;112:610–623.

93 **Tunkel AR, Scheld WM.** Pathogenesis and pathophysiology of bacterial meningitis. Clin Microbiol Rev 1993;6:118–136.

94 **Quagliarello V, Scheld WM.** Bacterial meningitis: pathogenesis, pathophysiology, and progress. N Engl J Med 1992;327: 864–872.

95 **Tuomanen E, Tomasz A, Hengstler B, Zak O.** The relative role of bacterial cell wall and capsule in the induction of inflammation in pneumococcal meningitis. J Infect Dis 1985;151:535–540.

96 **Tuomanen E, Liu H, Hengstler B, et al.** The induction of meningeal inflammation by components of the pneumococcal cell wall. J Infect Dis 1985;151:859–868.

97 **Syrogiannopoulos GA, Hansen EJ, Erwin AL, et al.** *Haemophilus influenzae* type b lipooligosaccharide induces meningeal inflammation. J Infect Dis 1988;157:237–244.

98 **Wispelwey B, Lesse AJ, Hansen EJ, Scheld WM.** *Haemophilus influenzae* lipopolysaccharide-induced blood brain barrier permeability during experimental meningitis in the rat. J Clin Invest 1988; 82:1339–1346.

99 **Mustafa MM, Ramilo O, Olsen KD, et al.** Tumor necrosis factor in mediating experimental *Haemophilus influenzae* type b meningitis. J Clin Invest 1989;84:1253–1259.

100 **Tunkel AR, Wispelwey B, Scheld WM.** Pathogenesis and pathophysiology of meningitis. Infect Dis Clin North Am 1990;4:555–581.

101 **Waage A, Halstensen A, Shalaby R, et al.** Local production of tumor necrosis factor alpha, interleukin 1, and interleukin 6 in meningococcal meningitis. Relation to the inflammatory response. J Exp Med 1989;170:1859–1867.

102 **Arditi M, Manogue KR, Caplan M, Yogev R.** Cerebrospinal fluid cachectin/tumor necrosis factor-α and platelet-activating factor concentrations and severity of bacterial meningitis in children. J Infect Dis 1990; 162:139–147.

103 **Saukkonen K, Sande S, Cioffee C, et al.** The role of cytokines in the generation of inflammation and tissue damage in experimental gram-positive meningitis. J Exp Med 1990;171:439–448.

104 **Seki T, Joh K, Os-Ishi T.** Augmented production of interleukin-8 in cerebrospinal fluid in bacterial meningitis. Immunology 1993;80:333–335.

105 **Tuomanen E, Hengstler B, Rich R, et al.** Nonsteroidal anti-inflammatory agents in the therapy for experimental pneumococcal meningitis. J Infect Dis 1987;155:985–990.

106 **Nolan CM, McAllister CK, Walters E, Beaty HN.** Experimental pneumococcal meningitis. IV. The effect of methylprednisolone on meningeal inflammation. J Lab Clin Med 1978;91:979–988.

107 **Scheld WM, Dacey RG, Winn HR, et al.** Cerebrospinal fluid outflow resistance in rabbits with experimental meningitis. Alterations with penicillin and methylprednisolone. J Clin Invest 1980;66:243–253.

108 **Täuber MG, Khayam-Bashi H, Sande MA.** Effects of ampicillin and corticosteroids on brain water content, cerebrospinal fluid pressure, and cerebrospinal fluid lactate levels in experimental pneumococcal meningitis. J Infect Dis 1985;151:528–534.

109 **Syrogiannopoulos GA, Olsen KD, Reisch JS, McCracken GH Jr.** Dexamethasone in the treatment of experimental *Haemophilus influenzae* type b meningitis. J Infect Dis 1987;155:213–219.

110 **Mustafa MM, Ramilo O, Mertsola J, et al.** Modulation of inflammation and cachectin activity in relation to treatment of experimental *Haemophilus influenzae* type b meningitis. J Infect Dis 1989;160:818–825.

111 **Lebel MH, Freij BJ, Syrogiannopoulos GA, et al.** Dexamethasone therapy for bacterial meningitis. Results of two double-blind, placebo-controlled trials. N Engl J Med 1988;319:964–971.

112 **Lebel MH, Hoyt MJ, Waagner DC, et al.** Magnetic resonance imaging and dexamethasone therapy for bacterial meningitis. Am J Dis Child 1989;143:301–306.

113 **Odio CM, Faingezicht I, Paris M, et al.** The beneficial effects of early dexamethasone administration in infants and children with bacterial meningitis. N Engl J Med 1991;324:1525–1531.

114 **Schaad UB, Lips U, Gnehm HE, et al.** Dexamethasone therapy for bacterial meningitis in children. Lancet 1993;342:457–461.

115 **Girgis NI, Farid Z, Mikhail IA, et al.** Dexamethasone treatment for bacterial meningitis in children and adults. Pediatr Infect Dis J 1989;8:848–851.

Cysticercosis

JULIO SOTELO
OSCAR H. DEL BRUTTO
GUSTAVO C. ROMAN

LIFE CYCLE OF TAENIASIS/CYSTICERCOSIS

The first observations on cysticercosis in humans were made in 1558 by Rumler in the brain of an epileptic person and in 1652 by Paranoli, who found some liquid-filled vesicles in the corpus callosum of an epileptic priest who died after a stroke, yet they did not identify the lesions as parasites. In the 17th century, Malpighi and Laennec among others recognized the correct nature of the disease. In 1803, Zeder named these vesicles cysticercus (from the Greek *Kystis*, cyst, and *Kerkos*, tail) because of their appearance (1). During the second half of 19th century, experiments by German investigators demonstrating that cysticercus is the larval stage of the tapeworm *Taenia solium* (2) spurred interest in this disease. Currently, cysticercosis is considered the most common parasitic disease of the central nervous system (3).

T. solium has a complex life cycle involving two hosts: humans and pork (Figure 12.1). In the usual cycle of transmission, humans harbor the adult worm *T. solium* as the only known definitive host in whom the adult sexually mature stage of the cestode develops; intestinal taeniasis is acquired by eating undercooked pork meat infected with cysticerci. The adult *T. solium* may live in the small intestine for many years; its length varies from 3 to 5 m. It has a globular rostellum with four suckers and a crown of hooks. The body is composed by hundreds of proglottids. Gravid proglottids, each containing around 80,000 viable eggs, are usually present in the stools of taenia carriers, explaining the contamination of water, vegetation, and food of communities living in poor hygienic conditions and the high frequency of infection of subjects in contact with taenia carriers. The life cycle of the cestode is completed when pork, the natural intermediate host, ingests *T. solium* eggs, which develop in brain and muscle resulting in cysticercosis, the embryonic stage of the parasite (4). Likewise, humans can also act as an intermediate host after ingesting *T. solium* eggs;

in this circumstance, human cysticercosis develops (3). The latter is a blind alley in the life cycle of *T. solium* because it does not contribute to the reproductive success of the cestode.

There are two main routes from which humans acquire cysticercosis: ingestion of food contaminated with human feces containing *T. solium* eggs and anus-to-mouth self-contamination in patients harboring the adult worm in their digestive tract (3). The latter is far less common than the former; therefore, it is quite unusual to find patients having both cysticercosis and taeniasis. Once in the human stomach, *T. solium* eggs lose their coat by action of the gastric juice liberating oncospheres (hexacanth embryos), which in turn cross the intestinal wall and enter the bloodstream to be carried to the tissues of the host where, after a period of 2 months, the larvae evolve forming a cysticercus (5). Several organs of the body may be infected by cysticerci. However, the most frequently affected are the eye, skeletal muscle, and the central nervous system (6). In the

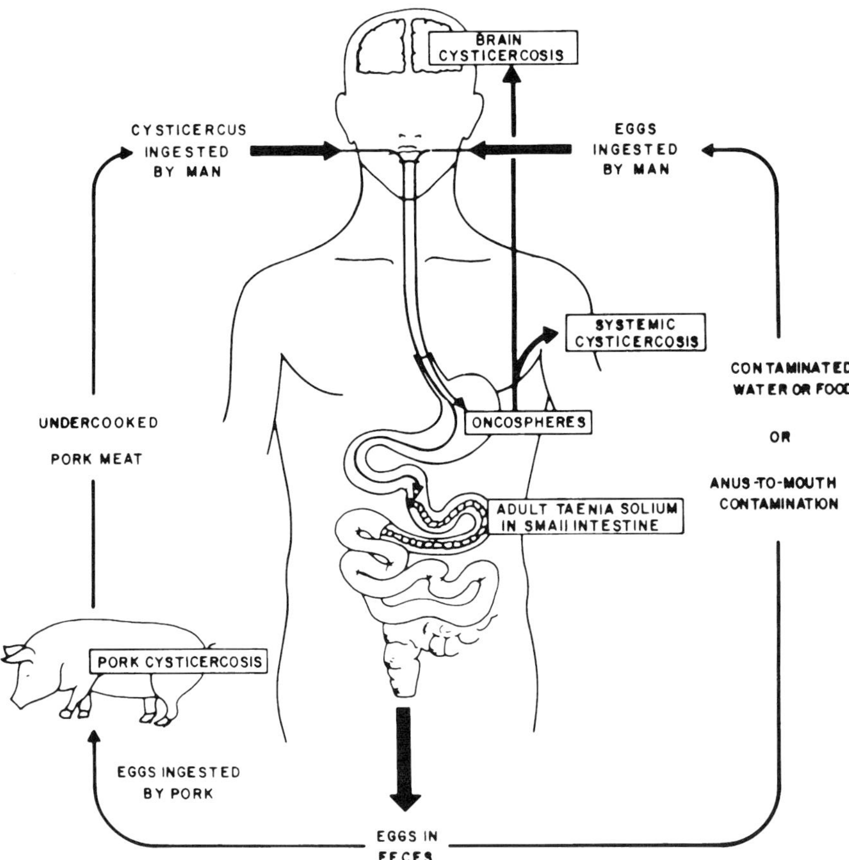

Figure 12.1. Life cycle of taeniasis/cysticercosis.

latter, parasites may lodge in brain parenchyma, subarachnoid space, ventricular system, or spinal cord (5).

Epidemiology

Cysticercosis has a worldwide distribution. However, its prevalence is highly variable, depending mainly on sociocultural and economic factors (7). Cysticercosis was endemic in several European countries during the first half of this century (6,8–10); however, with improved socioeconomic conditions, particularly in industrialized nations, its frequency progressively decreased (11). In contrast, it remains as a major public health problem in developing regions of the world (6,12,13–15). Today, massive immigration from endemic to nonendemic areas has produced a significant increase of cysticercosis in some countries where in past decades this disease was regarded as a medical curiosity (16). Although the causative agent of cysticercosis has been identified, its life cycle elucidated, and modern diagnostic tests and therapies have increased our knowledge of the disease and drastically changed its prognosis (3,17,18), cysticercosis control or eradication has been difficult. In some regions, it still presents a serious health problem with prevalence that may reach around 4% in the general population (3).

PATHOGENESIS

Natural Course

Cysticercus is a liquid-filled vesicle of variable size that may range from 0.5 to 5 cm or more in diameter. It has a wall composed of three layers: the outer cuticular layer, the middle cellular layer with pseudoepithelial structure, and inner reticular layer. Inside most vesicles there is an invaginated scolex with a morphology similar to the adult *T. solium*; the body, neck, and head are outfitted with four suckers and a crown of hooks (Figure 12.2). This formation can be readily identified in biopsy or necropsy material by placing the vesicle between two glass slides and pressing firmly until the scolex flattens; subsequent microscopic examination usually reveals the three-layered wall and the armed rostellum (5). The name *Cysticercus racemose* (from Lat. *racemus*, clusters) has been given to cysticercus in which the scolex cannot be identified; this form is composed either of giant cysts (more than 3 cm diameter) or by several large cysts attached to each other. It is most often encountered in the basal meninges (5). Apparently, these structures represent cysticerci in which the scolex has disappeared as a result of an hydatidiform degenerative process. The name *C. racemose* was used as a separate genus before it was known that this is the larval stage of *Taenia*. Sometimes it is still used for those cysts where the scolex can be identified (7). However, it seems that the above terminology is inadequate because both represent different stages of the same parasite rather than unrelated parasites originating from different cestodes.

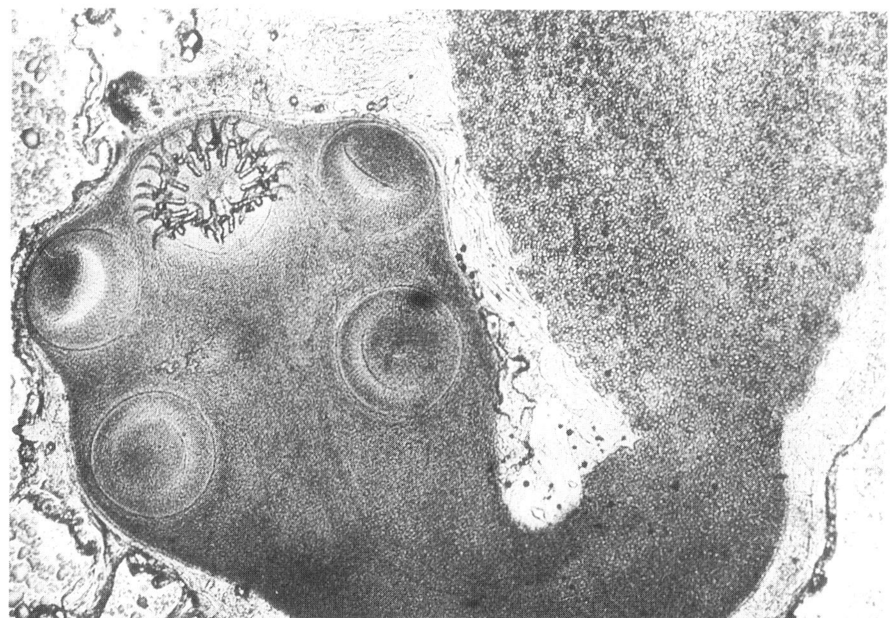

Figure 12.2. Scolex from a cysticercus showing the typical characteristics of *Taenia solium*—the rostellum with a row of hooks and four suckers (magnification ×4).

Localization of Parasites in the Brain

The macroscopic appearance of cysticerci depends on their location within the central nervous system (3,7). Brain parenchymal cysticerci are usually small cysts, single or multiple, that tend to lodge in areas with high vascular supply (Figure 12.3). Subarachnoid cysticerci may be small or large or may form large clumps of cysts within the subarachnoid cisterns; it is also frequent to observe abnormal thickening of leptomeninges more marked at the base of the skull (5). A rather common finding in microscopic examination of autopsy material from patients with meningeal cysticercosis is the presence of endarteritis in small arterial branches; in some cases it leads to complete occlusion of the vessel with subsequent brain infarction (19). The ventricular system is affected by cysticerci in two different ways: by the presence of intraventricular cysts or by the development of granular ependymitis. Intraventricular cysts are usually single and tend to lodge in the fourth ventricle, although they can be found in the third and lateral ventricles (20). In these cases the cysticercus reaches the ventricular system through the choroid plexus of the lateral ventricles and follows the cerebrospinal fluid (CSF) circulation. It seems that when the parasite arrives to the fourth ventricle, it has achieved a size large enough to prevent its passage to the subarachnoid space (5); this mechanism would explain the preferential

in patients with multiple cysts; these patients usually have a chronic and progressive neurologic disorder in which dementia and motor dysfunction predominate. In the past, this syndrome was occasionally found among long-stay patients in mental hospitals before the arrival of imaging studies.

A particular form of parenchymal NCC is cysticercotic encephalitis (32) in which the brain parenchyma is infested by countless cysticerci that elicit a severe inflammatory response leading to a picture of subacute encephalitis, indistinguishable from other forms of allergic or viral encephalitis. These patients present with signs and symptoms of increased intracranial pressure associated with mental disturbances, diminution of visual acuity, and generalized seizures; this rare form of NCC has a significant predilection for affected children and young females (32,33).

Subarachnoid NCC is often manifested by headache, vomiting, vertigo, cranial nerve dysfunction, gait disturbances, and mental deterioration. These manifestations are usually due to hydrocephalus caused by widespread inflammation of subarachnoid membranes and obstruction of the mechanisms of CSF absorption (34,35). In some cases, a large clump of cysts in the subarachnoid cisterns may induce a tumor-like syndrome (36). Differential diagnosis with other space-occupying lesions is difficult on clinical grounds. Infarction of the brain parenchyma is another complication of subarachnoid NCC (13). Such infarcts usually induce lacunar syndromes secondary to the occlusion of small terminal arteries (37). However, large infarcts produced by occlusion of the middle cerebral artery (38–40) or even the internal carotid artery (41) have been occasionally reported. Optic atrophy and visual field defects are frequently observed in patients with subarachnoid NCC. These clinical signs may be caused by hydrocephalus (42), optochiasmatic arachnoiditis, or large intrasellar cysts (43). The latter are usually associated with endocrine disturbances; differential diagnosis must be made with pituitary tumors, craniopharingiomas, or congenital cysts.

Intraventricular cysticercosis is generally associated with hydrocephalus resulting from obstruction of CSF circulation by cysts or by ependymitis (20,44,45). The most frequent presentation is a subacute or intermittent syndrome of intracranial hypertension. In some cases, acute hydrocephalus with sudden death has been documented (44). Patients with cysts in the fourth ventricle may present transient episodes of loss of consciousness due to sudden interruption of CSF flow related to movements of the head (Bruns' syndrome) (46). Granular ependymitis is also associated with hydrocephalus; it usually runs a chronic course and may be associated with focalizing signs of midbrain dysfunction, such as Parinaud's syndrome (42,45).

Clinical manifestations of spinal NCC are also nonspecific, and the differential diagnosis with other diseases of the spinal cord is difficult on clinical grounds alone. Leptomeningeal NCC is characterized by a combination of root pain and weakness of insidious onset and progressive course (47). Intramedullary spinal NCC is found more often in thoracic segments of the spinal cord, although it can be found in the lumbosacral region; clinical manifestations depend on the level of the lesion and usually include progressive motor deficits associated with sensory level and sphincter disturbances (21).

Cysticercosis also occurs outside the central nervous system (8), but it produces few clinical manifestations and is only occasionally diagnosed (48). Ocular cysticercosis may be associated with progressive decrease of visual acuity related either to the presence of the parasite in the eye or to an acute inflammatory reaction that causes vitritis, uveitis, or endophthalmitis (49). There are anecdotal reports of massive cysticerci infestation of striated muscles with a clinical picture of pseudohypertrophic myopathy (50) and cysticerci surrounding a peripheral nerve (51).

DIAGNOSIS

Modern neuroimaging techniques (52–55) and specific immunologic reactions in the CSF (56,57) have dramatically improved our diagnostic accuracy for NCC. These methods provide objective evidence about the topography of lesions and the degree of the inflammatory response to the parasite (see Figure 12.3). In our experience, the combination of these two types of studies offers a proper diagnostic evaluation and a means to individualize the therapeutic approach (13,58–60). Skull radiographs (59) or ventriculograms (10) can give additional information to complete the study of the patient but should not be taken as fundamental proof for the diagnosis of NCC. The efficacy of serum immune tests for diagnosis of NCC is controversial and apparently unreliable (57,60,61). False-positive results can be obtained in healthy individuals from endemic areas, perhaps due to frequent contact with the parasite or to subclinical forms of muscle cysticercosis without neurologic disease (56,62). On the other hand, patients with proved NCC may have false-negative serologic tests (61); these false-negative results in serum could be due to local production of specific antibodies within the central nervous system (63) without parallel increase in blood levels of antibodies, as has been observed in other neurologic disorders. In contrast, immunologic studies in the CSF provide highly reliable results.

Imaging Studies

Computed Tomography (CT) Almost two decades have elapsed since the first reports of NCC diagnosed by CT scan appeared (64,65). Since that time, the value of this imaging technique in the detection of patients with NCC has been confirmed, and currently CT is still the most useful diagnostic tool for this condition (3,26). CT provides reliable information about the topography of the lesions and disease activity (see Figure 12.3).

There are four CT patterns of parenchymal NCC: 1) small calcifications or granulomas that represent previous cysts destroyed by the host; patients with these lesions alone do not actually have NCC but carry its sequelae; 2) rounded areas of low density showing little or no enhancement after intravenous contrast; these lesions represent viable cysticerci (vesicular cysts) with immune tolerance from the host; 3) scattered hypodense or isodense lesions surrounded by edema and ring-like enhancement after contrast (colloidal cysts); these lesions represent the acute encephalitic phase of parenchymal NCC (53) in which the host's immune system is reacting against the parasite; and 4) diffuse brain edema associated with narrowing of the lateral ventricles and multiple nodular and ring-like areas of abnormal contrast enhancement in the parenchyma; this is the CT appearance of cysticercotic encephalitis (32).

Although the above described CT patterns are fairly characteristic of parenchymal NCC, in some cases the differential diagnosis with other diseases may be difficult. This is especially true for patients with cysticerci in the acute encephalitic phase, where abscesses or tuberculomas must be ruled out. In patients with acquired immune deficiency syndrome, toxoplasmosis and brain lymphoma give similar images. Also, in some cases of cysticercotic encephalitis, the CT scan appearance may be similar to that of multiple small brain metastases. In cases of large parenchymal cysts, the possibility of cystic tumors should be ruled out. In such cases, neuroimaging studies and CSF analysis usually provide clues for accurate diagnosis. Nevertheless, biopsy of a cortical lesion is sometimes necessary to confirm the diagnosis. With the advent of new, atoxic, and highly effective drugs for parenchymal NCC, a therapeutic trial can be attempted first in doubtful cases (66).

In subarachnoid NCC, the CT scan is also a valuable diagnostic method, although, as will be discussed below, CSF analysis is the cornerstone of diagnosis (59,67). CT findings in subarachnoid NCC include 1) communicating hydrocephalus secondary to inflammatory occlusion of CSF absorption at the subarachnoid membranes; 2) abnormal enhancement of tentorium and basal cisterns due to fibrous arachnoiditis; 3) hypodense lesions in the Sylvian fissure, cerebello-pontine angle cistern, or over the convexity of the cerebral hemispheres representing racemous cysticerci; 4) brain infarcts due to cysticercotic endarteritis; and 5) hypodense lesions in the sellar region that usually represent a single giant cyst bulging up the diaphragm sella and extending to the suprasellar cistern (43). A CT scan showing hydrocephalus and parenchymal brain infarction may be observed in patients with cysticercotic arachnoiditis, tuberculous meningoencephalitis, fungal meningitis, or carcinomatous meningitis. Again, proper integration of CT findings with CSF examination and the clinical course of the disease is decisive for accurate diagnosis (59). Large cysticerci in the Sylvian fissure, suprasellar cistern, or in posterior fossa cisterns may be occasionally confused with congenital arachnoid cysts or cystic tumors. In such instances, magnetic resonance imaging (MRI) may provide additional information about the nature of the lesion. In addition, a therapeutic course with cysticidal drugs could be attempted to clarify the diagnosis. Sometimes the proper diagnosis is reached only at surgery (36).

Intraventricular cysticerci appear in CT as rounded areas of low density that deform the ventricular system and interfere with CSF circulation causing obstructive hydrocephalus (20). In most cases, diagnosis cannot be made with conventional CT scans because granular ependymitis might give similar images of obstructive or asymmetric hydrocephalus (45). In these cases, CT scanning after intraventricular injection of contrast medium through a previously implanted ventricular shunt usually permits an accurate diagnosis (68). On conventional CT scans, intraventricular cysts fail to enhance after intravenous contrast unless there is associated granular ependymitis (44).

Myelography This method is still valuable for diagnosis of spinal NCC (64) because it reveals multiple filling defects in the case of leptomeningeal cysts or localized subarachnoid block in patients with intramedullary cysts (21). Postmyelogram CT adds valuable information. Currently, MRI has shown great sensitivity for the evaluation of patients with suspected spinal NCC and has replaced myelography as the procedure of choice (47).

MRI This imaging method provides useful information in the evaluation of NCC patients, especially when CT findings are not conclusive (54,55,69). The resolution obtained with MRI permits precise characterization of NCC in terms of disease activity and location of cysticerci. These advantages have important therapeutic implications (59). Live parenchymal cysticerci appear as small rounded areas with signal properties paralleling CSF. The three-layered wall of the parasite is not imaged on MRI but could be inferred from the sharp outline of the cyst fluid. On the T1-weighted sequences, the scolex is visualized within the cyst as a high-intensity nodule; this *hole-with-dot* imaging is characteristic of NCC (54). By contrast, the scolex is poorly visualized on T2-weighted images because it becomes isointense with the cyst fluid.

When the parasite begins to degenerate as a consequence of surrounding inflammation, proteins from the scolex and the cyst wall are added to the vesicular fluid. The T1 relaxation time of this proteinaceous solution is shorter than the T1 of pure vesicular fluid; therefore, these cysts show higher intensity than CSF. Additional evidence of dying cysts are the lack of scolex and an area of high signal intensity around parasites representing perilesional edema (54).

Subarachnoid cysticerci are more readily identified with MRI than with CT, particularly when they are located over the convexity of cerebral hemispheres or at the base of the brain. Large cysts within the subarachnoid cisterns are visualized by MRI as multilobular lesions with signal properties paralleling CSF. The high-intensity nodule representing the scolex is lacking in most of those cysts (59). Adhesive arachnoiditis is visualized by MRI as a diffuse and heterogeneous increase in the signal intensity of CSF cisterns around the brainstem and cerebellum, especially after administration of gadolinium contrast.

Noninvasive diagnosis of intraventricular cysticerci is probably one of the best advantages of MRI. As previously mentioned, conventional CT is insufficient for the diagnosis of intraventricular cysts and metrizamide CT ventriculography is frequently needed (68). Using MRI, detection of intraventricular cysts is possible in most patients by performing sagital and coronal scans that show distortion of the ventricular anatomy in association with an eccentric hyperintense nodular lesion and the membrane of the cyst which are usually undetected by CT (55). Cysticerci within the spinal cord are easily detected by MRI. In those cases, the signal properties of parasites are similar to those observed in the brain parenchyma. By contrast, MRI recognition of spinal leptomeningeal cysts may prove difficult, especially when they are scarce or unaccompanied by surrounding inflammation.

A shortcoming in the accuracy of MRI for the diagnosis of NCC is the poor disclosure of intracranial granulomas and calcifications (31). This is an important point because many patients with NCC have small calcifications as the only evidence of the disease (13,59). In our experience, many patients would have gone undetected had only MRI been performed. Granulomas and calcifications are seen by MRI as areas of reduced signal in one or more pulse sequences, particularly in T2-weighted images (70). This finding is nonspecific and CT always provides more information about the morphology of granulomas and calcifications.

Although some authors have considered MRI the best diagnostic method for patients with NCC (55,71), in our experience CT scan is still of paramount importance. Both CT and MRI are mutually complementary in providing optimal non-invasive diagnosis.

Immunodiagnosis

CSF All patients with suspected diagnosis of NCC should undergo CSF examination. This provides reliable evidence of degree of inflammation and precise diagnosis by immunologic methods. Pathologic changes in CSF vary in relation with the location of parasites. CSF results must be evaluated jointly with imaging studies and should not be used alone to confirm or exclude the diagnosis of NCC.

In parenchymal cysticercosis, CSF results may be within normal limits (57), and immunologic tests may be negative even when CT shows parenchymal cysts. This can be seen in cases where the parasites are not in contact with the subarachnoid space or in cases of remarkable immune tolerance to the parasite. Also, in some cases of ventricular cysticercosis, CSF may be normal because of lack of production of specific antibodies within the ventricular space. However, such cases are rare, and CSF analysis usually provides important information in most patients with active forms of NCC (72).

In general terms, the results of CSF can be separated into two groups, inflammatory and noninflammatory. Inflammation is manifested by elevation of proteins and cell count. When the CSF is not inflammatory, either NCC is inactive or the parenchymal or ventricular cysts are not in contact with the subarachnoid space. Even in the latter cases, immune tests sometimes confirm the diagnosis. Along with neuroimaging studies, CSF results provide evidence for proper classification (13). When the CSF is inflammatory, immune tests based on the complement fixation (CF) reaction (56) and enzyme-linked immunosorbent assay (ELISA) (57) are highly specific and sensitive for accurate diagnosis (greater than 90% in both sensitivity and specificity); CSF eosinophils are found in 50% of samples and low glucose in 25% (13). In our experience, the simultaneous use of CF and ELISA tests provide an accurate diagnosis in almost all cases of NCC with inflammatory CSF. Used in combination, each test detects few cases that are negative in the other, without reducing specificity. Currently, we have modified our previously reported method for ELISA (57) by using simultaneously anti-IgG and anti-IgM conjugates rather than either one alone.

It has been proposed that anticysticercal antibodies can be detected in serum by immunoblot (73) with high specificity and sensitivity. This test has been used to confirm or exclude the diagnosis of this disease (74). However, to assess the real value of serologic diagnosis of NCC by immunoblot, it must first be evaluated in a large and unbiased group of neurologic patients and controls in whom the diagnosis of NCC has been definitively proved or ruled out by neuroimaging studies in all subjects, patients, and controls (61). To our knowledge, such a study has not been performed. Our experience and that of other investigators using immunodiagnostic tests for testing serum has been disappointing, particularly due to a high proportion of false positives (about 30%) among healthy subjects from endemic areas (57,61,75).

TREATMENT

As stated above, NCC is a pleomorphic disease that runs a particular course in almost every patient. Therefore, a single therapeutic approach cannot be expected to be useful in each form of the disorder. Therapy of NCC, medical or surgical, must be chosen according to activity of the disease and location of cysticerci (76,77): as a rule, these are the main factors that determine the therapeutic approach.

Brain Parenchymal Cysticercosis

This form of the disease has provided the best opportunity to test the efficacy of newly introduced cysticidal drugs. Nevertheless, before planning a concise of therapy with such drugs, the characteristics of cysts and the degree of immune response to the parasite must be defined. CT or MRI and CSF analysis provide the necessary answers that allows for rational therapy in individual patients.

1. Cysticidal drugs have not been used in patients with granulomas or calcifications alone because these lesions represent only the sequelae of previous cysts which were destroyed by the host's immune system. Symptomatic treatment with antiepileptics is advised when calcifications are associated with seizures (78); therapy should follow the rules given by the International League Against Epilepsy. In these cases, a trial with cysticidals is justified in those patients in whom there is a suspicion of active forms of NCC sustained by imaging studies or CSF analysis.

2. Parenchymal cysts with little or no evidence of inflammation in imaging studies are especially favorably managed with specific therapy and such patients should receive a course with cysticidals (76). Two drugs, initially praziquantel (PZQ) and lately albendazole (ALB), have proved highly effective for parenchymal cysticercosis. PZQ is an isoquinoline with confirmed efficacy against a broad range of tapeworm infections (79). PZQ has been used for human NCC since 1979 when it was reported as the first truly effective treatment in a patient with parenchymal cysts (80). This preliminary finding was followed by other reports that stressed the usefulness of PZQ in NCC (81–83). Most studies, however, included a variety of forms of the disease and precise evidence of the effectiveness of PZQ was difficult to assess. In 1984, a controlled study in 26 patients with active parenchymal NCC showed that 67% of the cysts disappeared after a single course of PZQ in doses of 50 mg/kg/d for 2 weeks (84). One year later, the optimal time for accurate evaluation of the response to the drug was settled at 3 months (85). Quantification of the number and diameter of cysts on a control CT scan should be made 3 months after the end of treatment. Assessment of response to treatment before this time may be misleading, owing to residual signs of inflammation after destruction of cysticerci (85).

ALB is an imidazole with intense cysticidal properties. A preliminary study using this drug demonstrated its efficacy in patients with parenchymal NCC (86). ALB was administrated in doses of 15 mg/kg/d for 1 month and resulted in 86% disappearance of cysts after treatment. Proper evaluation of the effectiveness of ALB should also be made from the number and diameter of cysts on a control CT scan 3 months after the end of treatment. A subsequent prospective and controlled trial comparing the effectiveness of ALB versus PZQ for therapy of parenchymal NCC demonstrated that ALB was superior to PZQ (87), with the additional advantage that ALB is considerably less expensive than PZQ. Thus, ALB has become the drug of choice for initial therapy of NCC.

The initial length of 1 month of ALB therapy for NCC was settled after the experience with this drug in human hydatidosis (88) and toxicologic studies (89). However, we demonstrated that the length of therapy may be radically shortened to 1 week without lessening the efficacy of ALB (90,91). A short course with ALB increases the compliance of the patient, diminishes even further the cost of therapy, and limits the possibility of secondary reactions to the drug. Currently, we recommend a 1-week course of ALB as the initial form of treatment in all patients with active parenchymal NCC. If only a partial response to ALB is obtained, a new therapeutic course with PZQ may be initiated. There has been debate on whether cysticidal drugs actually improve the clinical status of the patients or if they only produce improvement of the brain images. This debate originated since the first studies of anticysticercal drugs due to the methodology used that only evaluated CT imaging before and after treatment, without detailed clinical evaluation or clinical follow-up. Recent studies with long-term clinical follow-up have shown that cysticidal drugs not only "cure" CT scans but markedly improve the clinical manifestations of NCC (92–94). This includes reversal of neurologic deficits and better control of seizures, providing a rational argument for the use of cysticidals.

During therapy with ALB or PZQ, some patients develop adverse reactions that are not related to drug toxicity. These drugs are remarkably safe as demonstrated in pharmacologic studies (89,95). Rather, the side effects are due to the strong inflammatory response induced by the host in response to the acute destruction of parasites. These reactions, therefore, may be considered reliable clinical predictors of drug effectiveness. Headache, vomiting, and exacerbation of seizures might be seen during treatment. These manifestations begin on the second or third day of therapy; are usually transient, lasting 1 or 2 days; and may be ameliorated with analgesics, antiemetics, or antiepileptics. Corticosteroids are highly effective for treatment of adverse reactions. Some authors have favored simultaneous use of corticosteroids and anticysticercal drugs (96). However, it has been demonstrated that plasma levels of PZQ are reduced by as much as 50% when dexamethasone is given simultaneously (97). In contrast, ALB plasma levels increase with simultaneous dexamethasone administration (98), which can be added with advantage to the ALB therapy. Nevertheless, most patients either do not have complaints during therapy or the side effects are mild and can be easily managed with nonsteroidal drugs. On the other hand, the use of intravenous dexamethasone bolus is advised for the treatment of intense reactions during therapy with anticysticercal drugs. Such complications may be anticipated in patients with multiple cysts or large lesions (18). In our experience, steroids are necessary only for a few days. Currently, only a few patients require hospitalization; most cases are treated as outpatients. It is important to advise the patient of the possibility of the discomforts associated with therapy and their meaning to prevent early discontinuation of treatment.

3. Patients with cysticerci in the acute encephalitic phase could also benefit from treatment with a cysticidal drug. However, because some of these lesions may show spontaneous remission without treatment (99), evaluation of the efficacy of drug therapy is difficult. Justification for ALB or PZQ therapy in these cases is that these drugs seem to shorten the time to involution of lesions. In some patients with intracranial hypertension due to brain edema, corticosteroids or immunosuppressant drugs should be given before cysticidal therapy to reduce brain edema (18). In addition, two studies have shown that control of seizures is better in patients with parenchymal NCC treated with cysticidals, providing a rational argument for their use in such cases (66,100).

4. Patients with cysticercotic encephalitis must be admitted to the hospital for initial management with high doses of steroids or immunosuppressants and osmotic diuretics to reduce the brain edema that accompanies this particular form of the disease (32). Follow-up CT or MRI studies help decide on the use of cysticidal therapy in cases that show persistence of lesions.

Subarachnoid Cysticercosis

Treatment for this form of NCC depends on several factors. When arachnoiditis is complicated by secondary hydrocephalus, a ventricular shunt must always be placed before attempting other measures. A therapeutic course with cysticidals may follow this surgical procedure when the CSF analyses show active disease. Unfortunately, the effectiveness of specific medical therapy in cysticercotic arachnoiditis is not as impressive as in parenchymal NCC (85). A recent study demonstrated a better prognosis for patients with cysticercotic arachnoiditis managed with both ventricular shunt and PZQ when compared with patients managed with ventricular shunt alone (101). Elevation of protein and cell count in the CSF is the major determinant for the protracted course and poor prognosis frequently observed in patients with arachnoiditis and hydrocephalus. In a long-term follow-up study of 92 patients with shunted hydrocephalus secondary to subarachnoid NCC, we found a mortality rate of 50% and severe disability in more than 20% of survivors (35). This study confirmed a direct relationship between inflammatory changes in the CSF, shunt obstruction and death, suggesting the need for better shunt design for the specific treatment of hydrocephalus secondary to inflammatory disorders of the subarachnoid space (102,103).

When active subarachnoid NCC is found in the absence of hydrocephalus, cysticidal treatment is also advised. Response to therapy should be guided by CSF findings before and after 3 months of the therapeutic trial. In addition, these patients should be followed with sequential CT scans to evaluate further development of hydrocephalus.

The treatment of racemous cysticerci in the subarachnoid cisterns is controversial. Some authors recommend surgical resection (104). However, it has recently been demonstrated that ALB induces the disappearance of subarachnoid cysts, obviating the need of surgery in many cases (105,106). Patients with subarachnoid cysts who are treated with ALB may develop an inflammatory reaction within the subarachnoid space; therefore, simultaneous administration of steroids is mandatory in such cases to avoid the risk of cerebral infarction (19,106).

Ventricular Cysticercosis

The therapeutic approach to intraventricular cysticerci has been based on surgical extirpation due to the low levels of cysticidal drugs in the ventricular fluid. Nevertheless, some cases of successful drug therapy of ventricular cysts have been reported (105,107). Patients with intraventricular cysts associated with hydrocephalus must also undergo a ventricular shunt before attempting other measures. Indeed, in most cases, cysts inside the lateral ventricles are diagnosed when asymmetric dilatation of the ventricular system persists after shunting and further CT ventriculography or MRI reveal the cyst. The latter tests also disclose cysts located in the third or fourth ventricles.

It has been reported that transoperative rupture of cysticerci with intraventricular liberation of its fluid could produce an irritative encephalopathy, ventriculitis, arachnoiditis (20). Such findings have not been confirmed by all authors, and we have not observed these complications in many patients in whom accidental rupture of cysticerci occurred during surgery.

Spinal Cysticercosis

Treatment for spinal forms of NCC also depends on the topography of the lesions and disease activity (76). For active leptomeningeal NCC, a trial with anticysticercal drugs may be attempted. Although there are no controlled studies on this therapy, a remission rate similar to that of intracranial subarachnoid cysticerci could be expected, on the basis of similarities between both forms of the disease. Response to treatment should be assessed by CSF findings 3 months after trial completion. If medical treatment is unsuccessful or if a single leptomeningeal cysticercus remains, cyst resection through a laminectomy is advised. Intramedullary spinal cysts are better removed at exploratory surgery.

Ocular Cysticercosis

Cysticerci may locate in the vitreus cavity or subretinal area. Until recently, its treatment was exclusively surgical. Unexpectedly, it has been shown that albendazole has strong cysticidal properties in ocular cysticercosis. After treatment with albendazole and dexamethasone, subretinal cysts are reduced to a small chorioretinal scar, whereas cysts in the vitreus cavity are killed and, once immobile, are easily extracted by surgery (108).

PREVENTION AND PUBLIC HEALTH ASPECTS

Eradication of taeniasis/cysticercosis is possible as demonstrated in countries that were endemic early in this century and are now free of the disease (1,2,8,9). The disease disappears with implementation of appropriate environmental sanitation and better sociocultural conditions. The main measures for prevention of cysticercosis are proper disposal of human waste, treatment of water contaminated with human feces before its use in irrigation of vegetable cultivation, proper cooking of pork, public education on the life cycle of *T. solium*, and sanitary breeding of porcine. In endemic areas, measures such as compulsory and repeated treatment of taenia carriers and domestic or industrial freezing of pork are effective methods (109). A further possibility for control of cysticercosis would be a vaccine produced by techniques of molecular biology (60). However, it is a more costly alternative than the abovementioned measures, and its feasibility for this parasitic diseases is still uncertain (22).

REFERENCES

1 **Nieto D.** Historical notes on cysticercosis. In: Flisser A, ed. Cysticercosis, present state of knowledge and perspectives. New York: Academic Press, 1982:1–7.

2 **Henneberg R.** Die tierischen parasiten des zentral nerven system. In: Bumke O, Foerster O, eds. Handbuch der neurologie. vol. 14. Berlin: Julius Springer, 1936:286.

3 **Sotelo J.** Neurocysticercosis. In: Kennedy PGE, Johnson RT, eds. Infections of the nervous system. London: Butterworths, 1987; 145–155.

4 **Faust EC, Russel PF, Jung RC.** Cysticercosis. In: Faust EC, ed. Clinical parasitology. Philadelphia: Lea & Febiger, 1970: 529–535.

5 **Escobar A, Nieto D.** Parasitic diseases. In: Minckler J, ed. Pathology of the nervous system. vol. 3. New York: McGraw-Hill, 1972:2503–2521.

6 **Flisser A.** Taeniasis and cysticercosis and to Taenia solium. In: Sun T, ed. Progress in Clinical Parasitology. Florida: CRC Press, 1994;4:77–116.

7 **Willms K.** Cestodes (tapeworms). In: Gorbach S, Bartlett JG, Blacklow NR, eds. Infectious diseases. Philadelphia: WB Saunders, 1992:2021–2037.

8 **Dixon HBF, Hargreaves WH.** Cysticercosis (*Taenia solium*): a further ten years' clinical study covering 284 cases. Q Med J 1944;13:107–121.

9 **Stepién L, Choróbski J.** Cysticercosis cerebri and its operative treatment. Arch Neurol Psychiatr 1949;61:499–527.

10 **Arana R, Asenjo A.** Ventriculographic diagnosis of cysticercosis of the posterior fossa. J Neurosurg 1945;2:181–190.

11 **Loo L, Braude A.** Cerebral cysticercosis in San Diego: a report of 23 cases and a review of the literature. Medicine (Baltimore) 1982;61:341–359.

12 **Acha PN, Aguilar F.** Studies on cysticercosis in Central America and Panama. Am J Trop Med Hyg 1964;13:48–53.

13 **Sotelo J, Guerrero V, Rubio F.** Neurocysticercosis: a new classification based on active and inactive forms. Arch Intern Med 1985;145:442–445.

14 **Gang-zhi W, Cun-jiang L, Jia-mei M, et al.** Cysticercosis of the central nervous system: a clinical study of 1400 cases. Chinese Med J 1988;101:493–500.

15 **Gajdusek C.** Introduction of *Taenia solium* into West New Guinea with a note on an epidemic of burns from cysticercus epilepsy in the Ekary people of the Wissel Lakes area. Papua New Guinea Med J 1978;21:329–342.

16 **Richards FO, Schantz PM, Ruiz-Tiben E, Sorvillo FJ.** Cysticercosis in Los Angeles county. JAMA 1985;254:3444–3448.

17 **Sotelo J.** Cysticercosis. In: Johnson RT, ed. Current therapy in neurologic disease. vol. 2. Philadelphia: Decker, 1987:114–117.

18 **Sotelo J, Del Brutto OH.** Therapy of neurocysticercosis. Child's Nerv Syst 1987; 3:208–211.

19 **Del Brutto OH.** Cysticercosis and cerebrovascular disease: a review. J Neurol Neurosurg Psychiatr 1992;55:252–254.

20 **Madrazo I, García JA, Sandoval M, López FJ.** Intraventricular cysticercosis. Neurosurgery 1983;12:148–152.

21 **Akiguchi I, Fujiwara T, Matsuyama H, et al.** Intramedullary spinal cysticercosis. Neurology 1979;29:1531–1534.

22 **Bloom BR.** Games parasites play: how parasites evade immune surveillance. Nature 1979;279:21–26.

23 **Correa D, Gorodezky C, Castro L, et al.** Detection of MHC products on the surface of *Taenia solium* cysticerci from humans. Rev Latiname Microbiol 1986;28:373–379.

24 **Del Brutto OH, Granados G, Talamás O, et al.** Genetic pattern of the HLA system: HLA, A, B, C, DR, and DQ antigens in Mexican patients with parenchymal brain cysticercosis. Human Biol 1991;63:85–93.

25 **Del Brutto OH, García E, Talamás O, Sotelo J.** Sex-related severity of inflammation in parenchymal brain cysticercosis. Arch Intern Med 1988;148:544–546.

26 **Del Brutto OH, Sotelo J.** Neurocysticercosis: an update. Rev Infect Dis 1988; 10:1075–1087.

27 **Sotelo J.** Cysticercosis. In: Vinken PJ, Bruyn GW, Klawans HL, eds. Handbook of clinical neurology. vol. 52. Amsterdam: Elsevier, 1988:529–534.

28 **McCormick GF, Zee CS, Heiden J.** Cysticercosis cerebri: a review of 127 cases. Arch Neurol 1982;39:540–544.

29 **Barry M, Kaldjian LC.** Neurocysticercosis. Semin Neurol 1993;13:131–143.

30 **Medina MT, Rosas E, Rubio F, Sotelo J.** Neurocysticercosis as the main cause of late-onset epilepsy in Mexico. Arch Intern Med 1990;150:323–325.

31 **Del Brutto OH, Noboa CA.** Late-onset epilepsy in Ecuador: aetiology and clinical features in 225 patients. J Trop Geogr Neurol 1991;1:31–34.

32 **Rangel R, Torres B, Del Brutto OH, Sotelo J.** Cysticercotic encephalitis: a severe form in young females. Am J Trop Med Hyg 1987;36:387–392.

33 **López-Hernández A, Garaizar C.** Childhood cerebral cysticercosis: clinical features and computed tomographic findings in 89 Mexican children. Can J Neurol Sci 1982;9:401–407.

34 **Lobato RD, Lamas E, Portillo JM, et al.** Hydrocephalus in cerebral cysticercosis: pathogenic and therapeutic considerations. J Neurosurg 1981;55:786–793.

35 **Sotelo J, Marín C.** Hydrocephalus secondary to cysticercotic arachnoiditis: a long-term follow-up review of 92 cases. J Neurosurg 1987;66:686–689.

36 **Ramina R, Hunhevicz SC.** Cerebral cysticercosis presenting as a mass lesion. Surg Neurol 1986;25:89–93.

37 **Barinagarrementería F, Del Brutto OH.** Lacunar syndrome due to neurocysticercosis. Arch Neurol 1989;46:415–417.

38 **Rodríguez J, Del Brutto OH, Penagos P, et al.** Occlusion of the middle cerebral artery due to cysticercotic angiitis. Stroke 1989;20: 1095–1099.

39 **TerPenning B, Litchman CD, Heier L.** Bilateral middle cerebral artery occlusions in neurocysticercosis. Stroke 1992;23:280–283.

40 **Monteiro L, Almeida-Pinto J, Leite J, et al.** Cerebral cysticercus arteritis: five angiographic cases. Cerebrovasc Dis 1994;4:125–133.

41 **McCormick GF, Giannotta S, Zee CS, Fisher M.** Carotid occlusion in cysticercosis. Neurology 1983;33:1078–1080.

42 **Keane JR.** Neuro-ophthalmologic signs and symptoms of cysticercosis. Arch Ophthalmol 1982;100:1445–1448.

43 **Del Brutto OH, Guevara J, Sotelo J.** Intrasellar cysticercosis. J Neurosurg 1988; 69:58–60.

44 **Zee CS, Segall HD, Apuzzo MLJ, et al.** Intraventricular cysticercal cysts: further neuroradiological observations and neurosurgical implications. AJNR 1984;5:727–730.

45 **Salazar A, Sotelo J, Martínez H, Escobedo F.** Differential diagnosis between ventriculitis and fourth ventricle cyst in neurocysticercosis. J Neurosurg 1983;59:660–663.

46 **Bickerstaff ER, Small JM, Woolf AL.** Cysticercosis of the posterior fossa. Brain 1956;79:622–634.

47 **Isidro-Llorens A, Dachs F, Vidal J, Sarrias M.** Spinal cysticercosis: case report and review. Paraplegia 1993;31:128–130.

48 Case records of the Massachusetts General Hospital. Case 26-1994. N Engl J Med 1994; 330:1887–1893.

49 **Kruger-Leite E, Jalkh AE, Quiroz H, Schepenz CL.** Intraocular cysticercosis. Am J Ophthalmol 1985;99:252–257.

50 **Sawnay BB, Chopra JS, Banerji AK, Wahi PL.** Pseudohypertrophic myopathy in cysticercosis. Neurology 1976;26:270–272.

51 **Nosanchuk JS, Agostini JC, Georgi M, Posso M.** Pork tapeworm of cysticerci involving peripheral nerve. JAMA 1980;244: 2191–2192.

52 **Mervis B, Lotz W.** Computed tomography (CT) in parenchymatous cerebral cysticercosis. Clin Radiol 1980;31:521–528.

53 **Rodríguez-Carbajal J, Salgado P, Gutiérrez R, et al.** The acute encephalitic phase of neurocysticercosis: computed tomographic manifestations. AJNR 1983;4: 51–55.

54 **Suss RA, Maravilla KR, Thompson J.** MR imaging of intracranial cysticercosis: comparison with CT and anatomopathologic features. AJNR 1986;7:235–242.

55 **Martínez HR, Rangel-Guerra R, Elizondo G.** MR imaging in neurocysticercosis: a study of 56 cases. AJNR 1989;10:1011–1019.

56 **García E, Sotelo J.** A new complement fixation test for the diagnosis of neurocysticercosis in cerebrospinal fluid. J Neurol 1991;238:379–382.

57 **Rosas N, Sotelo J, Nieto D.** ELISA in the diagnosis of neurocysticercosis. Arch Neurol 1986;43:353–356.

58 **Del Brutto OH.** Diagnosis and management of cysticercosis. J Trop Geogr Neurol 1992;2:1–9.

59 **Del Brutto OH.** Cysticercosis. In: Felamann E, ed. Current diagnosis in neurology. St Louis: Mosby, 1994:125–129.

60 **Sotelo J.** Neurocysticercosis. In: Roos KL, ed. Infections of the central nervous system. New York: Marcel Dekker (in press).

61 **Ramos-Kuri M, Montoya RM, Padilla A, et al.** Immunodiagnosis of neurocysticercosis. Disappointing performance of serology (enzyme-linked immunosorbent assay) in an unbiased sample of neurological patients. Arch Neurol 1992;49: 633–636.

62 **Coker-Van MR, Subianto DB, Brown P, et al.** ELISA antibodies to cysticerci of *Taenia solium* in human population in New Guinea, Oceania, and Southeast Asia. Southeast Asian J Trop Med Public Health 1981;12:499–505.

63 **Miller BL, Staugaitis SM, Tourtellotte WW, et al.** Intra-blood-brain-barrier IgG synthesis in cerebral cysticercosis. Arch Neurol 1985;42:782–784.

64 **Carbajal JR, Palacios E, Azar-Kia B, Churchill R.** Radiology of cysticercosis of the central nervous system including computed tomography. Radiology 1977;125: 127–131.

65 **Bentson JR, Wilson GH, Helmer E, Winter J.** Computed tomography in intracranial

cysticercosis. J Comput Assist Tomogr 1977;1:464–471.

66 **Del Brutto OH.** The use of albendazole in patients with single lesions enhanced on contrast CT. N Engl J Med 1993;328:356–357.

67 **Bandres JC, White C Jr, Samo T, et al.** Extraparenchymal neurocysticercosis: report of five cases and review of management. Clin Infect Dis 1992;15:799–811.

68 **Madrazo I, García JA, Paredes G, Olhagaray B.** Diagnosis of intraventricular and cisternal cysticercosis by computerized tomography with positive intraventricular contrast medium. J Neurosurg 1981;55: 947–951.

69 **Del Brutto OH, Zenteno MA, Salgado P, Sotelo J.** MR imaging in cysticercotic encephalitis. AJNR 1989;10:S18–S20.

70 **Oot RF, New PFJ, Pile-Spellman J, et al.** The detection of intracranial calcifications by MR. AJNR 1986;7:801–809.

71 **Ramos OM, Stiebel-Chin G, Altman N, Duchowny M.** Diagnosis of neurocysticercosis by magnetic resonance imaging. Pediatr Infect Dis 1986;5:470–475.

72 **Chang KH, Kim WS, Cho SY, et al.** Comparative evaluation of brain CT and ELISA in the diagnosis of neurocysticercosis. AJNR 1988;8:125–130.

73 **Tsang VCW, Brand J, Boyer AE.** Enzyme-linked immunoelectrotransferency blot assay and glicoprotein antigens for diagnosing human cysticercosis (taenia solium). J Infect Dis 1989;159:50–59.

74 **García HH, Gilman R, Martínez M, et al.** Cysticercosis as a major cause of epilepsy in Peru. Lancet 1993;341:197–200.

75 **Spina-Franca A, Livramento JA, Machado LR.** Cysticercosis of the central nervous system and cerebrospinal fluid. Immunodiagnosis of 1573 patients in 63 years (1929–1992). Arq Neuropsiquiatr 1993;51: 16–20.

76 **Del Brutto OH, Sotelo J, Román GC.** Therapy for neurocysticercosis: a reappraisal. Clin Infect Dis 1993;17:730–735.

77 **Del Brutto OH.** Medical management of neurocysticercosis. J Antimicrob Agents 1993;3:133–137.

78 **Del Brutto OH, Santibañez R, Noboa CA, et al.** Epilepsy due to neurocysticercosis: analysis of 203 patients. Neurology 1992; 42:389–392.

79 **Weniger BG, Schantz PM.** Praziquantel and refugee health. JAMA 1984;251:2391–2392.

80 **Robles C, Chavarría M.** Presentación de un caso de cisticercosis cerebral tratado médicamente con un nuevo fármaco, praziquantel. Sal Pub Mex 1979;21:603–618.

81 **Botero D, Castaño S.** Treatment of cysticercosis with praziquantel in Colombia. Am J Trop Med Hyg 1982;31:811–821.

82 **Spina-França A, Nobrega JPS, Livramento JA, Machado LR.** Administration of praziquantel in neurocysticercosis. Trop Med Parasitol 1982;33:1–4.

83 **Robles C, Serrano AM, Vargas-Tentori N, Galindo-Virgen S.** Long-term results of praziquantel therapy in neurocysticercosis. J Neurosurg 1986;66:359–363.

84 **Sotelo J, Escobedo F, Rodríguez J, et al.** Therapy of parenchymal brain cysticercosis with praziquantel. N Engl J Med 1984;310:1001–1007.

85 **Sotelo J, Torres B, Rubio F, et al.** Praziquantel in the treatment of neurocysticercosis: long-term follow-up. Neurology 1985;35:752–755.

86 **Escobedo F, Penagos P, Rodríguez J, Sotelo J.** Albendazole therapy for neurocysticercosis. Arch Intern Med 1987;147:738–741.

87 **Sotelo J, Escobedo F, Penagos P.** Albendazole versus praziquantel for therapy of neurocysticercosis: a controlled trial. Arch Neurol 1988;45:532–534.

88 **Saimot AG, Cremieux AC, Hay JM, et al.** Albendazole as a potential treatment for human hydatidosis. Lancet 1983;2:652–656.

89 **Rossignol JF.** Albendazol: estudios clínicos realizados en Francia y Africa Occidental. Informe sobre 1034 casos. Compendium de Investigaciones Clínicas Latinoamericanas 1981;(suppl 1):117–125.

90 **Sotelo J, Penagos P, Escobedo F, Del Brutto OH.** Short course of albendazole therapy for neurocysticercosis. Arch Neurol 1988;45:1130–1133.

91 **Sotelo J, Del Brutto OH, Penagos P, et al.** Comparison of therapeutic regimen of anticysticercal drugs for parenchymal brain cysticercosis. J Neurol 1990;237:69–72.

92 **Santoyo H, Corona R, Sotelo J.** Total recovery of visual function after treatment for cerebral cysticercosis. N Engl J Med 1991;324:1137–1139.

93 **Cruz M, Cruz I, Horon J.** Albendazole vs praziquantel in the treatment of cerebral cysticercus: Clinical evaluation. Trans Soc Trop Med Hyg 1991;85:244–247.

94 **Takayamagui OM, Jarsim E.** Therapy for neurocysticercosis: comparison between

albendazole and praziquantel. Arch Neurol 1992;49:290–294.

95 **Leopold GW, Ungethum W, Groll E.** Clinical pharmacology in normal volunteers of praziquantel, a new drug against schistosomes and cestodes: an example of a complex study covering both tolerance and pharmacokinetics. Eur J Clin Pharmacol 1978;14:281–291.

96 **Ciferri F.** Praziquantel for cysticercosis of the brain parenchyma. N Engl J Med 1984; 311:733.

97 **Vázquez ML, Jung H, Sotelo J.** Plasma levels of praziquantel decrease when dexamethasone is given simultaneously. Neurology 1987;37:1561–1562.

98 **Jung H, Hurtado M, Medina MT, et al.** Dexamethasone increases plasma levels of albendazole. J Neurol 1990;237:279–280.

99 **Miller B, Grinnell V, Goldberg MA, Heiner D.** Spontaneous radiographic disappearance of cerebral cysticercosis: three cases. Neurology 1983;33:1377–1379.

100 **Vázquez V, Sotelo J.** The course of seizures after treatment for cerebral cysticercosis. N Engl J Med 1992;327:696–701.

101 **Leblanc R, Knowles KF, Melanson D, et al.** Neurocysticercosis: surgical and medical treatment with praziquantel. J Neurosurg 1986;18:419–427.

102 **Sotelo J, Rubalcava MA, Gómez-Llata S.** A new shunt for hydrocephalus that relies on CSF production rather than on ventricular pressure. Initial clinical experiences. Surg Neurol 1995;43:324–332.

103 **Rubalcava MA, Sotelo J.** Differences between ventricular and lumbar CSF in hydrocephalus secondary to cysticercosis. Neurosurgery 1995;37.

104 **Colli BO, Martelli N, Assirati JA, et al.** Results of surgical treatment of neurocysticercosis in 69 cases. J Neurosurg 1986; 65:309–315.

105 **Del Brutto OH, Sotelo J.** Albendazole therapy for subarachnoid and ventricular cysticercosis. Case report. J Neurosurg 1990;72:816–817.

106 **Del Brutto OH, Sotelo J, Aguirre R, et al.** Albendazole therapy for giant subarachnoid cysticerci. Arch Neurol 1992;49:535–538.

107 **Allcut D, Couthard A.** Neurocysticercosis, regression of a fourth ventricular cyst with praziquantel. J Neurol Neurosurg Psychiatr 1991;54:461–462.

108 **Lozano-Elizondo D, Barbosa-Horta S.** Tratamiento con albendazol de la cisticercosis intraocular. Rev Mex Oftalmol 1990; 64:15–28.

109 **Sotelo J, Rosas N, Palencia G.** Freezing of infested pork muscle kills cysticerci. JAMA 1986;256:893–894.

Reactivation and Exogenous Reinfection: Their Relative Roles in the Pathogenesis of Tuberculosis

HANH QUOC LE
PAUL T. DAVIDSON

Endogenous reactivation versus exogenous reinfection in the pathogenesis of pulmonary tuberculosis have been debated for decades. Exogenous reinfection is thought to occur commonly in countries with a high prevalence of disease. In the United States where prevalence is low, the risk of being infected for a second or subsequent time is small, and most cases of pulmonary tuberculosis in adults appear to result from reactivation of healed primary infection. Exogenous reinfection appears to have a minimal role. This concept of pathogenesis has had a tremendous influence on tuberculosis control practice in the United States. Chemoprophylaxis (preventive therapy) is extensively recommended. The United States is probably the only country where chemoprophylaxis is given to infected individuals with a normal chest radiograph and no other risk factors. Tuberculosis control efforts in the United States also stress the detection and treatment of new cases, but considerable effort and resources are diverted to the prevention of reactivation.

A long period of declining rates of tuberculosis in the United States stopped in 1984, and the number of new cases actually increased through 1992 (1). This increase is partly attributed to the acquired immunodeficiency syndrome (AIDS) epidemic, but increases are found in other subpopulations, including the foreign-born, homeless, African American, and even certain white United States-born citizens. This is not explained by endogenous reactivation alone. Nearly 40% of tuberculosis cases investigated in San Francisco during 1991 to 1992 were the result of recent infection (2). Previously, evidence of reinfection required a pathologic demonstration. Now evidence for reinfection can be proven clinically by phage typing, drug susceptibility patterns, and DNA fingerprinting by restriction fragment length polymorphism (RFLP).

Reports of outbreaks due to reinfection in homeless and AIDS patients with multidrug-resistant bacilli suggest that the contribution of reinfection is no longer negligible (3,4).

The issue of exogenous reinfection versus endogenous reactivation is not only of academic interest. An understanding of the relative roles of each pathway will impact on tuberculosis control practice. If endogenous reactivation predominates, efforts should be directed toward chemoprophylaxis to prevent reactivation. If exogenous reinfection causes most cases of smear and culture positive pulmonary tuberculosis, the tuberculosis control objectives should be the prevention of transmission by early detection of infectious pulmonary tuberculosis cases and rendering them noninfectious with prompt and effective treatment.

This chapter briefly reviews the merits of both pathways. The main focus is on tuberculosis control practice when either one predominates or when both have a significant magnitude.

PATHOGENESIS OF PULMONARY TUBERCULOSIS—THE COMMON PATHWAY

Regardless of differences of opinion on the timing of genesis of a tuberculosis lesion in the lung, both the endogenous reactivation and exogenous reinfection concepts accept the first steps of the process.

Inhalation of the Infecting Particle

Apart from the rare situation when tuberculosis is transmitted by direct inoculation or through the gastrointestinal tract, the airborne route of transmission is widely accepted (5). The usual infecting dose contains one to three bacilli (6). The infecting particle must be less than 5 μm in size to reach the alveolus. Larger particles are stopped and rejected by a number of physical barriers in the airways.

Implantation of Infecting Bacilli

Tubercle bacilli are initially phagocytized by alveolar macrophages (AM) derived from circulating monocytes that are nonspecifically activated as they scavenge the alveolus surface ingesting organisms and other inhaled particles. These nonspecifically activated AM may be able to contain and kill the tubercle bacilli and prevent the implantation of a tuberculosis lesion. This containment depends on host genetic factors, the degree of nonspecific activation of AM, and the virulence of the bacilli. If the tubercle bacilli are not contained and killed, they grow intracellularly and eventually destroy the AM and burst out into the extracellular space where they are phagocytized again by other alveolar or bloodborne macrophages, and the cycle restarts. Bloodborne macrophages are attracted to the site by released mycobacterial antigens, cellular debris, and a variety of chemotactic factors. These newly arrived bloodborne macrophages are not activated, do not have bactericidal activity, and actually facilitate bacillary growth in their cytoplasm. The cytokines released by macrophages attract bloodborne T lymphocytes, which in turn activate the macrophage. It is at this point the tuberculous lesion is initiated and the *M. tuberculosis* organism is implanted (7,8).

Lymph Node Invasion and the Gohn Complex

The bacilli-ladden macrophages escape the local lesion and invade the satellite lymph node of drainage. The local parenchymal lesion and the satellite lymph node form the so-called Gohn complex characteristic of primary tuberculosis infection (8). The infected satellite lymph node may grow larger than the primary lesion. It is common to see large calcified lymph nodes with minimal calcification in the lung parenchyma on chest radiographs after primary infection.

During this time, two basic independent but interrelated phenomena develop. Cell-mediated immunity (CMI) appears, which is a beneficial host-response characterized by an expanded population of specific T lymphocytes. These cells, sensitized and stimulated by mycobacterial antigens presented by the macrophages, release lymphokines that activate macrophages and make them bactericidal. Delayed—type hypersensitivity (DTH) appears and has the same immunologic process as CMI involving T cells with their lymphokines and macrophages but is pathologic because it induces a local caseous necrosis or a remote cutaneous tuberculin reaction. Both CMI and DTH inhibit multiplication of tubercle bacilli. CMI does so by activating macrophages to kill the bacilli they have ingested and DTH does so by killing the bacilli-laden nonactivated macrophages and necrosing the nearby tissues, thereby creating an unfavorable environment for bacillary growth (7,8).

Hematogenous Dissemination

Tubercle bacilli in the lymph node may escape via the thoracic duct and the systemic venous system and be disseminated to other areas of the lung. Tubercle bacilli may also escape into the pulmonary venous system and directly into the aorta where they are disseminated to other organs.

The occurrence of extrapulmonary tuberculosis, particularly in organs that cannot be reached by direct inoculation (e.g., liver brain, bone, etc.) is direct proof of hematogenous dissemination. It may occur as a result of the progressive primary infection or with activation of an earlier infection (9). Evidence of hematogenous dissemination was found in only 9% of cases of calcified primary complex at autopsy. The disease was strictly limited to the parenchymal focus and the lymph nodes in the path of drainage in 91% of cases (10). Although AIDS patients with tuberculosis frequently have positive blood cultures for tubercle bacilli (11), tuberculosis bacillemia is exceedingly rare in immunocompetent individuals.

Persistence of Tubercle Bacilli in Pulmonary Lesions

Opie et al (12) reported that 20% of calcified lung nodules and 26% of mediastinal and pulmonary calcified lymph nodes (primary or childhood type lesions) and 24% of fibrous scars of the apex (reactivation or adult type lesions) contained living bacilli. Sweany et al (13) reported that 13% to 16% of occult or healed lesions were culture positive for tubercle bacilli. Canetti (14,15) and Saenz et al (16) included data from other authors with their own and reported that 18% of calcified pulmonary and lymph node lesions contained virulent bacilli. They concluded that most primary tuberculous lesions are rapidly sterilized.

Vulnerable Region of the Lung

Sweany et al (17) noted that the first observable parenchymal excavations of the lung are most likely located in the superior and posterior lung fields. Medlar (10) studied 1225 autopsies of individuals dying of other causes than tuberculosis. He found 105 calcified parenchymal lung foci from a single primary complex distributed uniformly in both lung fields. However, the distribution of 96 minimal lesions were apical-posterior, 55 without satellite lymph nodes and 41 with a primary lesion with lymph nodes. Medlar concluded that this distribution does not fit with either hematogenous or lymphohematogenous dissemination because 82% were unilateral. His data indicated that in adults, certain areas of the lung, particularly apical posterior segments, are especially sensitive to the development of tuberculosis. This concept is shared by many others (9,12,18–20).

Endogenous Reactivation Stead (21,22) proposed a unitary concept of endogenous reactivation based primarily on the following:

1 A hematogenous dissemination of tubercle bacilli during the process of primary infection occurs with seeding to the apex of the lungs and to other organs with a high oxygen content such as kidneys and the growing ends of long bones. This concept is not supported by the data as presented earlier that hematogenous spread was observed in only 9% of cases (10).

2 There is a persistence of living bacilli in healed lesions of the apex. This is supported by the fact that 24% of fibrous scars of the apex from autopsies of sudden and unexpected deaths contained living tubercle bacilli (12).

3 There is reactivation of apical foci in later years; this is supported by the clinical observation of such reactivation of old fibrous scars of the apex (23,24).

The strongest support for a unitary concept is a statistical one. Palmer et al (25) reported a higher rate of tuberculosis in Navy recruits who were tuberculin positive compared with those who were tuberculin negative, even though both groups had the same life style and no tuberculosis exposure. Heimbeck (26),

Madsen et al (27), and Daniels et al (28) reported that nursing or medical students who were tuberculin reactors were protected against tuberculosis when compared with tuberculin nonreactor colleagues. It is suggested that previous tuberculosis infection gives some protection in a heavy exposure situation (21).

Hyge (29) reported that tuberculin-positive school girls exposed to an infectious teacher developed tuberculosis sporadically during 12 years of follow-up. Tuberculin-negative school girls with the same exposure developed tuberculosis mostly during the 1 to 2 years postexposure.

Although Stead is not the first proponent of endogenous reactivation, he is undoubtly the most enthusiastic. From this and other statistical information, he draws these conclusions: in tuberculin negative subjects, clinical pulmonary tuberculosis develops proportionately to the degree of exposure; tuberculin reactors enjoy a distinct protection from development of clinical pulmonary tuberculosis when heavily exposed; and the development of clinical tuberculosis in tuberculin reactors does not appear to be influenced by further exposure.

Stead proposed the unitary concept and concluded that most cases of clinical pulmonary tuberculosis derive from the reactivation of latent foci engendered by a primary infection and dismissed the role of exogenous reactivation as negligible (21,22).

Styblo (30) supported the endogenous reactivation theory in older persons by reporting that in the Netherlands between 1973 and 1975, the estimated annual rate of infection of the population was 30 in 100,000 but that the tuberculosis disease incidence rate for those aged 65 to 74 and for those older than 75 years were 14 in 100,000 and 25 in 100,000, respectively. Such rates cannot be explained by recent infection alone. Thus, to a large extent he concluded they must be from endogenous reactivation.

Exogenous Reinfection Arguments in support of exogenous reinfection are based on two simple questions: 1) Because most persons have a primary infection at a younger age but transmission of tuberculosis still persists in the population, why would reinfection not occur? 2) Because immunity engendered by the primary infection is not complete, why would not some of these reinfections produce tuberculosis disease (14)? To answer these two basic questions, the early proponents of exogenous reinfection, mostly pathologists, assumed that 1) the maturity of a lesion is time dependent. In the lungs of the same person, an ossified scar is older than a calcified one, which itself is older than a caseous lesion. 2) The lesion of reinfection progresses without homologous lymph node involvement. Therefore, if there are two lesions in the lung, one with a lymph gland component and the other without, then the later is the reinfection lesion. Canetti (31) calculated that over 80% of calcified (ossified) lesions and 55% of calcific or chalky foci were sterile. In subjects who died of other causes than tuberculosis, 24% to 62% had reinfection foci. The older the subject, the larger the number of reinfection foci (14). In adults dying of pulmonary tuberculosis, Canetti found that 42% of cases under 30 years of age had postprimary tuberculosis due to exogenous reinfection. In those adults over 30 years of age, 60% had evidence of exogenous reinfection. Terplan (32) found evidence of exogenous reinfection in 44% of those dying under age 40 years and in 85% of those over 40 years old. These studies suggest that during the period of study (1940 to 1950), adults over 30 to 40 years of age had a high prevalence of postprimary tuberculosis due to exogenous reinfection (31).

New technics to identify infecting strains have helped to consolidate the concept of exogenous reinfection. Phage typing and susceptibility patterns have been used to differentiate tuberculosis strains during different episodes of pulmonary tuberculosis in the same patient (4,32,34). Phage typing has also been used to identify different strains from different sites of disease in the same patient (35,36). RFLP has been used to document reinfection in patients with both tuberculosis and AIDS. It has also helped to link cases with a source case (3).

Experimental airborne infections with tuberculosis support the reinfection concept. Guinea pigs preinfected with a low virulence tubercle bacilli strain can be reinfected when challenged by the airborne route even with a small number of infecting organisms. This reinfection can even disseminate to the spleen if the challenging organism is highly virulent (37). Recently reported statistical data also support the role of reinfection. Stead et al (38) reported that 80% of tuberculosis cases in the elderly of Arkansas occurred in persons living at home and 20% in nursing homes. Because only 5% of the elderly in Arkansas live in nursing homes, he calculated that the elderly in the nursing homes had a tuberculosis rate almost five times higher than those living at home. The Centers for Disease Control and Prevention (CDC) reported that in 1984 and 1985 the incidence rate of tuberculosis in the elderly living in nursing homes was 39.2 of 100,000 compared with 21.5 of 100,000 in elderly living at home (39). If one assumes that the elderly have the same infection rate, this difference can be explained only if many of the elderly living in nursing homes have recently been infected or reinfected with tuberculosis.

PATHOGENESIS OF TUBERCULOSIS IN HUMAN IMMUNODEFICIENCY VIRUS (HIV) INFECTED INDIVIDUALS

HIV is a terrible threat to human health. This new epidemic, however, provides a unique opportunity to observe the natural evolution of many infectious diseases, including tuberculosis in human beings with various degrees of immunodeficiency. This situation can otherwise be observed only in artificially bred and treated animals.

HIV specifically infects CD4 T cells upon which the immunologic defense against tuberculosis depends. HIV infection progressively depletes and causes the dysfunction of CD4 T cells. The release of lymphokines that stimulate the reproduction of T cells and activate macrophages is disturbed. Macrophages apparently become malfunctional from both a direct effect of HIV and by lack of T-cell lymphokine stimulation.

Tubercle bacilli engulfed by malfunctional macrophages continue to reproduce unchecked, leading to rapid and progressive primary tuberculosis. Thirty-seven percent of HIV-infected individuals who were close contacts to infectious tuberculosis patients developed tuberculosis disease within 5 months in one study (40).

Tuberculosis bacteremia is common in patients with AIDS (11,41). Disseminated and extrapulmonary tuberculosis frequently occur in AIDS patients (42,43,44). In Los Angeles county, 32% of HIV/AIDS patients with tuberculosis have extrapulmonary sites versus 18% of total cases (43). HIV-infected individuals who are previously infected with tuberculosis reactivate at an estimated rate of 8% to 10% per year (45–47).

Patients with confirmed AIDS are at higher risk than HIV-infected individuals without AIDS to exhibit tuberculosis due to recent infection. This probably reflects the greater immunosuppression of the former group (2). Because of the rapid progression to infectious pulmonary tuberculosis, tubercle bacilli can be rapidly isolated and strains can be identified with RFLP and susceptibility patterns facilitating the establishment of a link with a source case. This permits documentation of exogenous reinfection in AIDS patients already infected with a previous episode of tuberculosis (3,48). This rapid progression is frequently lethal when HIV/AIDS patients are infected with multidrug-resistant tubercle bacilli (MDR) (49). Effective treatment requires knowledge of the drug susceptibility test results that may take many weeks to complete.

The patterns of tuberculosis in AIDS patients once diagnosed are similar to that of non-AIDS patients in terms of rate of positive sputum smear, rate of positive sputum cultures, and the rate of drug resistance (50). The marked increase of drug resistant tuberculosis in AIDS patients observed in New York City probably reflects a cluster effect (3,48).

THREE PATHOGENIC PATHWAYS OF TUBERCULOSIS

Progressive primary tuberculosis after a first infection, reactivation of an old healed infection, and exogenous reinfection are three accepted pathogenic pathways for developing clinical pulmonary tuberculosis. What is the contribution of each of them to the tuberculosis prevalence in a given population?

The definition of progressive primary tuberculosis needs to be clarification. During what period of time after the estimated first contact with the tubercle bacillus and the development of disease should the process be called progressive primary? Is there a continuum during this period of time? The clinical definition is facilitated when the moment of contact can be pinpointed or closely estimated and clinical observation has been continued from the time of tuberculin skin test conversion and the first radiologic evidence of a primary complex to an overt progressive disease such as tuberculosis pnuenomia, pleural effusion, or miliary tuberculosis. An epidemiologic definition is likely to be more arbitrary. It has been proposed that for epidemiologic purposes, clinical pulmonary tuberculosis occurring within 5 years of the estimated first contact, by definition, is progressive primary tuberculosis. This is an acceptable definition because it has been estimated that 80% of cases of clinical tuberculosis will develop during 10 years of observation starting within 2 years of the estimated date of infection. Nearly all occur within 5 years (30). Chiba (51) reported similar results during 30 years of observation of tuberculosis convertors.

In 1967 the United States Public Health Services (USPHS) conducted an isoniazid (INH) chemoprophylaxis trial for household contacts. After the first year, the rate of clinical tuberculosis in the group that received INH was 1.4 in 1000 and the rate in the placebo group was 6.2 in 1000. During 8 years of follow-up, the difference narrowed to 0.2 for the INH group and 0.8 for the placebo group. The rate of 1.4 in 1000 in the INH group remained stable until the eighth year of observation. These data suggest that INH given to household contacts mostly cures the inapparent progressive primary tuberculosis (52).

A clinical differentiation between endogenous reactivation and exogenous reinfection in tuberculosis cases is impossible unless the source of infection is recognized, the history of a previous episode of tuberculosis infection is documented, and the tubercle bacillus strains can be identified (3,4).

The contribution of each of the three pathways to the pool of tuberculosis cases is difficult to assess clinically. Sutherland and associates (53) designed a mathematical model linking the risk of annual infection with the rate of tuberculosis in different age groups (15 to 69 years of age), both sexes, and by calendar years in the Netherlands. Their results are particularly interesting. In the early 1950s when the annual risk of infection was high, the majority of cases in older persons appeared to be exogenous in origin. By 1970, with the decrease in the risk of infection, the exogenous contribution had decreased markedly but remained substantial (15%), particularly in males. Table 13.1 is a simplification

Table 13.1. Percentage of Progressive Primary Tuberculosis, Exogenous Reinfection, and Endogenous Reactivation Contributing to Tuberculosis Incidence

Age Group (yr)	*Progressive Primary Tuberculosis*[a] *1951/1970*	*Exogenous Reinfection*[b] *1951/1970*	*Endogenous Reactivation*[c] *1951/1970*
15–19	86/95	10/1	4/4
35–39	36/48	46/8	18/44
65–69	0.3/2	72/15	28/83

[a] Pulmonary tuberculosis within 5 years of estimated primary infection.
[b] Distant tuberculosis infection plus recent infection (within 5 years of estimated recent infection).
[c] Distant tuberculosis more than 5 years from estimated infection.
SOURCE: Sutherland I, Svandova E, Radhakrishna S. The development of clinical tuberculosis following infection with tubercle bacilli. Tubercle 1982;63:255–268.

of information from this study to illustrate the contribution of the three pathways.

The risk of developing all forms of pulmonary tuberculosis is high with the progression of primary infection (Table 13.2). It may be as high as 5% per year for a 5-year period. This is much higher than the currently used estimates of 10% lifetime risk but fits well with the actual rate noted during clinical follow-up by Chiba (51). There is also an apparent high risk of infectious tuberculosis with recent infection, including progressive primary and exogenous reinfection (4,8) (Table 13.3).

It must be emphasized that Sutherland et al's elegant mathematical model is based on the annual risk of infection in a very stable population with an almost uniform living standard. Immigrants were eliminated from the calculations. The results are estimates and should be regarded as indicating an order of magnitude rather than precise numerical values.

This mathematical model suggests conclusions that could influence future tuberculosis control practice. The contribution of exogenous reinfection is substantial even when there is a low annual risk of infection. Progressive primary tuberculosis in adolescents is often infectious. It is estimated that 25% of newly developed tuberculosis resulting from a primary infection acquired after age 15 years is smear positive (30). With a case rate of 1.4% annually and with 86% to 95% of the cases in the age group 15 to 19 years having progressive primary tuberculosis, the potential contribution of a large number of infectious pulmo-

Table 13.2. Estimates of the Risk of Development of All Forms of Clinical Pulmonary Tuberculosis According to History of Infection for Males and Females in the Netherlands from 1950 to 1970

Class of Clinical Pulmonary Tuberculosis	*Risk of Development of Tuberculosis (% per year)*	
	Males	*Females*
Progressive primary[a]	5.06	5.85
Exogenous reinfection[b]	1.91	1.10
Endogenous reactivation[c]	0.0253	0.0020

[a] Within 5 years of estimated primary infection.
[b] From distant primary infection plus recent reinfection (within 5 years).
[c] Distant primary infection (more than 5 years from estimated primary infection) and no recent infection.
SOURCE: Sutherland I, Svandova E, Radhakrishna S. The development of clinical tuberculosis following infection with tubercle bacilli. Tubercle 1982;63:255–268.

Table 13.3. Estimates of Risk of Development of Infectious Pulmonary Tuberculosis According to History of Infection for Males and Females in Netherlands from 1950 to 1970

Class of Clinical Pulmonary Tuberculosis	*Risk of Development of Infectious Pulmonary Tuberculosis (% per year)*	
	Males	*Females*
Progressive primary[a]	1.39	1.33
Exogenous reinfection[b]	1.18	0.45
Endogenous reactivation[c]	0.0161	0.0029

[a] Within 5 years of estimated primary infection.
[b] From distant primary infection plus recent reinfection (within 5 years).
[c] Distant primary infection (more than 5 years from estimates of primary infection) and no recent infection.
SOURCE: Sutherland I, Svandova E, Radhakrishna S. The development of clinical tuberculosis following infection with tubercle bacilli. Tubercle 1982;63:255–268.

nary tuberculosis cases is evident. Recent infection, including progressive primary tuberculosis and exogenous reinfection, produce a large number of infectious tuberculosis cases. Primary infection may not provide protection against active tuberculosis arising from a recent infection.

EPIDEMIOLOGIC INDICES FOR THE UNITED STATES

The World Health Organization advocates using the annual risk of tuberculosis infection as an epidemiologic index. This index indicates the proportion of the population that will be infected or reinfected with tubercle bacilli during a period of 1 year. It is derived from the result of tuberculosis skin testing. The accuracy of the annual risk depends on the significance of the tuberculin skin test and how well it can differentiate between atypical mycobacterial infection and true tuberculosis infection. It also depends on the stability of the population.

The United States has a high prevalence of atypical mycobacterial infection and a very mobile and complex population. Seventy percent of new cases of tuberculosis in the United States are from racial and ethnic minorities (54). This is particularly true in urban areas where most of the cases of tuberculosis are reported.

Even with data from an ongoing annual skin testing program for first-time school entrants from grades K to 12 Los Angeles County, a workable annual risk of infection cannot be calculated because of the diversity of the population. This is generally true of the United States as a whole. Consequently, the index used in the United States is the notification of new cases. This index depends largely on the quality and extent of case finding methods.

Sputum smear positivity is also used as a rough index of risk of infection. Even though the imperfections are similar to that of case finding, it remains a good index of potential tuberculosis transmission in the community. A decrease in the number of smear-positive cases should occur if cases are detected earlier by intensified contact investigations, particularly of smear-positive cases. Styblo (30) estimates that there are 10 infected individuals as a result of one unknown smear positive case during a 1-year period.

Application of these two indices in Los Angeles County reflects the kind of information that results in the United States. For the most part, case finding is passive. The patient presents to the health care system when symptomatic. Transmission of infection to others has frequently already occurred. The number of new cases reported each year was not declining in Los Angeles County but fluctuated around an average of 1400 new cases for many years. In 1989, an increasing trend in number of new cases began and peaked at 2198 in 1992. Subsequently, there has been a 2-year downward trend reaching 1796 cases in 1994. Presumably, the risk of infection in the population was increasing during the upward trend but is now declining. This cannot be directly documented, however. There is no data to substantiate how much disease was due to recent infection and how much was due to reactivation. There is also no data regarding how aggressively or accurately cases were found and reported. Notification of new cases obviously has considerable limitation but does reflect in general terms whether tuberculosis control is better or worse.

The characteristics of positive sputum smear cases also shows variability that may confound the ability to calculate an accurate risk of infection. In Los Angeles County for 1994, HIV-positive tuberculosis patients were more often smear positive than HIV-negative patients (63% versus 44%). This is different than previously published data that showed no significant difference and remains unexplained (44,50,55,56). There were less smear-positive cases among Hispanics and Asians in Los Angeles County in 1994 than whites and blacks (Hispanic 48%, Asian 35%, white 50%, blacks 55%). Case finding among Hispanics and Asians may be more aggressive because these two groups are mostly foreign-born and constitute more than 80% of the tuberculosis cases in this jurisdiction. Whites and blacks are U.S.-born and case finding may be less aggressive. Tuberculosis may be more likely diagnosed later in whites and blacks and is therefore more likely to be symptomatic and smear positive. The fact that the overall smear-positive rate is around 50% suggests that considerable tuberculosis transmission has occurred by the time of diagnosis, indicating a significant risk of infection in certain subpopulations. A decline or increase in the number of smear positive cases is a rough index that tuberculosis control is better or worse.

REFOCUSING TUBERCULOSIS CONTROL

A major objective of tuberculosis control programs for years has been to stop transmission of tuberculosis within the community. Since 1989, the USPHS has had the objective of eliminating tuberculosis from the United States (57). Whatever the objective, the strategy is to first find tuberculous patients, give them treatment, render them noninfectious, and prevent them from relapsing. A second strategy is to detect individuals with tuberculosis infection and give them isoniazid chemoprophylaxis to prevent them from developing clinical tuberculosis.

These relatively straightforward objectives and strategies are enormously difficult to achieve. The tuberculosis incidence in the United States steadily declined for decades until 1984. Because of the decline in incidence and the apparent prevalence of endogenous reactivation, considerable tuberculosis control efforts since the 1960s have been placed on preventing reactivation. There is now increasing evidence that a larger percentage of tuberculosis in the United States is due to recent infection. Estimates of up to 40% or greater in some populations have been made (2,58). Maintaining programs to prevent reactivation of tuberculosis is important. It is also essential, however, that tuberculosis control efforts in the United States focus more effectively on identifying population groups where the risk for transmission and infection with tuberculosis is increased. This is done by intensifying case finding and improving case holding.

Identifying Populations at Increased Risk for Transmission of Tuberculosis

Academic debates on exogenous or endogenous origin of pulmonary tuberculosis aside, most U.S. tuberculosis control officials agree that the populations at higher risk of tuberculosis transmission and infection can be identified. They include the poor and homeless; the foreign-born; African Americans; residents of facilities for long-term care, including correctional institutions, nursing homes, and mental institutions; HIV infected; and migrant agricultural workers (57).

Intensification of Case Finding Effective and proactive case finding in the United States is generally a failure. A significant percentage of tuberculosis cases in the United States as well as elsewhere are diagnosed after death (59,60). A good tuberculosis control program was able to find only 10% of the cases connected by a cluster of infection during contact investigation (2). Passive case finding, that is, waiting for the patient to seek medical care when symptomatic for tuberculosis, is not good public health practice. Unfortunately, various strategies for case finding have had mixed results. Active case finding focusing on symptomatic patients was not effective in a developing country (61,62). Using the tuberculin skin test for case finding is also ineffective because of the low yield and poor return for reading.

Radiography screening, which was discontinued on the grounds of inefficiency, should be reconsidered at least for populations at high risk (63). Chest radiography should be included upon admission to long-term care facilities such as nursing homes, AIDS hospices, mental institutions, and jails or prison in areas of the United States where tuberculosis is more common. In Los Angeles County, chest radiography screening with a 70-mm minifilm has been incorporated into the County Jail incarceration procedure. Two to 300 cases of pulmonary tuberculosis are identified each year by this process. Recently, Los Angeles County has done a chest radiography screening in selected shelters for the homeless. The preliminary result is that 437 tuberculosis-related abnormal films have been identified from 8500 chest x-rays done. Thirty-three new cases of tuberculosis have been found and 208 are pending suspects, many of whom are likely to be old disease. Simultaneous skin testing, sputum examination, and chest radiography screening have been used effectively in the homeless shelters of Boston (64). In most settings, contact investigation appears to be the most cost effective case-finding tool (62,65). It requires skilled well-trained investigators, however.

Improving Case Holding An effective treatment program includes a good drug regimen and strategies that promote the completion of the prescribed course of medication. Directly observed therapy (DOT) must be available and used when medication noncompliance is likely. It should include field delivery of medicine to home or workplace by public health workers. Incentives can be helpful in holding the patient on therapy.

Housing and food vouchers as incentives for DOT are very effective in holding homeless tuberculosis patients. When outreach workers alone were used to follow-up homeless patients in Los Angeles County, the treatment completion rate was about 75% or less. When housing and food vouchers are added, the completion rate reaches 95% or better. Housing for the homeless during treatment of tuberculosis should be considered part of the treatment regimen and not a social service. Hospitalization or incarceration are costly but effective ways to hold certain tuberculosis patients who remain contagious, cannot participate or cooperate with outpatient care, or are too sick for a different level of care. This is a necessary backup and must be available if tuberculosis is ever to be eliminated.

CONCLUSIONS

Stopping the transmission of tuberculosis is a paramount objective of tuberculosis control and eventual eradication. It is incumbent upon public health officials to constantly assess the epidemiologic factors influencing the course of tuberculosis in a particular environment of people. The role of exogenous reinfection and recent infection, particularly in adults, must be revisited.

Strengthening programs to identify infectious cases early and broaden contact investigations should take precedence over preventive treatment of persons with old infection in certain populations. New epidemiologic studies must continue to reassess the factors that lead to tuberculosis transmission and control the pathogenesis of this complex and persistent infectious disease.

The changing tuberculosis incidence rate beginning in 1984 in the United States was initially attributed to the AIDS epidemic. However, an increasing rate had been noted in New York City beginning in 1979 before AIDS had been identified. Dismantling of the tuberculosis control program due to budget cuts, socioeconomic decline, and the HIV epidemic all contributed to the resurgence of tuberculosis in New York City (66). A similar phenomenon has been noted in Europe, Asia, and Africa (55,67). It could be that the success of tuberculosis control efforts in the past has been a significant contributing cause to the present failure. Euphoria over the effectiveness of chemotherapy stimulated the scientific and public health communities to support transferring the management of tuberculosis into the mainstream of medicine. As a consequence, the management of tuberculosis was often placed in primary care settings. Active case finding has been reduced to a minimum, and tuberculosis infection has been allowed to progress to active smear-positive disease before patients reach medical care. Contact investigations have been restricted with few or no contacts identified for each case. Follow-up is shortened. Treatment completion rates have dropped, and more relapses with smear-positive disease and drug resistance have occurred.

Because of concern with the tuberculosis problem in the United States and elsewhere, the scientific and public health communities have reacted, and federal and state governments have begun to provide more money to control tuberculosis. Some tuberculosis services have been restored. Tuberculosis patient treatment and follow-up is improving with DOT and the use of incentives to improve compliance. Treatment completion rates are improving. National centers for tuberculosis have been funded to restore tuberculosis training and education that have been long neglected. Tuberculosis has started to decline again in the United States. There may be a second wave of danger, however, for tuberculosis control as health care reform embraces managed care and cost containment. Managed care systems are unlikely to pay for surveillance, case finding, DOT, or housing and other incentives. If public health programs and officials are not given the necessary continuing resources for tuberculosis control and management, there is great risk of another tuberculosis crisis, and the goal of tuberculosis elimination will again become remote.

ACKNOWLEDGEMENT

We thank Bonnie S. Cooley for help in preparation of the manuscript.

REFERENCES

1 **Centers for Disease Control and Prevention**. 1992 Tuberculosis statistics in the United States. U.S. Department of Health and Human Services Public Health Service. July 1994.

2 **Small PM, Hopewell PC, Singh SP, et al.** The epidemiology of tuberculosis in San Francisco. N Eng J Med 1994;330:1703–1709.

3 **Small PM, Shafer RW, Hopewell PC.** Exogenous reinfection with multidrug-resistant *Mycobacterium tuberculosis* in patients with advanced HIV infection. N Eng J Med 1993:328:1137–1144.

4 **Nardell E, McInnis B, Thomas B, Weidhass S.** Exogenous reinfection with tuberculosis in a shelter for the homeless. N Eng J Med 1986;315:1570–1575.

5 **Riley RL.** Transmission and environmental control of tuberculosis. In: Reichman LB, Hershfield ES, eds. Tuberculosis, a comprehensive international approach. Lung biology in health and disease. vol. 66. New York: Marcel Decker, 1993:123–135.

6 **Ratcliffe, HL.** Tuberculosis induced by droplet nuclei infection: pulmonary tuberculosis of predetermined initial intensity in mammals. Am J Hyg 1952;55:36–48.

7 **Dannenberg AR Jr.** Pathogenesis and immunology: basic aspects. In: Schossberg D ed. Tuberculosis. New York: Springer-Verlag, 1994:17–39.

8 **Nardell EA.** Pathogenesis of tuberculosis. In Reichman LB, Hershfield ES, ed. Tuberculosis, a comprehensive international approach. Lung biology in health and disease. vol. 66, New York: Marcel Decker, 1993:123–135.

9 **Rich A.** The pathogenesis of tuberculosis. Springfield Illinois: Charles C. Thomas, 1951.

10 **Medlar EM.** The pathogenesis of minimal pulmonary tuberculosis: a study of 1225 necropsies in cases of sudden and unexpected death. Am Rev Tuber 1948;58:583–611.

11 **Shafer RW, Goldberg R, Sierra M, Glatt AE.** Frequency of *Mycobacterium tuberculosis* bacteremia in patients with tuberculosis in an area endemic for AIDS. Am Rev Respir Dis 1989;140:1611–1613.

12 **Opie EL, Aronson, JD.** Tubercle bacilli in latent tuberculous lesions and in lung tissue without tuberculous lesions. Arch Pathol Lab Med 1927;4:1–21.

13 **Sweany HC, Levinson SA, Stadnichenko, AMS.** Tuberculous infection in people dying of causes other than tuberculosis. Am Rev Tuber 1953;48:131.

14 **Canetti G.** Exogenous reinfection and pulmonary tuberculosis a study of the pathology. Tubercle 1950;31:224–233.

15 **Canetti G.** Primo-infection et reinfection dans la tuberculose pulmonaire. Collection de l' Institut Pasteur. Editions Medicales Flammarion, Paris-6e, 1954.

16 **Saenz A, Canetti G.** Recherches sur le sort du bacille de Koch chez les sujets cliniquement non tuberculeux. Ann Inst Pasteur 1939;62:4.

17 **Sweany HC, Cook CE, Kegerreis R.** A study of the position of primary cavities in pulmonary tuberculosis. Am Rev Tuber 1931;24:558–582.

18 **Medlar EM.** The behavior of pulmonary tuberculous lesions. Medlar monograph. Am Rev Tuber Pulm Dis 1955.

19 **Smith DT, Abernathy RS, Smith GB, Jr, Bondurant S.** The apical location of reinfection pulmonary tuberculosis. Am Rev Tuber 1954;70:547–556.

20 **Balasubramanian V, Wiegeshaus EH, Taylor BT, Smith DW.** Pathogenesis of tuberculosis: pathway to apical localization. Tubercle Lung Dis 1994;75:168–178.

21 **Stead WW.** Pathogenesis of a first episode of chronic pulmonary tuberculosis in man: recrudescence of residuals of the primary infection or exogenous reinfection? Am Rev Respir Dis 1967;95:729–745.

22 **Stead WW.** The unitary concept of tuberculosis in man. Bull Int Union Tuberc Lung Dis 1974;49:318–322.

23 **Rasmussen KN.** The apical localization of pulmonary tuberculosis. Acta Tuberc Scand 1957;34:245.

24 **Stead WW.** The pathogenesis of pulmonary tuberculosis among older persons. Am Rev Respir Dis 1965;91:811.

25 **Palmer CE, Jablon S, Edward PQ.** Tuberculosis morbidity of young men in relation to tuberculin sensitivity and body build. Am Rev Tuber 1957;76:517.

26 **Heimbeck J.** Incidence of tuberculosis in young adult women with special reference to employment. Br J Tuberc 1938;32:154.

27 **Madsen T, Holm J, Jensen KA.** Study on the epidemiology of tuberculosis in Denmark. Acta Tuberc Scand 1942;(suppl 6).

28 **Daniels M, Ridehaligh F, Springett VH, Hall IM.** Tuberculosis in young adult: report on the prophit tuberculosis survey, 1935–1944. London: H.K. Lewis, 1948.

29 **Hyge TV.** The efficacy of BCG vaccination: epidemic of tuberculosis in a state school with an observation of 12 years. Acta Tuber Scand 1957;32:89.

30 **Styblo K.** Epidemiology of tuberculosis. Bull Int Union Tuber 1978;53:141.

31 **Canetti G.** Endogenous reactivation and exogenous reinfection: their relative importance with regard to the development of non-primary tuberculosis. Bull Int Union Tuber 1972;47:116–122.

32 **Terplan K.** Pathogenesis of post-primary tuberculosis, in relation to chronic pulmonary tuberculosis (Phtisis). Adv Tuber Res 1951;4:186–219.

33 **Mankiewicz E, Liivak M.** Phage types of *Mycobacterium tuberculosis* in cultures isolated from Eskimo patients. Am Rev Respir Dis 1975;111:307–312.

34 **Raleigh JW, Wichelhausen RH, Rado TA, Bates J.** Evidence for infection by two distinct strains of *Mycobacterium tuberculosis* in pulmonary tuberculosis: report of 9 Cases. Am Rev Respir Dis 1975;112:497–503.

35 **Bates JH, Stead WW, Rado TA.** Phage type of tubercle bacilli isolated from patients with two or more sites of organ involvement. Am Rev Respir Dis 1976;114:353–358.

36 **Raleigh JW, Wichelhaussen R.** Exogenous reinfection with *Mycobacterium tuberculosis* confirmed by phage typing. Am Rev Respir Dis 1973;108:639–642.

37 **Ziegler JE, Edwards ML, Smith DW.** Exogenous reinfection in experimental airborne tuberculosis. Tubercle 1985;66:121–128.

38 **Stead WW, To T.** The significance of tuberculin skin test in elderly persons. Ann Intern Med 1987;107:837–842.

39 **Center for Disease Control.** Prevention and control of tuberculosis in facilities providing long-term care to the elderly: recommendation of the Advisory Committee for Elimination of Tuberculosis (ACET). MMWR 1990;39:7–20.

40 **Daley CL, Small PM, Schecter GF, et al.** An outbreak of tuberculosis with accelerated progression among persons infected with the human immunodeficiency virus. N Engl J Med 1992;326:231–235.

41 **Barnes P.** Six cases of *Mycobacterium tuberculosis* bacteremia. J Infect Dis 1987;156:377–378.

42 **Hill AR, Premkumar S, Brustein S, Vaidya K, et al.** Disseminated tuberculosis in the acquired immunodeficiency syndrome era. Am Rev Respir Dis 1991;144:1164–1170.

43 **Barnes PF, Le HQ, Davidson PT.** Tuberculosis in patients with HIV infection. Med Clin North Am 1993;77:1369–1390.

44 **Chaisson RE, Schecter GF, Theuer CP, et al.** Tuberculosis in patients with the acquired immunodeficiency syndrome. Am Rev Respir Dis 1967;136:570–574.

45 **Narain JP, Raviglione MC, Kochi A.** HIV-associated tuberculosis in developing countries: epidemiology and strategies for prevention. Tubercle Lung Dis 1992;73:311–321.

46 **Selwyn PA, Sckell BM, Alcabes P, et al.** High risk of active tuberculosis in HIV-infected drug users with cutaneous anergy. JAMA 1992;268:504–509.

47 **Moreno S, Baraia-Etxabura J, Bouza E, et al.** Risk for developing tuberculosis among anergic patients infected with HIV. Ann Intern Med 1993;119:194–198.

48 **Edlin BR, Tokars JI, Grieco MH, et al.** An outbreak of multidrug-resistant tuberculosis among hospitalized patients with the acquired immunodeficiency syndrome. N Engl J Med 1992;326:1514–1521.

49 **Centers for Disease Control.** Nosocomial transmission of multidrug resistant tuberculosis among HIV infected patients. MMWR 1991;40:585–591.

50 **Githui W, Nunn P, Juma E, et al.** Cohort study of HIV-positive and HIV-negative tuberculosis, Nairobi, Kenya: comparison of bacteriological results. Tuberc Lung Dis 1992;73:203–209.

51 **Chiba Y.** Significance of endogenous reactivation, 30 year follow-up of tuberculin positive converters. Bull Int Union Tuberc 1974;49:321–325.

52 **Ferebee SH.** Controlled chemoprophylaxis trials in tuberculosis, a general review. Adv Tuberc Res 1970;17:28–106.

53 **Sutherland I, Svandova E, Radhakrishna, S.** The development of clinical tuberculosis following infection with tubercle bacilli. Tubercle 1982;63:255–268.

54 **Raviglione MC, Snider DE, Kochi A.** Global epidemiology of tuberculosis: morbidity and mortality of a worldwide epidemic. JAMA 1995;273:220–226.

55 **Pitchenik AE, Cole C, Russell BW, et al.** Tuberculosis, atypical mycobacteriosis and the acquired immunodeficiency syndrome among Haitian and non-Haitian patients in

South Florida. Am Intern Med 1984;101:641–645.

56 **Theuer CP, Hopewell PC, Elias D, et al.** Human immunodeficiency virus infection in tuberculosis patients. J Infect Dis 1990;162:8–12.

57 **Centers for Disease Control.** A strategic plan for the elimination of tuberculosis in the United States. MMWR 1989;38(suppl.): 1–25.

58 **Alland D, Kalkut GE, Moss AR, et al.** Transmission of tuberculosis in New York City. N Engl J Med 1994;330:1710–1716.

59 **Rieder HL, Kelly GD, Bloch AB, et al.** Tuberculosis diagnosed at death in the United States. Chest 1991;100:678–681.

60 **Szopinski J, Remiszewski P, Szymanska D, Rowinska-Zakrzewska E.** Tuberculosis found in autopsies done in the institute of tuberculosis and lung disease 1972–1991. Pneumonol Pol 1993;61:275–279.

61 **Nsanzumuhire H, Aluoch JH, Karuga WK, et al.** A study of the use of community leaders in case finding for pulmonary tuberculosis. Tubercle 1977;58:117–128.

62 **Aluoch JA, Karuga WK, Nsanzumuhirre H, et al.** A second study of the use of community leaders in case finding for pulmonary tuberculosis in Kenya. Tubercle 1978;59: 233–243.

63 **Davidson PT.** Tuberculosis control. In: Tierney DF, ed. Current pulmonology. vol. 15. Mosby Yearbook, 1994:309–339.

64 **Barry MA, Wall C, Shirley L, et al.** Tuberculosis screening in Boston's homeless shelters. Public Health Rep 1986;101:487–494.

65 **Rieder HL, Cauthen GM, Comstock GW, Snider DE, Jr.** Epidemiology of tuberculosis in the United States. Epidemiol Rev 1989;11:89–95.

66 **Brudney K, Dobkin J.** Resurgent tuberculosis in New York City. Am Rev Respir Dis 1994;144:745–749.

67 **Rieder HL.** Misbehaviour of a dying epidemic: a call for less speculation and better surveillance. Tuberc Lung Dis 1992;73:181–183.

Diagnosis and Management of Invasive Aspergillosis

DAVID W. DENNING

Aspergillus was first recognized as an organism by Micheli in 1729. The first description of disease due to *Aspergillus* was in the air sacs and lungs of a jackdaw in 1815, and the first human case of aspergillosis was described in 1842 in Edinburgh, Scotland (1). This was almost certainly an example of an aspergilloma in a tuberculous cavity. Various superficial forms of aspergillosis were described in the late 1800s, and from 1890 to 1897 *Aspergillus* tracheobroncitis, renal aspergillosis, and both maxillary and sphenoid sinus aspergillosis were described. The first case of invasive pulmonary aspergillosis as an opportunistic infection was described in a patient with aplastic anemia in Britain in 1953 (2). Attempts to treat invasive aspergillosis began with amphotericin B in 1959. The first comprehensive description of the pathology of invasive aspergillosis was published in 1970 from the National Institutes of Health (3). The first multicentre trial of therapy for invasive aspergillosis was commenced in 1989 and published in 1994 by the NIAID Mycoses Study Group (4).

There are a number of different diseases produced by *Aspergillus* and these can be classified as shown in Table 14.1. The incidence of invasive aspergillosis is rising, whereas that of aspergilloma is falling in the developed world. *Aspergillus* is regarded as an opportunistic pathogen. However, there are many reports on record of invasive aspergillosis in nonimmunocompromised patients, and it is a primary pathogen of a large number of different mammals and birds and the honey bee. Thus, it is a rare primary pathogen and an increasingly common opportunistic pathogen in humans.

Aspergillus fumigatus causes approximately 85% of all forms of aspergillosis, followed by *Aspergillus flavus* (5% to 10%), *Aspergillus niger* (2% to 3%), and *Aspergillus terreus* (2% to 3%). Certain forms of aspergillosis are more common due to particular species, for example otitis externa due to *A. niger*, sinusitis due to *A. flavus*, and joint disease due to *A. glaucus*. Many other rare species of *Aspergillus* have caused disease.

Table 14.1. Classification of *Aspergillus* Infection

- I. Disease in the normal host
  - A. Allergic diseases
    1. Allergic bronchopulmonary aspergillosis
    2. Allergic *Aspergillus* sinusitis
  - B. Superficial infection
    1. Otomycosis, onychomycosis
  - C. Invasive infection
    1. Pulmonary aspergillosis, invasive sinusitis
- II. Saprophytic disease
  - A. Aspergilloma
  - B. *Aspergillus* sinusitis
- III. Infection associated with tissue damage, surgery, or foreign body
  - A. Superficial infection, e.g. keratitis and/or endophthalmitis
    1. Burn wound aspergillosis
  - B. Operative site infection
    1. Prosthetic valve endocarditis, empyema and pleural aspergillosis, osteomyelitis
  - C. Foreign body associated
    1. Hickman or other intravenous line, chronic ambulatory peritoneal dialysis catheter
- IV. Infection in the immunocompromised host
  - A. Primary cutaneous aspergillosis
  - B. Pulmonary aspergillosis
    1. Acute invasive
    2. Chronic necrotising aspergillosis
  - C. Airways aspergillosis
    1. Invasive *Aspergillus* tracheobronchitis
    2. Obstructing bronchial aspergillosis
  - D. Rhinosinusitis
  - E. Disseminated
    1. Cerebral, renal, cutaneous aspergillosis

PATHOGENESIS

Aspergillus almost certainly has a substantial number of different pathogenicity factors. The small size of the conidia of *A. fumigatus* are probably one reason why it causes pulmonary infection. The ability of the pathogenic aspergilli to grow at 37°C is clearly another factor that is important for human disease. *A. fumigatus* can bind to various molecules, including laminin, fibrinogen, complement, and lactoferrin. This binding may be important in allowing adherence to epithelial surfaces and possibly endothelial surfaces.

As a eucaryotic organism that thrives on dead organic matter, *Aspergillus* spp. produce a large number of extracellular products. Various proteolytic factors have been described, in particular, elastase, which are of dubious importance as a pathogenicity factors. Other proteins, which may be toxic to the mammalian cells include restrictocin, fumigatoxin, and various cellular lytic enzymes, may or may not contribute to pathogenicity. A poorly characterized lipid component produced by *A. fumigatus* inhibits the alternative pathways of complement, but its role in pathogenicity is not yet fully evaluated. A number of other products may also be important, such as gliotoxin, which causes apoptosis and impairs macrophage and neutrophil function, and mannitol, which acts as a hydroxyl radical scavenger. Much work remains to be done to establish which, if any, of these factors are or are not relevant to disease. There are probably other factors of importance yet to be identified.

INCIDENCE OF INVASIVE ASPERGILLOSIS

The incidence of invasive aspergillosis is increasing substantially in the Western world. A multicentre autopsy study of cancer patients from 12 centers in North America and Japan from 1980 to 1988 demonstrated that 30% of all fungal infections were due to *Aspergillus* (5). A large study of autopsies in two Frankfurt hospitals from 1978 to 1992 showed an increase of all mycoses at autopsy from 1.5% to 6% and a proportional increase due to *Aspergillus* from 17% to 60% (6).

The range of incidence of invasive aspergillosis in different host groups is substantial as shown in Table 14.2.

RISK FACTORS

Asthma and cystic fibrosis appear to be the only risk factors for allergic bronchopulmonary aspergillosis. Only cavitary lung disease is important for

Table 14.2. Incidence of Invasive Aspergillosis in Different Host Groups

	Range (%)
Allogeneic/autologous BMT	0.5–9
Acute leukemia	5–24
AIDS	0–12
Liver transplantation	1.5–10
Heart and renal transplantation	0.5–10
Heart and lung or lung transplantation	19–26[a]
Chronic granulomatous disease	25–40[b]

[a] Both colonization and disease.
[b] Lifetime incidence.
SOURCE: Denning DW. *Aspergillus*, aspergilloma and invasive aspergillosis. In: Mitchell TG, Cutler JE, Deepe GS, Hazen KC. Principles of Medical Mycology, 1st Edition. American Society for Microbiology, Washington DC 1996. In press.

pulmonary aspergilloma, and local anatomic features appear to be most important for saprophytic *Aspergillus* sinusitis.

The key risk factors for invasive aspergillosis in decreasing order of importance are profound neutropenia (<100 × 10^6/l), prolonged neutropenia (7), neutrophil function deficits (8) (usually combined with macrophage or other cellular immune deficits) as in chronic granulomatous disease and AIDS, supraphysiologic corticosteroid therapy, graft-versus-host disease (9,10), and/or rejection in transplantation (11) (which may or may not be an independent variable as it reflects additional immunosuppression), and probably CMV disease and advanced human immunodeficiency virus infection (12) (Table 14.3). Less important risk factors appear to be diabetes mellitus, influenza, alcohol excess, prematurity, and exposure to *Aspergillus* in large quantities, (e.g., marijuana smoking or living in a rural or farm environment). Ambulatory outpatients with chronic respiratory disease treated with corticosteroids are also at higher than average risk of invasive aspergillosis but probably not at great risk. Particular groups of patients colonized with *Aspergillus* are at increased risk; this particularly includes patients with nasal colonization before chemotherapy for acute leukemia (12) and colonization of the tracheobronchial tree before lung transplantation.

There are other factors that probably do not contribute to disease. These include antibiotic therapy, cyclosporin therapy (which probably reduces risk by acting as a corticosteroid sparing agent), and use of corticosteroid aerosols in patients with respiratory disease.

Corticosteroid therapy is a risk factor by virtue of its effect to reduce pulmonary macrophage killing of *Aspergillus* conidia and neutrophil killing of *Aspergillus* hyphae (13). In addition, corticosteroids directly increase the growth rate of *A. fumigatus* and *A. flavus*. Under the influence of hydrocortisone, *Aspergillus* hyphae extend at the astonishing rate of 1 to 2 cm/h (14). The detrimental effect of corticosteroids on neutrophil function can be reversed in vitro by granulocyte colony stimulating factor and gamma interferon (15).

Table 14.3. Major Risk Factors for Invasive Aspergillosis*

Neutropenia, <500 and especially <100 × 10^6/l
Prolonged neutropenia, e.g., >12 days
Neutrophil ± other cellular immune deficits
Corticosteroid therapy*
Graft-versus-host disease after bone marrow transplantation*
Acute rejection after solid organ transplants*
Cytomegalovirus disease after transplantation
Advanced AIDS

*These factors are probably not independent of each other.

CLINICAL FEATURES OF INVASIVE ASPERGILLOSIS

Pulmonary Aspergillosis

At least 25% to 33% of patients initially have no symptoms attributable to invasive pulmonary aspergillosis. As the disease progresses, symptoms appear but this may be close to the time of death. Early symptoms are cough, usually dry, and fever. In corticosteroid-treated patients, fever is often absent. Chest pain is common and may be pleuritic or more commonly is mild and nonspecific. Hemoptysis can occur, although it is rarely a presenting feature. Dyspnea is more common in patients with diffuse disease. The presentation in some patients is akin to pulmonary embolism. In neutropenic patients, pneumothorax is an occasional presenting feature and sharp chest pain with dyspnoea is typical (16).

In chronic granulomatous disease, acquired immunodeficiency syndrome (AIDS), and other less immunocompromised patients, a more indolent course is typical and local extension of disease into the chest wall, brachial plexus, or vertebral column is occasionally seen.

Apart from a raised respiratory rate and a fever, there are usually no signs attributable to invasive aspergillosis. Auscultation of the chest is usually unrewarding. A pleural rub is sometimes heard.

In patients with diffuse disease, hypoxemia and hypocapnea is usually present. White cell counts are usually normal as is plasma biochemistry. A raised bilirubin and lactate dehydrogenase are occasionally seen but are nonspecific. If the disease is disseminated, coagulation defects are seen that include those typical of disseminated intravascular coagulation.

In the lung, the radiographic appearances of invasive aspergillosis are extremely heterogenous (17). Nodular shadows (Figures 14.1, A and B), with and without cavitation, thin-walled cavities (in AIDS and chronic necrotizing pulmonary aspergillosis) and "alveolar" consolidation that coalesces over time to form small nodules are typical. Perhaps the most distinctive appearance of invasive aspergillosis, aside from cavitation, is the pleural-based wedge-shaped lesion, but these are uncommonly seen on plain radiographs and may be late manifestations. More commonly, diffuse, usually lower lobe, fine shadowing is seen (Figure 14.2). Pleural effusions are rare. In the context of neutropenia, a spontaneous pneumothorax is also highly suggestive of invasive aspergillosis or zygomycosis.

Early in the course of progressive invasive pulmonary aspergillosis, plain chest radiographs are falsely negative, and thus high quality computed tomography (CT) scans of the chest can play a major role in early diagnosis (18). The following comments apply mostly to hematology patients. The most distinctive early lesions on CT scan are small nodules and small pleural based lesions with straight edges. There may be only one lesion, but often there are several. The "halo" sign is common (low attenuation surrounding the lesion) (Figure 14.3). As the disease progresses, the nodules may cavitate (often as the neutrophil count recovers), revealing the "air crescent" sign (19) (Figure 14.4).

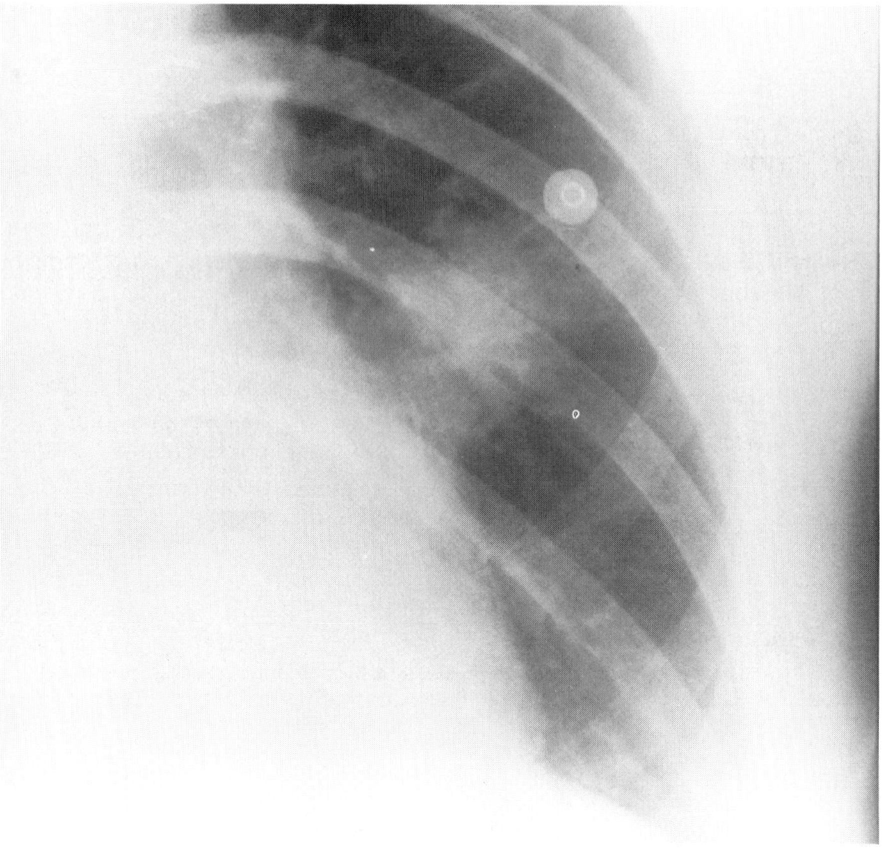

FIGURE 14.1A

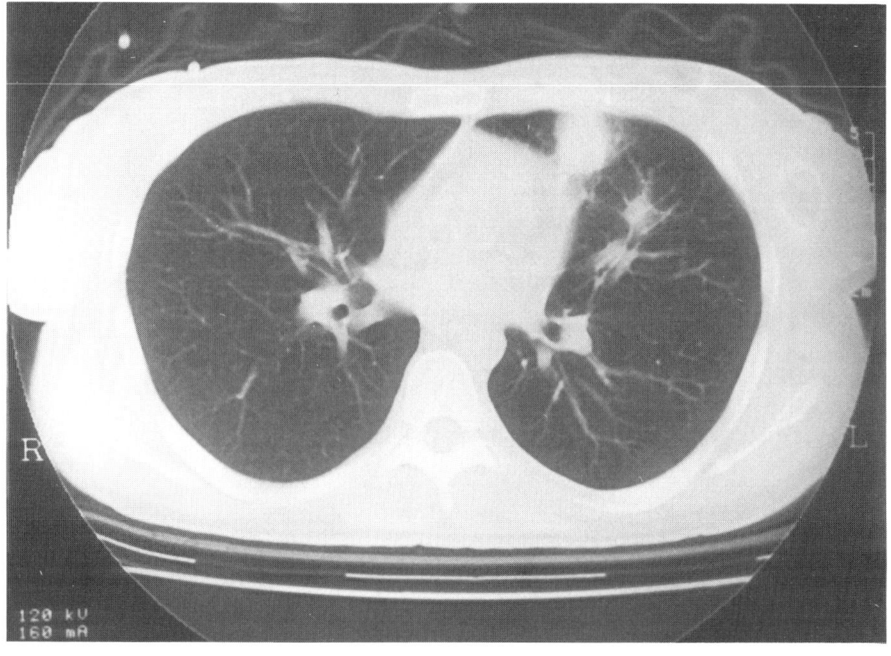

FIGURE 14.1B

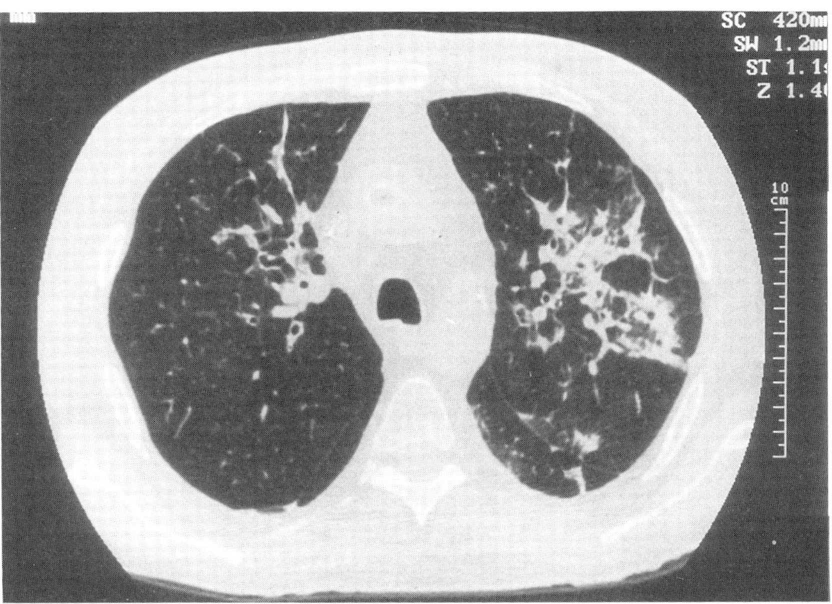

Figure 14.2. CT scan appearance of the midzones of an allogeneic BMT patient with diffuse pulmonary aspergillosis.

These lesions are highly distinctive for invasive fungal disease of the lung and are usually due to *Aspergillus* but may occasionally be due to a Mucorales, *Trichosporon*, *Blastoschizomyces*, or *Fusarium*. Pathoradiologic correlative studies have conclusively shown these lesions to represent infarcted lung tissue full of hyphae (20).

Aside from the halo and air crescent signs, consolidation is frequently seen. This is usually initially pleural based, but extensive disease can involve whole lobes. An early characteristic feature is a sharp demarcation line against the pleura, be it on the chest wall or one of the fissures. Sometimes these lesions are complicated by large or small pneumothoraces.

In solid organ transplant patients, both nodular and diffuse disease is seen. The major differential diagnoses of nodular disease in these patients are nocardial infection or lymphoma (21). There is a wider differential diagnosis for diffuse disease including *Pneumocystis carinii* pneumonia, strongyloidiasis, bacterial, or cytomegalovirus pneumonia if early after transplantation and rejec-

Figure 14.1. (**A**) An example of a focal lesion in the midzone of a neutropenic leukemic patient. (**B**) The CT scan appearance of the same patient demonstrating three lesions in the same vicinity that are superimposed on each other on the chest radiograph.

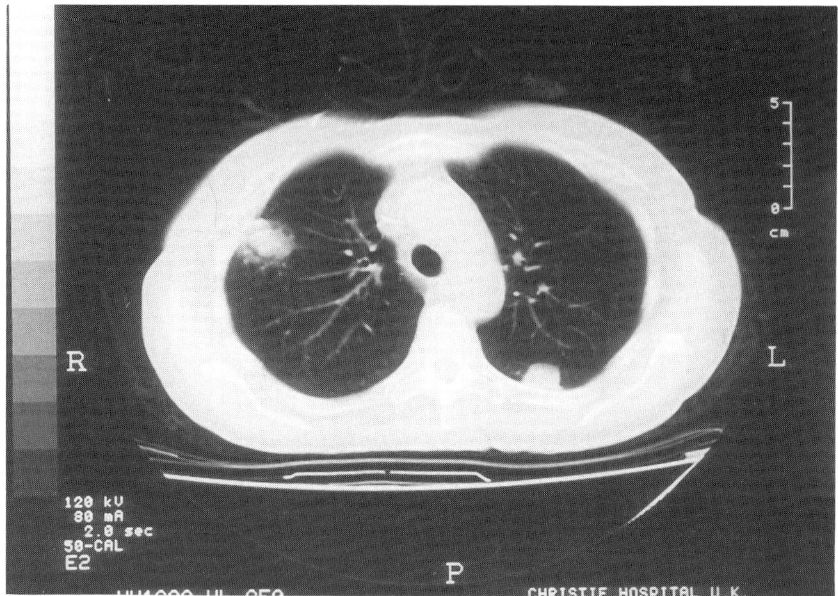

Figure 14.3. CT scan appearance of a neutropenia leukaemic patient showing a focal lesion with characteristic lower attenuation surrounding area (the "halo" sign).

tion in lung transplant recipients. The appearances of invasive aspergillosis in diffuse disease are rarely distinctive enough to obviate the need for diagnostic studies. Sometimes mixed appearances in invasive aspergillosis are seen, for example, pleural-based consolidation in one area with diffuse disease elsewhere. In the first 1 to 2 weeks after heart, lung, or liver transplantation, interpretation of radiologic abnormalities may also be confounded by postsurgical changes.

In patients with chronic granulomatous disease, AIDS, or on corticosteroid therapy, pulmonary lesions alone may be present or there may be extension into local structures such as rib. Thin- or thick-walled cavitary lesions are relatively frequent in AIDS patients with invasive aspergillosis (17,22). In addition, direct local extension from the airways into surrounding lung parenchyma, in a multifocal fashion, has also been described in AIDS (23).

Aspergillus Tracheobronchitis

Aspergillus airway disease ranges from a relatively mild tracheobronchitis with excess mucus production and inflammation to pseudomembraneous *Aspergillus* tracheobronchitis in which a shaggy greyish lining of the whole trachea and bronchial wall is apparent at autopsy (24, 25). Intermediate forms include those with ulcers of or plaques on the bronchial lining. Some 80% of the

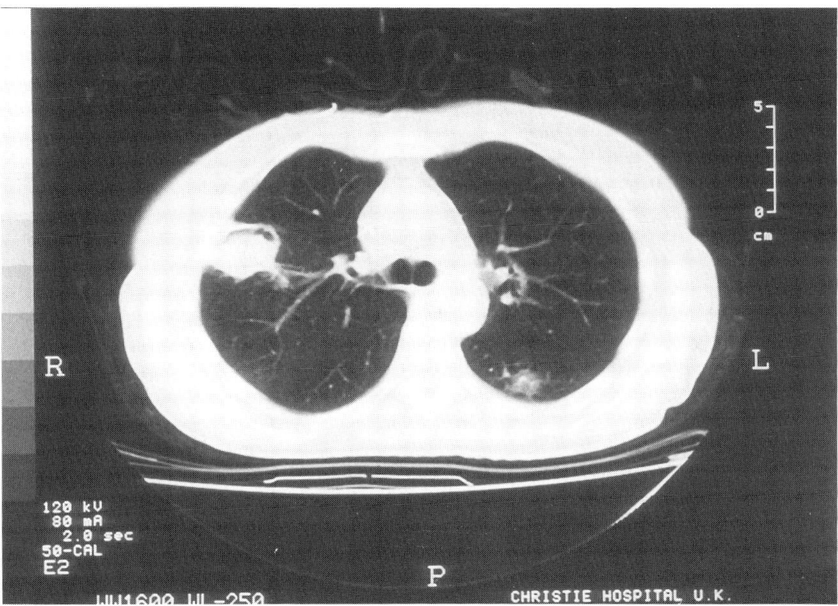

Figure 14.4. CT scan appearance of a neutropenic leukemic patient showing two lesions. The one on the right side exhibits the characteristic "air crescent" sign. It is a pleural-based lesion with at least two sharp borders, both features typical of invasive pulmonary aspergillosis. The other smaller lesion on the left posteriorly demonstrates the "halo sign".

patients are symptomatic, although symptoms may be mild. Symptoms include cough, fever and dyspnea, chest pain, and hemoptysis (25). At least 20% of patients are asymptomatic or, if symptomatic, other causes for these symptoms were identifiable (e.g., lung rejection). Almost all patients had a normal chest radiograph early in the course of disease. As the disease progresses, symptoms become more common and more severe. Those with very extensive involvement (pseudomembranous *Aspergillus* tracheobronchitis) may develop a unilateral monophonic wheeze or stridor reflecting obstruction of the lumen of the airway with necrotic material. Many patients die of respiratory insufficiency as a result of occlusion of the airway. Others develop disseminated disease in the last few days of life. Occasionally, perforation of the trachea or a bronchus occurs. About 60% of patients with tracheobronchitis have a positive respiratory culture for *Aspergillus* before death.

Bronchoscopy is essential for diagnosis (see below).

Acute Invasive *Aspergillus* Rhinosinusitis

Acute invasive *Aspergillus* rhinosinusitis occurs almost exclusively in leukemia patients after cytotoxic chemotherapy (26,27), bone marrow transplant recipients (28), in aplastic anemia, or in AIDS (9). Invasive *Aspergillus* sinusitis appears to be extremely uncommon in solid organ transplant patients.

The clinical features of acute invasive *Aspergillus* rhinosinusitis during neutropenia are variable but include fever, cough, epistaxis, headache, nasal discharge, sinus or eye pain, nasal congestion, or toothache. Early symptoms are nonspecific and easily mistaken for possible bacterial infection. Examination of the nose will show crusting of the nasal mucosa in about half the patients and a nasal or oral ulcer in about a third and either hyperemic, necrotic, or dusky nasal mucosa in 15% to 20%. About a third of the patients have sinus, facial, or nasal tenderness.

Plain radiology of the sinus is often unrevealing or merely shows opacification of the sinus. CT scanning is an essential tool to evaluate the extent of the disease and usually shows bony invasion in more advanced cases. Extension of injection from the sinuses through the roof of the mouth or into the orbit and brain is frequent.

Cerebral Aspergillosis

Cerebral aspergillosis occurs in 10% to 20% of all cases of invasive aspergillosis but is particularly common in disseminated aspergillosis. Allogeneic BMT and liver transplant recipients in particular are at high risk of dissemination (29). As with pulmonary aspergillosis, the clinical presentation and pace of progression of cerebral aspergillosis varies remarkably with the host group. Alteration in mental status is frequent (90%) as are seizures (50%) (30). Only 30% have focal neurologic deficit and less than a quarter have headache or meningeal signs. In granulocytopenic patients, focal neurologic features and seizures are more frequent. Fever may be present, but other infections are usually coexistent, including CMV disease, peritonitis, or pneumonia.

The majority of patients with cerebral aspergillosis has disease elsewhere, usually in the lungs, which implies hematogenous spread, but occasionally in the ear or sinuses.

Differential diagnoses depend on the host group. In BMT patients with a brain abscess visualized on CT scan, *Aspergillus* accounts for about half the cases and *Candida* a quarter; bacterial causes were seen in only 10% (31). In liver transplant recipients, *Aspergillus* is the most common infectious cause of brain abscess, but cerebral infarction and hemorrhage are more common (29). In other solid organ transplant recipients, cerebral aspergillosis and nocardiosis are seen with approximately equal frequency with toxoplasmosis, cryptococcosis, and lymphoma being less frequent. In AIDS patients, cerebral toxoplasmosis is a much more common cause of cerebral abscess as is lymphoma with cerebral aspergillosis being only rarely identified before death. Unfortunately, cerebrospinal fluid examination is usually abnormal but is not specific (30).

In highly immunocompromised patients, the CT appearances of cerebral

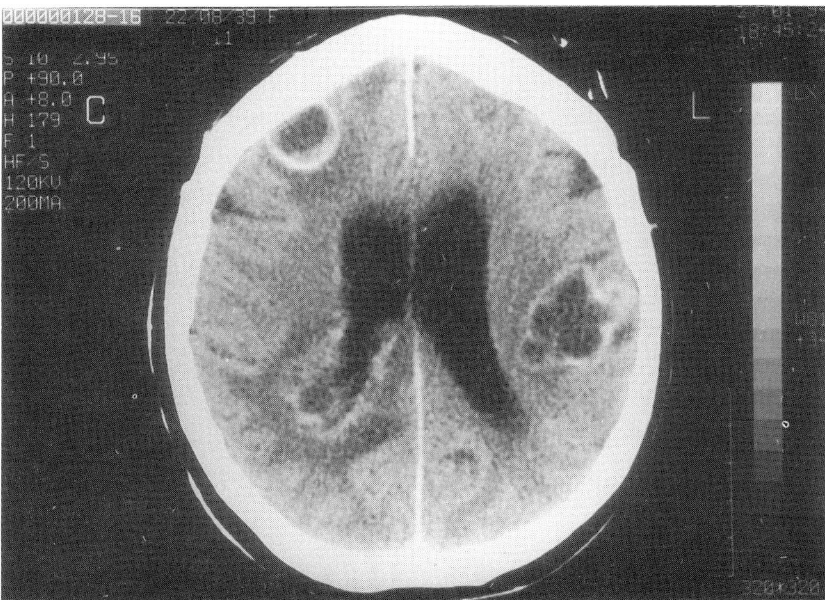

Figure 14.5. The typical appearance of multiple cerebral abscesses due to *A. fumigatus* in a renal transplant recipient. In an AIDS patient, such lesions would much more likely represent toxoplasmosis, which is also a significant differential diagnosis in the transplant population. Other filamentous fungi such as *Pseudallescheria boydii* would be a consideration in the BMT, neutropenic, and transplant patient.

aspergillosis are hypodense well-demarcated lesions (Figure 14.5). Hemorrhage and mass effect are unusual. Sometimes, clearer definition of the hypodense lesion is obtained with intravenous contrast. Magnetic resonance (MR) scans often reveal additional lesions but without distinctive features. The location of lesions are usually deep in the brain and difficult to access surgically.

DIAGNOSTIC PROCEDURES

In highly immunocompromised patients, particularly neutropenic patients, the CT scan of the chest should be the first definitive investigation when the suspicion of invasive pulmonary aspergillosis has been raised. A simple algorithm indicates the reasoning behind this (Figure 14.6). Some radiographic lesions are virtually diagnostic in this context. For less immediately diagnostic features, the optimal diagnostic (and therapeutic) approach can then be taken.

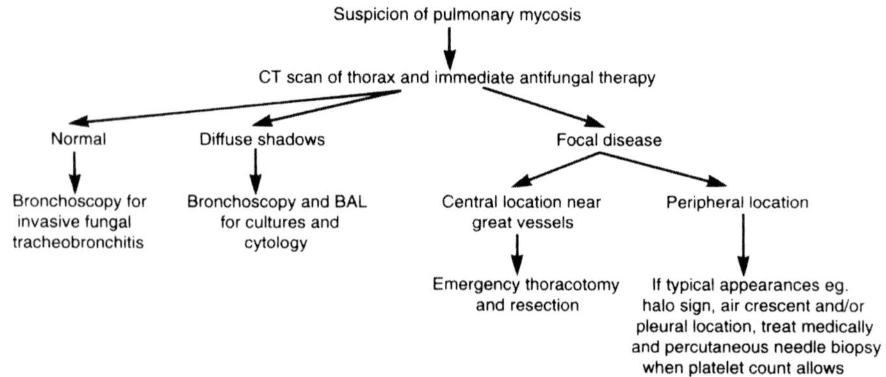

Figure 14.6. Management algorithm on suspicion of pulmonary mycosis.

Culture

The significance of *Aspergillus* cultured from sputum can be difficult to assess (32). A positive culture of *Aspergillus* from the sputum of healthy people occurs in 1% to 16%. Chronic lung disease increases the frequency of colonisation. In one British study, *Aspergillus* species were cultured from sputum, for example, 7% of 2080 hospitalized patients with various chest diseases and 57% in a group of patients with cystic fibrosis. Increased rates are also seen in those living in rural settings.

In most patients with *Aspergillus* in the sputum, no disease is present. However, a positive sputum culture in an immunocompromised patient is highly significant: all 17 leukemia patients with positive sputum cultures were subsequently shown to have invasive aspergillosis by lung biopsy. Thus, the positive predictive value for sputum culture is high, but unfortunately the negative predictive value is low in most immunocompromised patients with features suggestive of invasive aspergillosis (Table 14.4). Similar studies in other solid organ transplant patients other than liver transplant recipients are needed. In solid organ transplant patients, *Aspergillus* tracheobronchitis has been described with no symptoms and normal chest x-ray, and thus a positive *Aspergillus* culture should prompt immediate bronchoscopy. Invasive aspergillosis occurs in about 4% of patients with AIDS, but recovery of *Aspergillus* from respiratory sites in such patients may reflect colonization.

Studies examining the sensitivity and specificity of combinations of positive findings in immunocompromised patients, for example, a positive respiratory culture *and* an abnormal chest radiograph, are urgently needed.

Positive cultures of nasal swabs for *Aspergillus* are uncommon but useful in leukemia. Isolation of *Aspergillus* from the nose has a 90% correlation with invasive pulmonary aspergillosis in leukemia. A positive nasal culture before

Table 14.4. Respiratory Tract Cultures Positive for *Aspergillus* in Patients with Invasive Pulmonary Aspergillosis

Host Group	*Frequency of Positivity in IPA (%)*	*Specificity (%)*
Acute leukemia	8–34	>95
No BMT	25–38	70–95
Liver transplantation	≈80	70
AIDS	≈33%	10–20

SOURCE: Barnes AJ, Denning DW. *Aspergillus*—significance as a pathogen. Rev Med Microbiol 1993;4:176–180.

chemotherapy for leukaemia carries a high risk of invasive pulmonary aspergillosis (12). However surveillance swabs have a low yield. A positive nasal swab for *Aspergillus* in a context other than leukemia may or may not be significant unless there is overt sinus or nasal disease.

Aspergillus may be isolated in blood cultures and may represent genuine *Aspergillus* fungemia (33) or *Aspergillus* pseudofungemia. Genuine *Aspergillus* fungemia usually occurs in typical at-risk patients or patients who have received prosthetic heart valves. Many different culture systems have yielded *Aspergillus*. In a recent series of fungemia in leukemia, *Aspergillus* fungemia comprised 8% of all cases (34). *Aspergillus* pseudofungemia is more likely if the patient is not in a typical host group and/or the clinical course is not compatible. In most retrospective analyses, a laboratory source for the contamination is identified, and this has often followed a change in the usual blood culture handling procedure.

Bronchoscopy

Fibreoptic bronchoscopy is now an essential component of the diagnostic approach for pulmonary aspergillosis. It may diagnose *aspergillus* airways disease or diffuse (e.g., nonfocal) invasive pulmonary aspergillosis (Table 14.5). In addition to diagnosing aspergillosis, other important diagnoses can be made such as cytomegalovirus pneumonitis or *P. carinii* pneumonia. In the context of leukemia and bone marrow transplantation, the most useful procedure is bronchoalveolar lavage (BAL) or a bronchial wash (9,10,35–38). Samples should be processed for both culture and microscopy (or cytology). Transbronchial biopsy is simple and extremely productive if airways disease is present but has limited value for invasive pulmonary aspergillosis. Brushings contribute little to diagnosis above BAL and/or biopsy.

The positive yield for *Aspergillus* varies depending on the pattern of disease

Table 14.5. BAL for Diagnosis of Invasive Pulmonary Aspergillosis

Patients	*% Positive Result in All Those with Definitive or Probable Aspergillosis*		
	BAL culture	*BAL cytology*	*Either or both*
Leukemia	ND	ND	50
Leukemia	23	53	59
Acute leukemia	0	0	0
Leukemia, BMT, oncology	40	64	67
BMT			
Localized disease	0	0	0
Diffuse disease	100	?	100

ND, not done.
SOURCE: Reference 10,35–38.

and the host group. In leukemia and bone marrow transplantation, cytology and culture of BAL fluid will yield the diagnosis in 30% to 67% of patients (see Table 14.5). In solid organ transplant patients, the yield is probably lower, except in lung transplant patients in whom airways disease is probably more frequent (24). Diffuse disease radiologically is more likely to yield a positive result than focal disease (9). The utility of BAL for diagnosing invasive aspergillosis in AIDS is unclear.

Transbronchial biopsy is often falsely negative in cases of invasive pulmonary aspergillosis. This may be due to sampling error and in particular the depth of the biopsy. For example, in three series of AIDS patients with invasive aspergillosis that included 18 patients, transbronchial biopsy established the diagnosis in only 4; the others were confirmed by other means, usually autopsy.

Bronchoscopy with bronchial biopsy and culture is the only means of making the diagnosis of *Aspergillus* airways disease antemortem. Biopsy of loose material in the tracheal lumen, plaques, or ulcers will often reveal necrotic cartilage invaded by hyphae.

Percutaneous Lung Biopsy

Percutaneous lung biopsy or aspiration is best done with a 16–18 gauge needle; fine needle aspiration is less likely to be diagnostically useful. Percutaneous needle biopsy is indicated in patients with focal disease, particularly in the periphery of the lung, because these lesions are not accessible to the bronchoscope and BAL is often negative. The platelet count should be above 30 $\times 10^9/l$ or platelet transfusions should be given. Significant bullous or emphysematous lung disease in the area of interest is a contraindication. Specimens should be processed for culture and cytology or histology. The yield with respect to *Aspergillus* has not been accurately assessed in prospective studies, but it yielded the diagnosis in five AIDS patients with invasive aspergillosis in whom BAL was negative (22). It is also helpful in establishing the diagnosis of nocardiosis, lymphoma, *Pseudomonas*, and other rare lung mycoses. The incidence of radiologically apparent pneumothorax after percutaneous biopsy is about 10%, but only 2% of patients require a chest drain if the procedure is carefully done.

Thoracoscopy

Another approach used little to date has been thoracoscopy. This involves inserting a rigid fibreoptic instrument in the pleural cavity to visualize and biopsy any pleural or pulmonary lesions. As pleural localization is common in invasive aspergillosis, this approach is likely to be highly successful if the patient is not hypoxic or thrombocytopenic.

Open Lung Biopsy

Open lung biopsy is less frequently used to establish the diagnosis of invasive pulmonary aspergillosis, except when the diagnosis is thought to be a malignancy or other infection such as *Pneumocystis*. Studies of the usefulness of open lung biopsy for the diagnosis of invasive aspergillosis have not been done, and its role in the diagnostic cascade is presently unclear. However, when positive, it yields unequivocal evidence of invasive aspergillosis.

Serology

Aspergillus antibody is rarely detectable at the time of diagnosis of invasive aspergillosis during neutropenia but may be positive in patients after solid organ transplantation, depending on the test used. Data on the frequency of antibody positivity in other host groups, such as chronic granulomatous disease or AIDS, is lacking. The antibody response to *Aspergillus* infection has been well characterized in allergic bronchopulmonary aspergillosis and aspergilloma. More than 95% of patients with an aspergilloma have detectable precipitating immunoglobulin (Ig)G antibodies. Some have IgM antibodies as well. Successful surgical removal of an aspergilloma will result in a fall of *Aspergillus* antibody to low or undetectable levels subsequently.

Several antigen tests have been developed using galactomannan, complex protein antigens, and heat shock proteins. Only in leukemia and bone marrow transplant patients has any antigen test system been carefully examined. Reproducibility of the galactomannan latex test in serum is less than ideal, and sensitivity is around 30%. Several samples may have to be tested before positive results are obtained because antigenemia is often shortlived. Antigen positivity increases closer to time of death with progressive invasive aspergillosis. Unfortunately, many studies on antigen detection for invasive aspergillosis have not accurately described the temporal relationship of a positive antigen test and the

Table 14.6. *Aspergillus* Serology: Key Points

- Antibody is almost always detectable in cases of aspergilloma and allergic bronchopulmonary aspergillosis.
- Antibody is occasionally positive in leukemia patients with invasive aspergillosis.
- Studies of the utility of antibody for diagnosis of invasive aspergillosis in AIDS and transplant recipients have not been done.
- Antigen is detectable in about 30% of leukemic patients and or bone marrow transplant patients with invasive aspergillosis at suspicion of diagnosis.
- Multiple antigen tests necessary during neutropenia to detect positives.

early symptoms of invasive aspergillosis and initiation of treatment. The present position regarding serology for aspergillosis is shown in Table 14.6.

Sinus Aspergillosis

Invasive *Aspergillus* sinusitis requires a biopsy for diagnosis. Usually, part of the nose is affected in addition to the sinuses, and this is accessible externally. Cultures of any nasal discharge or of any crusted lesions should also be taken.

Cerebral Aspergillosis

Cerebral aspergillosis is usually confirmed at death. Aspiration of a suspicious lesion in the brain will usually yield *Aspergillus* on culture or the presence of hyphae on histologic examination. Unfortunately, histologic appearances alone may not be distinctive enough to diagnose *Aspergillus* as the hyphae are similar to those of many other pathogens, including *Pseudallescheria boydii.*

TREATMENT

Invasive aspergillosis carries a nearly 100% mortality if untreated. The only exception are patients whose immunocompromising factors are removed (e.g., permanent cessation of corticosteroids).

The pace of progression of invasive aspergillosis varies widely. In patients such as liver and bone marrow transplant recipients and patients with profound neutropenia, the course of disease from first clinical or radiologic abnormality to death is typically 10 to 14 days. The diagnosis is often difficult to establish and several days usually elapse between consideration of the diagnosis and partial or complete confirmation. A critical window of opportunity may have been missed if treatment is not started early, with fatal consequences for the patient. There is therefore room for discussion about exactly when treatment should be initiated for invasive aspergillosis.

Table 14.7 shows appropriate criteria for the initiation of therapy in the

Table 14.7. Criteria for Initiation of Therapy for Invasive Aspergillosis or Increasing the Dose of Amphotericin B to ≥1 mg/kg/d in Neutropenia (<1000 × 10^6/l) Including Aplastic Anemia

1. Isolation of *Aspergillus* from any site including nose swab, blood, BAL etc.
2. New pulmonary infiltrates on chest x-ray.
3. Infiltrates on CT scan of chest showing characteristic features, e.g.,
   a. Halo/crescent sign
   b. Pleural based sharply angulated lesion
   c. Pleural based lesion with pneumothorax
4. Persistent fevers (>7 days) with any localizing clinical features and not responding to antibiotics, e.g.,
   a. Chest pain
   b. Dry cough
   c. Facial/sinus pain
   d. Epistaxis
   e. Hoarseness
   f. New skin lesions consistent with aspergillosis
5. Any sudden intracranial event including stroke or fit with or without fever

Table 14.8. Criteria for Initiation of Therapy for Invasive Aspergillosis in Solid Organ Transplantation or Allogeneic Bone Marrow Transplantation

1. Radiologic infiltrate with isolation of *Aspergillus* from respiratory secretions, BAL, or blood.
2. Evidence of ulcers/bronchitis on bronchoscopy with hyphae visualized in BAL.
3. Histologic or cytologic evidence of hyphae from any tissue.
4. Any sudden intracranial event, including stroke or fit with or without fever.

neutropenic patient (39). In many such patients, empiric amphotericin B therapy will have been given because of persistent fever despite after 3 to 7 days of broad-spectrum antibiotics. If a dose of less than 1 mg/kg/d of conventional amphotericin B has been used for empiric therapy then the criteria given will constitute a reason to increase the dose to 1 to 1.25 mg/kg/d. If, however, empiric amphotericin B therapy is started at 1 mg/kg/d, as is more frequent these days, then a decision must be made about whether to switch therapy from this treatment to alternative therapies using the criteria stated in Table 14.7.

In solid organ or allogeneic bone marrow transplantation, the criteria for initiation of therapy are slightly different than they are during neutropenia (Table 14.8) (39). This is because there is a higher frequency of *Aspergillus* tracheobronchitis in this population and also a much wider differential diagnosis of cases of pneumonitis. If it occurs months after transplantation, the presentation is more likely to be of nodular disease that may represent *Aspergillus*, nocardia, or development of lymphoma (21). Immediately after liver transplantation, interpretation of the chest x-ray is difficult because of changes after surgery. In addition, solid organ transplantation patients are more likely to get *Aspergillus* in operative sites (e.g., mediastinitis, wound drainage, wound infection), which are problems that do not occur in the leukemic population. After allogeneic bone marrow transplantation, invasive aspergillosis occurs during or immediately after the short period of aplasia or more often with graft-versus-host disease, weeks or months after transplantation. Progression of disease in these patients may be extremely rapid.

In the context of AIDS, invasive aspergillosis tends to be a relatively subacute disease, and there is usually time to make a positive diagnosis without having to embark upon empiric therapy (Table 14.9) (39). The major exception to this is intracranial disease. Many patients and their physicians are not willing for the patient to undergo a brain biopsy or aspiration and therefore empirical therapy may be appropriate if there is a single lesion or small number of lesions not responding to anti-*Toxoplasma* therapy.

The standard therapeutic agent for the treatment of invasive aspergillosis is conventional amphotericin B (Fungizone). The success rate of amphotericin B therapy varies substantially between different host groups. There are two major considerations in the initial choice of therapy: Can the patient take oral medication and is he/she likely to absorb it? Is the patient taking cyclosporin or is renal dysfunction already present? If the patient is able to take oral therapy and the patient is not taking drugs that induce the metabolism of P450 enzymes (e.g., rifampin, phenytoin, carbamazepine, phenobarbitone), then itraconazole would be a reasonable first choice (Table 14.10). Other factors that might reduce absorption and therefore efficacy include H2 blockers and patients with intestinal problems (such as graft-versus-host disease) and patients with AIDS. The dose of itraconazole should be 200 mg three times a day for 4 days followed by 200 mg twice daily. All doses should be taken with food or an acid drink. Itraconazole serum concentrations should be done after 5 to 10 days. Typical target concentrations of itraconazole should be at least 1 μg/mL if measured by HPLC and at least 5 μg/mL if measured by bioassay.

If the patient is not a suitable candidate for oral therapy as outlined above, intravenous therapy is necessary. Conventional amphotericin B should be used in a minimum dose of 0.8 to 1.0 mg/kg/d regardless of renal dysfunction,

Table 14.9. Criteria for Initiation of Therapy for Invasive Aspergillosis in AIDS

1. Respiratory symptoms, abnormal chest x-ray or bronchoscopy, and isolation of *Aspergillus* or visualization of hyphae in BAL.
2. Cerebral lesions unresponsive to therapy for toxoplasmosis or a single enhancing lesion consistent with aspergillosis.
3. Histologic or cytologic evidence of hyphae from any site (culture not obtained or pending).

except in neutropenic patients in whom 1 to 1.25 mg/kg/d is appropriate (see Table 14.10). If renal dysfunction is, or is likely to be, a major problem, then one of the new preparations of amphotericin B in doses of 4 to 5 mg/kg/d may be appropriate (see Table 14.10). These dosage levels should be continued for at least 2 weeks until a therapeutic response has been obtained.

The apparent severity of illness of the patient should not be a guide as to whether to give oral itraconazole or intravenous amphotericin B. Responses have been obtained in profoundly neutropenic patients with extensive disease using oral itraconazole alone, and amphotericin B therapy is often ineffective.

There has been much discussion in case reports about the relative role of adjunctive therapy with either rifampicin or flucytosine. The use of amphotericin B with flucytosine does seem to improve clinical response rates marginally (40) and may be appropriate for sites of disease in which amphotericin B may penetrate poorly (e.g., brain, meninges, heart valve, and eye). There is a potential for antagonism in vitro, and it would be wise to have the isolate checked for this, if possible. Flucytosine serum concentrations should always be checked in patients to prevent toxicity, especially if dual therapy is prolonged, given the frequency of renal impairment with amphotericin B. The use of flucytosine for invasive aspergillosis during neutropenia has shown benefit in one or two small series but has not met with universal acceptance partly because of concern about prolonging neutropenia or thrombocytopenia (unproven).

The addition of rifampicin to amphotericin B may be synergistic in vitro (40).

Table 14.10. First- and Second-Line Therapy for Invasive Aspergillosis*

Agent	*Initial Dose*	*Comments*
Amphotericin B (Fungizone)	0.8–1.25 mg/kg/d (IV)	Considered first-line therapy but high failure rate. Significant interaction with cyclosporin.
Itraconazole (Sporonox)	200 mg tds for 4 d; then 200 mg bd (PO)	Useful if patient eating and not on P450 inducers. Significant interaction with cyclosporin. Levels should be measured to ensure adequate absorption.
Amphotericin B colloidal dispersion (Amphocil)	4 mg/kg/d (IV)	Less toxicity than Fungizone.
Liposomal amphotericin B (AmBisome)	4–5 mg/kg/d (IV)	Less toxicity than Fungizone.

*None of these agents or regimens have been compared in controlled trials, but all have been shown to be partially effective.

However, it is not appropriate in the context of transplantation because rifampicin induces the metabolism of many immunosuppressants and rejection or graft-versus-host disease may result (39). In addition, because rifampicin is a powerful inducer of P450 enzymes, its use (for more than 3 days) absolutely precludes subsequent use of itraconazole, which may be useful subsequently in patients failing amphotericin B or for continued therapy after amphotericin B (39).

There has also been debate about whether combinations of amphotericin B and itraconazole are appropriate. There are theoretical reasons for considering antagonism because itraconazole inhibits the production of ergosterol and the mode of action of amphotericin B requires binding to ergosterol. There is some limited animal model work (some unpublished by the author) suggesting that antagonism may be a real phenomenon, although the magnitude of this effect is difficult to ascertain. The present recommendations are that it is better to treat with one or other drug alone. If itraconazole is the desired agent but there is concern about its absorption, then initial use of both agents until itraconazole levels have been obtained and absorption confirmed is a reasonable therapeutic strategy.

Switching Therapy

Unfortunately, a substantial proportion of patients fail the first therapy selected for them. In patients with rapidly progressive disease, failure of the first regimen means a fatal outcome, and therefore a good initial choice for these patients is critical. However, for patients with more slowly progressive disease, the evaluation of response after 10 to 20 days of therapy can be made using clinical, radiologic and other criteria to decide whether they are or are not improving and whether therapy should or should not be changed. The less immunocompromised the patient, the longer it takes to make an evaluation of response. Many patients will respond to alternative therapy if they fail the primary therapy, and therefore all patients should be offered more than one form of therapy if their response is suboptimal.

Many patients and doctors prefer to switch from initial intravenous amphotericin B as primary therapy to oral itraconazole as follow up therapy and maintenance therapy. This is reasonable strategy if the patient has no problems with absorbing itraconazole.

Duration of Therapy

Patients should be treated for as long as they are immunocompromised and until there has been either complete or near complete resolution of disease. In the neutropenic patient, this certainly means treatment until the neutrophil count is above $1000 \times 10^6/l$. If at that time there is residual evidence of disease, treatment should be continued. Eradication of disease may require surgery. In patients whose immune status improves gradually over a long period of time (e.g., a solid organ transplant patient treated for many months), therapy should be continued until there is a complete clinical response. AIDS patients and patients who have received an allogeneic bone marrow transplant should probably receive treatment for years if they can tolerate and absorb itraconazole. If they cannot, long-term intermittent amphotericin B would be their only alternative (apart from surgical resection).

Surgical Excision

In invasive pulmonary aspergillosis, surgery has several roles (40). One group has advocated immediate surgical resection of one or more localized *Aspergillus* lesions in the lung during neutropenia. Most clinicians reserve lung resection for patients with persisting lung shadows who must undergo subsequent bone marrow transplantation or more aggressive chemotherapy, those with significant haemoptysis (19), or those with lesions impinging on the great vessels or major airways. This last point has been only recently emphasized. Erosion of invasive aspergillosis into the pulmonary vessels is not rare and is a rapidly fatal complication that can be averted by surgery.

In patients with invasive sinus aspergillosis, a biopsy of the affected area is necessary for diagnosis. Surgical debridement is useful for therapy but should not be done during neutropenia as hemorrhage and other operative complications are frequent (40).

With respect to cerebral aspergillosis, resection of the lesions is often impossible without causing untoward cerebral damage because most of the lesions are deep in the brain. For there patients, surgery has no role other than diagnostic aspiration or biopsy.

Surgery is an essential part of the management of patients with *Aspergillus* endophthalmitis, endocarditis, and probably osteomyelitis.

OUTCOME

The attributable mortality of invasive aspergillosis is from 50% to 100% in collected series (40). There are substantial variations from host group to host group and within each host group. In leukemia, achieving complete remission is critical to survival (41). Cerebral aspergillosis still has a mortality exceeding 95% in the immunocompromised patient. Many of the factors influencing the outcome of invasive aspergillosis are shown in Table 14.11.

Clearly, new agents for the treatment of invasive aspergillosis are urgently required. The role of G-CSF and other cytokines as adjunctive therapy is unclear at present. The efficacy of the primary therapeutic choice is going to be critical for improving mortality rates.

Table 14.11. Factors Influencing Outcome in Invasive Aspergillosis

Better Outcome	*Poor Outcome*
Host factors	
Resolution of neutropenia	Persistent neutropenia
Leukemia in remission	Leukemic relapse
Heart or kidney transplantation	Bone marrow transplantation
	Liver transplantation
	AIDS
Organ involvement	
Focal pulmonary disease	Diffuse pulmonary disease
	Cerebral aspergillosis
Therapeutic issues	
Early initiation of therapy	Delayed diagnosis/therapy
Switch of therapy if initial choice unsuccessful	
Appropriate surgery	

REFERENCES

1 **Bennett JH.** On the parasitic vegetable structures found growing in living animals. Trans R Soc Edinburgh 1842;15:277–279.

2 **Rankin NE.** Disseminated aspergillosis and moniliasis associated with agranulocytosis and antibiotic therapy. Br Med J 1953;25: 918–919.

3 **Young RC, Bennett JE, Vogel CL, et al.** Aspergillosis the spectrum of the disease in 98 patients. Medicine (Baltimore) 1970;49: 147–173.

4 **Denning DW, Lee JY, Hostetler JS, et al.** NIAID Mycoses Study Group multicenter trial of oral itraconazole therapy of invasive aspergillosis. Am J Med 1994;97:135–144.

5 **Bodey G, Bueltmann B, Duguid W, et al.** Fungal infections in cancer patients: an international autopsy survey. Eur J Clin Microbiol Infect Dis 1992;11:99–109.

6 **Groll A, Shah PM, Mentzel CH, Schneider M.** Changing pattern of invasive mycoses at autopsy. Presented at the Interscience Conference on Antimicrobial Agents and Chemotherapy, Orlando, FL, October, 1994.

7 **Gerson SL, Talbot GH, Hurwitz S, et al.** Prolonged granulocytopenia: the major risk factor for invasive pulmonary aspergillosis in patients with acute leukemia. Ann Intern Med 1984;100:345–351.

8 **Mouy R, Fischer A, Vilmer E, et al.** Incidence, severity, and prevention of infections in chronic granulomatous disease. J Pediatr 1989;114:555–560.

9 **Khoo S, Denning DW.** Aspergillus infection in the acquired immune deficiency syndrome. Clin Infect Dis 1994;19(suppl 1): 541–548.

10 **McWhinney PHM, Kibbler CC, Hamon MD, et al.** Progress in the diagnosis and management of aspergillosis in bone marrow transplantation: thirteen years experience. Clin Infect Dis 1993;17:397–404.

11 **Gustafson TL, Schaffner W, Lavely GB, et al.** Invasive aspergillosis in renal transplant recipients: correlation with corticosteroid therapy. J Infect Dis 1983;148:230–234.

12 **Martino P, Raccah R, Gentile G, et al.** *Aspergillus* colonization of the nose and pulmonary aspergillosis in neutropenic patients: a retrospective study. Haematologica 1989;74: 263–265.

13 **Schaffner A, Douglas H, Braude A.** Selective protection against conidia by mononuclear and against mycelia by polymorphonuclear phagocytes in resistance to *Aspergillus*. J Clin Invest 1982;69:617–631.

14 **Ng TTC, Robson GD, Denning DW.** Hydrocortisone-enhanced growth of *Aspergillus* spp.: implications for pathogenesis. Microbiology 1994;140:2475–2480.

15 **Roilides E, Unlig K, Venzon D, et al.** Prevention of corticosteroid-induced suppression of human polymorphonuclear leukocyte-induced damage of *Aspergillus fumigatus* hyphae by granulocyte colony-

stimulating factor and gamma interferon. Infect Immun 1993;61:4870–4877.

16 **Martino P, Girmenia C, Venditti M, et al.** Spontaneous pneumothorax complicating pulmonary mycetoma in patients with acute leukemia. Rev Infect Dis 1990;12:611–617.

17 **Miller WT Jr, Sais GJ, Frank I, et al.** Pulmonary aspergillosis in patients with AIDS. Clinical and radiographic correlations. Chest 1994;105:37–44.

18 **Kuhlman JE, Fishman EK, Siegelman SS.** Invasive pulmonary aspergillosis in acute leukemia: characteristic findings on CT, the CT halo sign, and the role of CT in early diagnosis. Radiology 1985;157:611–614.

19 **Kibbler CC, Milkins SR, Bhamra A, et al.** Apparent pulmonary mycetoma following invasive aspergillosis in neutropenic patients. Thorax 1988;43:108–112.

20 **Orr DP, Myerowitz RL, Dubois PJ.** Pathoradiologic correlation of invasive pulmonary aspergillosis in the compromised host. Cancer 1978;41:2028–2039.

21 **Haramati LB, Schulman LL, Austin JHM.** Lung nodules and masses after cardiac transplantation. Radiology 1993;188:491–497.

22 **Denning DW, Follansbee S, Scolaro M, et al.** Pulmonary aspergillosis in AIDS. N Engl J Med 1991;324:654–662.

23 **Lortholary O, Meyohas M-C, Dupont B, et al.** Invasive aspergillosis in patients with acquired immunodeficiency syndrome: report of 33 cases. Am J Med 1993;95:177–187.

24 **Kramer MR, Denning DW, Marshall SE, et al.** Ulcerative tracheobronchitis following lung transplantation: a new form of invasive aspergillosis. Am Rev Respir Dis 1991;144: 552–556.

25 **Kemper CA, Hostetler JS, Follansbee S, et al.** Ulcerative and plaque-like tracheobronchitis due to infection with *Aspergillus* in patients with AIDS. Clin Infect Dis 1993; 17:344–352.

26 **Talbot GH, Huang A, Provencher M.** Invasive *Aspergillus* rhinosinusitis in patients with acute leukemia. Rev Infect Dis 1991;13:219–232.

27 **Voillier A-F, Peterson DE, de Jongh CA, et al.** *Aspergillus* sinusitis in cancer patients. Cancer 1986;58:366–371.

28 **Drakos PE, Nagler A, Or R, et al.** Invasive fungal sinusitis in patients undergoing bone marrow transplantation. Bone Marrow Transplant 1993;12:203–208.

29 **Martinez AJ, Ahdab-Barmada M.** The neuropathology of liver transplantation: Comparison of main complications in children and adults. Modern Pathol 1993;6:25–32.

30 **Walsh TJ, Hier DB, Caplan LR.** Aspergillosis of the central nervous system: clinicopathological analysis of 17 patients. Ann Neurol 1985;18:574–582.

31 **Hagansee M, Bauwens JE, Kjos B, Bowden RA.** Presented at the etiology of Brain abscess bone marrow transplant: experience at the Fred Hutchinson Cancer Research Center 1984–1992. Clin Infect Dis 1994; 19:402–408.

32 **Barnes AJ, Denning DW.** *Aspergillus*—significance as a pathogen. Rev Med Microbiol 1993;4:176–180.

33 **Duthie R, Denning DW.** *Aspergillus* fungemia. Two cases and review. Clin Infect Dis 1995;20:598–605.

34 **Martino P, Girmenia C, Micozzi A, et al.** Fungemia in patients with leukemia. Am J Med Sci 1993;306:225–232.

35 **Albelda SM, Talbot GH, Gerson SL, et al.** Role of fibreoptic bronchoscopy in the diagnosis of invasive pulmonary aspergillosis in patients with acute leukemia. Am J Med 1984;76:1027–1034.

36 **Kahn FW, Jones JM, England DM, et al.** The role of bronchoalveolar lavage in the diagnosis of invasive pulmonary aspergillosis. Am J Clin Pathol 1986;86:518–523.

37 **Levy H, Horak DA, Tegtmeier BR, et al.** The value of bronchoalveolar lavage and bronchial washings in the diagnosis of invasive pulmonary aspergillosis. Respir Med 1992;86:243–248.

38 **Saito H, Anaissie EJ, Morice RC, et al.** Bronchoalveolar lavage in the diagnosis of pulmonary infiltrates in patients with acute leukemia. Chest 1988;94:745–749.

39 **Denning DW.** The treatment of invasive aspergillosis. J Infect 1994;28(suppl 1):25–33.

40 **Denning DW, Stevens DA.** Antifungal and surgical treatment of invasive aspergillosis: review of 2121 published cases. Rev Infect Dis 1990;12:1147–1201.

41 **Ribrag V, Dreyfus F, Venot A, et al.** Prognostic factors of invasive pulmonary aspergillosis in leukemic patients. Leuk Lymph 1993;10:317–321.

Index

C